T0227224

Infectious Disease

Editor

MICHAEL A. MALONE

PRIMARY CARE: CLINICS IN OFFICE PRACTICE

www.primarycare.theclinics.com

Consulting Editor
JOEL J. HEIDELBAUGH

September 2013 • Volume 40 • Number 3

ELSEVIER

1600 John F. Kennedy Boulevard • Suite 1800 • Philadelphia, Pennsylvania, 19103-2899

http://www.theclinics.com

PRIMARY CARE: CLINICS IN OFFICE PRACTICE Volume 40, Number 3
September 2013 ISSN 0095-4543, ISBN-13: 978-0-323-18868-5

Editor: Yonah Korngold

© 2013 Elsevier Inc. All rights reserved.

This periodical and the individual contributions contained in it are protected under copyright by Elsevier, and the following terms and conditions apply to their use:

Photocopying
Single photocopies of single articles may be made for personal use as allowed by national copyright laws. Permission of the Publisher and payment of a fee is required for all other photocopying, including multiple or systematic copying, copying for advertising or promotional purposes, resale, and all forms of document delivery. Special rates are available for educational institutions that wish to make photocopies for non-profit educational classroom use. For information on how to seek permission visit www.elsevier.com/permissions or call: (+44) 1865 843830 (UK)/(+1) 215 239 3804 (USA).

Derivative Works
Subscribers may reproduce tables of contents or prepare lists of articles including abstracts for internal circulation within their institutions. Permission of the Publisher is required for resale or distribution outside the institution. Permission of the Publisher is required for all other derivative works, including compilations and translations (please consult www.elsevier.com/permissions).

Electronic Storage or Usage
Permission of the Publisher is required to store or use electronically any material contained in this periodical, including any article or part of an article (please consult www.elsevier.com/permissions). Except as outlined above, no part of this publication may be reproduced, stored in a retrieval system or transmitted in any form or by any means, electronic, mechanical, photocopying, recording or otherwise, without prior written permission of the Publisher.

Notice
No responsibility is assumed by the Publisher for any injury and/or damage to persons or property as a matter of products liability, negligence or otherwise, or from any use or operation of any methods, products, instructions or ideas contained in the material herein. Because of rapid advances in the medical sciences, in particular, independent verification of diagnoses and drug dosages should be made.

Although all advertising material is expected to conform to ethical (medical) standards, inclusion in this publication does not constitute a guarantee or endorsement of the quality or value of such product or of the claims made of it by its manufacturer.

Primary Care: Clinics in Office Practice (ISSN: 0095–4543) is published quarterly by Elsevier Inc., 360 Park Avenue South, New York, NY 10010-1710. Months of issue are March, June, September, and December. Periodicals postage paid at New York, NY and additional mailing offices. Subscription prices are $216.00 per year (US individuals), $353.00 (US institutions), $108.00 (US students), $264.00 (Canadian individuals), $415.00 (Canadian institutions), $169.00 (Canadian students), $329.00 (international individuals), $415.00 (international institutions), and $169.00 (international students). Foreign air speed delivery is included in all *Clinics* subscription prices. All prices are subject to change without notice. POSTMASTER: Send address changes to *Primary Care: Clinics in Office Practice*, Elsevier Periodicals Customer Service, 11830 Westline Industrial Drive, St. Louis, MO 63146. Customer Service Health Sciences Division, Subscription Customer Service, 3251 Riverport Lane, Maryland Heights, MO 63043. **Customer Service: 1-800-654-2452 (U.S. and Canada); 314-447-8871 (outside U.S. and Canada). Fax: 314-447-8029. E-mail: journalscustomerservice-usa@elsevier.com (for print support); journalsonlinesupport-usa@elsevier.com (for online support).**

Reprints. For copies of 100 or more, of articles in this publication, please contact the Commercial Reprints Department, Elsevier Inc., 360 Park Avenue South, New York, NY 10010-1710. Tel. (212) 633-3812; Fax: (212) 482-1935; E-mail: reprints@elsevier.com.

Primary Care: Clinics in Office Practice is covered in *MEDLINE/PubMed (Index Medicus) and EMBASE/ Excerpta Medica, Current Contents/Clinical Medicine, and ISI/BIOMED.*

Printed and bound by CPI Group (UK) Ltd, Croydon, CR0 4YY

Transferred to digital print 2012

Contributors

CONSULTING EDITOR

JOEL J. HEIDELBAUGH, MD, FAAFP, FACG
Clinical Associate Professor, Departments of Family Medicine and Urology, Clerkship
Director, University of Michigan Medical School, Ann Arbor, Michigan; Ypsilanti Health
Center, Ypsilanti, Michigan

EDITOR

MICHAEL A. MALONE, MD
Assistant Professor, Department of Family Medicine, Penn State College of Medicine,
Hershey, Pennsylvania

AUTHORS

LYLA BLAKE-GUMBS, MD, MPH
Assistant Professor, Department of Family Medicine and Community Health, University
Hospitals Case Medical Center, Case Western Reserve University School of Medicine,
Cleveland, Ohio

JOEL V. CHUA, MD
Staff Infectious Diseases Specialist, Infusion Solutions of Delaware; Staff Infectious
Diseases Specialist, Kent General Hospital - Bayhealth Medical Center, Dover, Delaware

TRACEY CONTI, MD
Clinical Assistant Professor, Family Medicine, University of Pittsburgh School of Medicine,
Pittsburgh, Pennsylvania; Residency Program Director, UPMC McKeesport Family
Medicine Residency, McKeesport, Pennsylvania

WANDA CRUZ-KNIGHT, MD, MBA
Associate Professor, Department of Family Medicine and Community Health, University
Hospitals Case Medical Center, Case Western Reserve University School of Medicine,
Cleveland, Ohio

NANCY S. GRAVES, MD
Assistant Professor, Department of Family and Community Medicine, Milton S. Hershey
Medical Center, Penn State Hershey, Hershey, Pennsylvania

SAMUEL N. GRIEF, MD, FCFP
Associate Professor of Clinical Family Medicine, Department of Family Medicine,
University of Illinois at Chicago, Chicago, Illinois

KAREN HAYANI, MD
Associate Professor of Pediatrics, Division of Pediatric Infectious Diseases,
Children's Hospital of University of Illinois, University of Illinois at Chicago, Chicago, Illinois

ESTHER DAN-PHUONG HO, MD
Associate Clinical Professor, Assistant Family Medicine Residency Program Director, Hospitalist Program, Department of Family Medicine, University of California, Irvine, Orange, California

MANJUSHA KAD, MD
Primary Care Physician and Faculty Member, UPMC McKeesport Family Medicine Residency, McKeesport, Pennsylvania

JEFFREY KIM, MD
Assistant Professor, Department of Family Medicine, Loma Linda University, Loma Linda, California

HOBART LEE, MD
Assistant Professor, Department of Family Medicine, Loma Linda University, Loma Linda, California

MICHAEL A. MALONE, MD
Assistant Professor, Department of Family Medicine, Penn State College of Medicine, Hershey, Pennsylvania

WILLIAM MARKLE, MD, DTM&H
Clinical Associate Professor, Family Medicine, University of Pittsburgh School of Medicine, Pittsburgh, Pennsylvania; Sr. Associate Residency Director, UPMC McKeesport Family Medicine Residency, McKeesport, Pennsylvania

VAN NGUYEN, DO
Resident Physician, Department of Family Medicine, Loma Linda University, Loma Linda, California

PARMINDER NIZRAN, MD
Penn State Department of Family and Community Medicine, Hershey, Pennsylvania

GEORGE G.A. PUJALTE, MD, CAQSM
Assistant Professor, Primary Care Sports Medicine, Departments of Family and Community Medicine, Orthopaedics and Rehabilitation, Penn State Milton S. Hershey Medical Center, Hershey, Pennsylvania

KATHERINE PUTZ, MD
Resident Physician, Department of Family Medicine, University of Illinois at Chicago, Chicago, Illinois

TIMOTHY RILEY, MD
Assistant Professor, Penn State Department of Family and Community Medicine, Hershey, Pennsylvania

JARRETT K. SELL, MD
Assistant Professor, Penn State Hershey Department of Family and Community Medicine, Penn State Milton S. Hershey Medical Center, Hershey, Pennsylvania

ABRAHAM R. TAYLOR, MD
Assistant Professor, Department of Family and Community Medicine, Penn State Milton S. Hershey Medical Center, Hershey, Pennsylvania

ALINA WANG, MD
Penn State Department of Family and Community Medicine, Hershey, Pennsylvania

FRED ARTHUR ZAR, MD, FACP
Professor of Clinical Medicine, Program Director, Internal Medicine Residency, Director, M2 Clinical Pathophysiology Course, Vice Chair for Education, Department of Medicine, College of Medicine, University of Illinois Hospital and Health Sciences System, Chicago, Illinois

Contents

Sexually transmitted infections (STIs), also referred to as sexually transmitted diseases, remain a growing worldwide problem and public health issue. This article covers the epidemiology of STIs, the history and physical findings, screening guidelines, and the general plan to combat STIs. Prevention is discussed using the latest information from the Centers for Disease Control and Prevention and other references. Infections discussed from the standpoint of cause, epidemiology, risk factors, clinical disease, diagnosis, and treatment include gonorrhea, *Chlamydia trachomatis*, *Trichomonas vaginalis*, syphilis, chancroid, *Herpes simplex*, lymphogranuloma venereum, granuloma inguinale, *Herpes papilloma* virus, *Molluscum contagiosum*, and pubic lice.

This article presents an overview of current human immunodeficiency (HIV) management for primary care practitioners. Discussion is focused on appropriate screening, antiretroviral treatment, opportunistic infection prophylaxis, laboratory testing and prevention. Improved screening can identify the 20–25% of persons living with HIV in the United States who remain undiagnosed. Expansion of treatment recommendations to include all HIV-infected persons and expanded opportunities for prophylaxis will likely significantly increase the number of persons who receive antiretroviral treatment. Understanding of opportunistic infection prophylaxis, proper vaccination, and comorbid risk factor modification can improve life expectancy for many patients living with chronic stable HIV infection.

Patients with illnesses caused by ticks may present with flulike symptoms. Physicians should learn how to recognize these illnesses by specific aspects in the patients' histories and physical examinations. Prevention of mortality and morbidity may depend on correct early diagnosis and treatment. Illness prevention may result with early removal of the tick, because infection usually requires 24 to 48 hours of attachment to the host. A bite from one tick may transmit several different pathogens leading to concurrent infections. The prevention of tick-borne illnesses can start with advice on how to prevent tick bites, especially during summer time.

Methicillin-resistant *Staphylococcus aureus* (MRSA) is an increasingly common multidrug-resistant clinical pathogen responsible for increasing health costs and for patient morbidity and mortality. Presented in this review, the definition, cell and molecular biology, epidemiology, prevention, diagnosis, and treatment of MRSA infections, including skin and soft tissue infections, bacteremia and endocarditis, pneumonia, bone and joint infections, and central nervous system infections, are addressed. In the treatment of MRSA, this article highlights several common antibiotics that retain activity against different strains of MRSA.

This article provides an overview of community-acquired pneumonia in adults and children. The epidemiology, causes, clinical presentation, diagnostic testing, site-of-care decisions, treatment, possible complications, and prevention of pneumonia are discussed.

This article reviews the diagnosis and treatment of acute otitis externa and acute otitis media, and will be helpful to primary care physicians who diagnose and treat these common diseases in the clinic. The pathophysiology, microbiology, clinical features, diagnosis, treatment, prognosis, and complications are discussed.

Clinical presentation helps differentiate between upper and lower urinary tract infections (UTIs). UTIs are classified as either complicated or uncomplicated. A complicated UTI is associated with an underlying condition that increases the risk of failing therapy. Primary laboratory tests for UTIs consist of urinalysis and urine culture. The most common pathogen for uncomplicated cystitis and pyelonephritis is *Escherichia coli*. Nitrofurantoin, fosfomycin, and trimethoprim-sulfamethoxazole are first-line therapies for acute uncomplicated cystitis. Decisions regarding antibiotic agents should be individualized based on patients' allergies, tolerability, community resistance rates, cost, and availability.

Meningitis is defined as inflammation of the meninges, in almost all cases identified by an abnormal number of white blood cells in the cerebrospinal fluid and specific clinical signs/symptoms. Onset may be acute or chronic, and clinical symptoms of acute disease develop over hours to days. This article reviews the epidemiology, pathophysiology, clinical manifestations, diagnosis, and management of acute meningitis, and provides a list of key points for primary care practitioners. Aseptic and bacterial meningitis vary significantly and are discussed separately.

Acute gastroenteritis is a common infectious disease syndrome, causing a combination of nausea, vomiting, diarrhea, and abdominal pain. There are more than 350 million cases of acute gastroenteritis in the United States annually and 48 million of these cases are caused by foodborne bacteria. Traveler's diarrhea affects more than half of people traveling from developed countries to developing countries. In adult and pediatric patients, the prevalence of Clostridium difficile is increasing. Contact precautions, public health education, and prudent use of antibiotics are necessary goals in decreasing the prevalence of Clostridium difficile. Preventing dehydration or providing appropriate rehydration is the primary supportive treatment of acute gastroenteritis.

Tuberculosis (TB) is still a public health issue; it continues to reign as one of the world's deadliest diseases. One-third of the world's population has been infected with TB. Identified cases of mycobacterium must be notified in an attempt to reduce the public health impact of TB on the population. TB transmission occurs via inhalation of droplet nuclei. The most common site for the development of TB is the lungs. Treatment of TB depends on whether latent TB or active TB is treated.

Upper respiratory infections (URIs) are infections of the mouth, nose, throat, larynx (voice box), and trachea (windpipe). This article outlines the epidemiology, etiology, diagnosis, and management of URIs, including nasopharyngitis (common cold), sinusitis, pharyngitis, laryngitis, and laryngotracheitis.

PRIMARY CARE:
CLINICS IN OFFICE PRACTICE

DOWNLOAD
Free App!

Review Articles
THE CLINICS

NOW AVAILABLE FOR YOUR iPhone and iPad

Foreword

Beware—Use Universal Precautions for Everything!

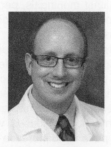

Joel J. Heidelbaugh, MD, FAAFP, FACG
Consulting Editor

STOP! Go wash your hands with boiling hot (already purified and filtered) water and soap for at least an hour prior to reading this volume of *Primary Care: Clinics in Office Practice*! Please don a full-body plastic gown, two pairs of nonlatex gloves, an N-95 mask, plastic goggles... a respirator and space boots... and please ensure that you read this volume of *Primary Care: Clinics in Office Practice* in a negative-pressure room. When you finish, please incinerate the medium that contains this volume and wash your hands again. (*Note to readers: this is an evidence-based recommendation on how to eliminate all forms of infectious disease to be discussed in this volume....*)

With all of the attention toward infectious diseases, focusing on strategies for prevention, why aren't we winning the war? Are the bacteria, viruses, parasites, and other organisms just always one step ahead of us in the chess game of elimination versus victory? Are universal precautions not working? Are our patients simply ignoring our pleas toward prevention? As a father of two school-aged children, I do everything short of sending them to school in a bubble, and they still get sick. What am I doing wrong?

Back in the mid-1990s, I can remember how MRSA was viewed as sort of a "joke" in medical school. A medical school classmate would ask, "What rotation were you on last month?" When I replied, "Surgery at the VA," the standard response was commonly, "well [laughs...], I'll bet if I swabbed your lab coat, you'd have a 50% chance of testing positive for MRSA!" While likely true, I don't remember seeing a single MRSA infection in my medical school or residency training. Now, MRSA haunts our practices with increasing incidence of cellulitis and abscesses, along with the challenges of choosing appropriate antibiotic regimens without inducing complications such as *Clostridium difficile*–associated diarrhea, or antibiotic resistance.

Recent guidelines have posited that we should increase screening for hepatitis C, predominantly in our patients born during the "baby-boomer" generation. While we are likely to find more cases, we can't yet predict the costs associated with screening relative to potential improvements in outcomes. Nonetheless, decades of mass

Prim Care Clin Office Pract 40 (2013) xi–xii
http://dx.doi.org/10.1016/j.pop.2013.07.001
0095-4543/13/$ – see front matter © 2013 Published by Elsevier Inc.

screening for highly communicable viral sexually transmitted infections, including HIV, have proven to allow for both increased awareness and opportunity to treat, coupled with better strategies to manage these conditions as major public health problems.

This volume of *Primary Care: Clinics in Office Practice* comprises vast amounts of portable data for immediate use in our daily practices. In reading these articles, I again realized that I probably overprescribe antibiotics for upper respiratory tract infections and otitis media; likely miss opportunities to immunize against meningitis, pertussis, and pneumonia, as well as screen for tuberculosis; and underestimate the incidence and potential complications associated with gastroenteritis.

Congratulations to Dr Malone and his panel of talented experts who compiled this very detailed and evidence-based compendium of articles on common infectious diseases encountered in primary care practices. It is with these epidemiological statistics, as well as diagnostic and treatment paradigms, that we can best educate our patients on how to prevent concerning infectious diseases. While universal precautions have greatly reduced the transmission of many infectious diseases, we can all raise the proverbial bar in augmenting education to our patients to increase efforts toward prevention. I sincerely hope that you find this volume of *Primary Care: Clinics in Office Practice* as informative and enjoyable as I have.

Joel J. Heidelbaugh, MD, FAAFP, FACG
Departments of Family Medicine and Urology
Department of Family Medicine
University of Michigan Medical School
Ann Arbor, MI 48109, USA

Ypsilanti Health Center
200 Arnet Suite 200
Ypsilanti, MI 48198, USA

E-mail address:
jheidel@umich.edu

Preface

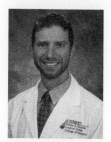

Michael A. Malone, MD
Editor

Primary care providers are often the initial or sole provider for the evaluation and management of infectious diseases. Therefore, I am pleased to present the 2013 issue of *Primary Care: Clinics in Office Practice* devoted to the topic of Infectious Diseases. The eleven infectious disease topics covered in this issue were selected to cover topics that would be easily utilized in a busy primary care setting. Each article of this issue is set up for quick and practical use during patient care, including key points, boxes, and tables that summarize essential information for each topic. Current evidence-based guidance on assessment and treatment are included for topics seen in everyday inpatient and outpatient practice, such as UTI, pneumonia, and upper respiratory tract infections. However, primary care providers can also improve outcomes for less common infections encountered in their practice. Therefore, topics such as human immunodeficiency virus, tick-borne illnesses, and tuberculosis have also been included in this issue for clinical reference.

Although set up for quick reference, each article provides a thorough overview each topic, including Epidemiology, Microbiology, Clinical Presentation, Diagnostic Testing, Treatment, and Complications.

I hope you enjoy reading this issue and find it evidence-based and clinicially relevant.

Michael A. Malone, MD
Department of Family Medicine
Penn State College of Medicine
845 Fishburn Road
Hershey, PA 17033, USA

E-mail address:
mmalone@hmc.psu.edu

Prim Care Clin Office Pract 40 (2013) xiii
http://dx.doi.org/10.1016/j.pop.2013.07.002
0095-4543/13/$ – see front matter © 2013 Published by Elsevier Inc.

Sexually Transmitted Diseases

William Markle, MD, DTM&H[a,b],*, Tracey Conti, MD[a,b],
Manjusha Kad, MD[b]

KEYWORDS

- Gonorrhea • Syphilis • *Chlamydia* • Chancroid • Herpes
- Lymphogranuloma venereum • Lice • Genital warts

KEY POINTS

- Many patients with sexually transmitted disease are asymptomatic. Targeted screening of at-risk populations is the most cost-effective measure to reduce the burden of disease.
- The most sensitive tests for gonorrhea and *Chlamydia* are the nucleic acid amplification tests.
- In the United States, most cases of syphilis are found in men who have sex with men (MSM). The incidence peaked around 1990 but is again on the increase.
- Genital herpes can be caused by *Herpes simplex* virus type 1 and type 2 and is a chronic, lifelong disease.
- Proctitis in the MSM population should raise the suspicion of lymphogranuloma venereum.
- Human papilloma virus is the most common sexually transmitted disease, with a worldwide point prevalence of around 10%.
- Prevention measures include education, rapid diagnosis and treatment, partner notification and treatment, condoms, and vaccinations.

INTRODUCTION

Sexually transmitted diseases (STDs) or sexually transmitted infections (STIs) remain a growing worldwide problem and public health issue. In 2002, it was estimated there were 15 million cases of STDs in the United States.[1] By 2010, there were 19 million cases and growing.[2] Half of these cases are among young people aged 15 to 24 yrs. STDs add 17 billion dollars to the health care costs of the country. The family physician is frequently confronted by patients with symptoms of a possible STD, at-risk behavior, or worry about STD exposure. It is important for them to be

[a] Family Medicine, University of Pittsburgh School of Medicine, Pittsburgh, PA, USA; [b] UPMC McKeesport Family Medicine Residency, 2347 Fifth Avenue, McKeesport, PA 15132, USA
* Corresponding author. UPMC McKeesport Family Medicine Residency, 2347 Fifth Avenue, McKeesport, PA 15132.
E-mail address: marklew@upmc.edu

Prim Care Clin Office Pract 40 (2013) 557–587
http://dx.doi.org/10.1016/j.pop.2013.05.001
0095-4543/13/$ – see front matter © 2013 Elsevier Inc. All rights reserved.

knowledgeable about the signs and symptoms of these diseases and the diagnosis, treatment, and prevention.

There is often a large population of people at risk for STDs in a practice, and this is not always appreciated. One study, conducted among women aged 16 to 29 years presenting to a family planning clinic, found that 8.1% or 1 in 12 of the women had a lifetime history of trading sex for money or other resources.[3] Several studies have shown a need for better provider understanding of STD risk assessment, recognition, legal knowledge of reporting requirements, and counseling.[4–6]

There are differences in STD rates among ethnic and racial groups that are important to consider. High rates of poverty, income inequality, unemployment, and low educational attainment make it more difficult for individuals to protect their sexual health.[7] In 2009, poverty rates, unemployment rates, and high school drop-out rates for blacks, American Indians/Alaska natives, and Hispanics were higher than for whites and these differences were commensurate with observed disparities in STD burden.[8] Even when health care is available, fear and distrust of institutions negatively affect the health care–seeking experience for many minorities.[9] Acknowledging the inequity in STD rates by race or ethnicity is one of the first steps in empowering affected communities to organize and focus on this problem. Detailed data can be found on the Centers for Disease Control and Prevention (CDC) STD Surveillance Report.[10]

Adolescents, in particular, are at high risk of contracting STDs. In the United States and United Kingdom, the average age of first coitus is about 16 years.[11,12] About half of all new STDs in the United States are acquired by those in the 15-year to 24-year age group.[13] Adolescent females have a higher incidence of cervical ectopy, which makes them more susceptible to some STDs such as *Chlamydia*. In 2003, 24% of female adolescents aged 14 to 19 years had laboratory evidence of an STD, specifically, human papilloma virus (HPV), *Chlamydia, Trichomonas, Herpes simplex,* or gonorrhea. Of those who reported ever having sex, 40% had laboratory evidence of a STD.[11]

There are barriers for adolescents, such as lack of health insurance, lack of transportation, discomfort of facilities and services, and concerns about confidentiality. Behavioral factors have also been shown to be important for adolescents acquiring an STD:

- Sexual activity in early and middle adolescence, especially for *Chlamydia*
- Multiple partners
- New partners
- Partners with multiple other partners
- Inconsistent use of condoms
- Alcohol and other drug consumption[14–17]

Although the diagnosis and treatment of adolescents is the same as adults, there are special counseling issues that affect adolescents. Privacy and confidentiality are important. Although state laws vary as to notification, all 50 states have self-consent laws for diagnosis and treatment of STDs.[18]

Another group that should be screened includes men requesting prescriptions for erectile dysfunction (ED) drugs. A study looking at insurance claims data of 1,410,806 men older than 40 years found 33,968 men who had filled a prescription for an ED drug. These men had higher rates of STDs, especially human immunodeficiency virus (HIV), both in the year before and after use of these drugs. Counseling about safe sexual practices and screening for STDs should accompany the prescription of ED drugs.[19] A higher prevalence of sexually risky behaviors and STDs has been found in patients with borderline personality disorder (BPD), especially those who were opiate dependent.[20] There is a clear need for interventions aimed at decreasing sexual risk behaviors among individuals with BPD.

SCREENING

The approach to STD diagnosis has been based on disease or symptom-specific syndromes. However, many patients are asymptomatic, which sustains transmission within the community. Targeted screening of at-risk populations is the most cost-effective measure to reduce the burden of disease and has been shown to be effective.[21]

The history is the first step in risk assessment. It should be undertaken in a private setting, be nonjudgmental, and include:

- Symptoms and duration
- Any treatment taken
- Past history of STDs
- Allergies
- Menstrual and obstetric history
- Sexual history, including new sexual partners, history of multiple partners, history of genital ulceration, history of sexual intercourse with trauma, types and locations of sexual exposures, frequency of condom use.

Special attention should be paid to risk factors such as:

Age between 15 and 24 years, African American race, unmarried status, new sex partner in past 60 days, multiple partners, history of a previous STD, illicit drug use, admission to a correctional facility, meeting partners on the Internet, and contact with sex workers.[17,22]

On physical examination, the physician needs to inspect the mouth, palms, and skin in addition to the genital area. The urethra can be milked to show discharge. The inguinal areas, scrotum (for epididymitis), perianal area, and the pelvic examination for signs of pelvic inflammatory disease (PID) should all be part of the routine examination.

Patients with 1 STD should be screened for others, especially HIV, and they should be rescreened after about 3 months, because reinfection is common.[23]

Screening recommendations in general:

- Hepatitis B vaccine is appropriate for all adolescents and all adults at risk of hepatitis B, including men who have sex with men (MSM). Screening should be offered to MSM, injection drug users (IDU), persons infected with HIV, persons attending an STD clinic or requesting treatment, and persons with a history of multiple sex partners. Pregnant women should be screened with the hepatitis B surface antigen.
- Hepatitis A screening should be offered to MSM, IDU, and those with chronic liver disease. Vaccination should be offered if not immune.
- Hepatitis C screening is offered to anyone with exposure to an infected partner or multiple partners, IDU, those on hemodialysis, those receiving a blood transfusion before 1992, and pregnant women if at high risk. Anyone with a new diagnosis of HIV infection should be screened for hepatitis C. The US Preventive Services Task Force (USPSTF) now recommends screening for all adults born between 1945 and 1965 because of a high incidence in this population (http://www.uspreventiveservicestaskforce.org/uspstf12/hepc/hepcdraftrec.htm).
- HIV screening is now recommended for all adults age 15 to 65 years by the USPSTF (http://www.uspreventiveservicestaskforce.org/uspstf13/hiv/

hivdraftrec.htm). Younger adolescents and older adults should also be screened if at high risk. Groups such as MSM, IDU, commercial sex workers, those with multiple partners, those with an HIV-positive partner, people presenting with another STD, and anyone who required a blood transfusion between 1978 and 1985 are at high risk and should be screened. MSM account for about 60% of cases in the United States. Pregnant women should be screened, preferably in the first and third trimesters.

- Syphilis screening is recommended for commercial sex workers or those who trade sex for drugs, MSM, women who have sex with women, people with another STD including HIV, persons in correctional facilities, and others with high-risk behaviors. Pregnant women should be screened in the first and third trimesters.
- Gonorrhea screening is recommended for those with multiple partners or partners with multiple sexual contacts, those with partners with a culture-proven STD or HIV, those with repeated episodes of STDs, commercial sex workers, illicit drug users, and in pregnancy if at risk. Risk includes those younger than 25 years or those living in an area with a high incidence of gonorrhea. Current recommendations call for screening of all women younger than 25 years if at risk, including all those factors already mentioned plus inconsistent condom use. For MSM, the nucleic acid amplification test (NAAT) test can be performed on urine, but swabs must be obtained from the rectum and the oral cavity.
- Screening for *Chlamydia trachomatis* is recommended for all sexually active women 25 years of age and younger annually. Women older than 25 years should be screened if they have risk factors, including more than 1 partner, a new partner in the past 60 days, inconsistent condom use, a history of STDs, unmarried sexually active women, and women who have sex with women. All women in correctional facilities or juvenile detention facilities should be screened up to age 35 years. Screening is recommended for all pregnant women. Men should be screened in correctional facilities and STD clinics, and MSM can be screened with a NAAT urine test and a rectal swab. Oral swabs are not recommended for *Chlamydia*. All patients with HIV should be screened for *Chlamydia*.
- *Trichomonas* screening is recommended in women with new or multiple partners, those with a history of STD, IDU, and those who trade sex for drugs.
- HPV tests are available with cervical cancer screening for women older than 30 years. They are not general tests for STDs, but regular Pap tests are recommended for all women, and screening for high-risk HPV types can be helpful. The HPV vaccine is recommended for all persons between 9 and 26 years of age.
- No screening is recommended for *Herpes simplex*.
- The public health authorities should be notified of cases of gonorrhea, *Chlamydia*, chancroid, acute hepatitis A, acute hepatitis B, acute hepatitis C, HIV, and syphilis.
- Partners should be notified, examined, and treated.

Current screening recommendations from the CDC are outlined in the 2010 STD treatment guidelines.[24]

INDIVIDUAL STDS
Diseases with Urethral or Vaginal Discharge

Gonorrhea
Cause and epidemiology Gonorrhea is caused by a gram-negative coccus, *Neisseria gonorrhea.*

It is found worldwide and is the second most common STD reported in the United States caused by a bacterium. In the United States, in the year 2011, a total of 321,849 cases of gonorrhea were reported to the CDC.[25] Cases of gonorrhea were reported to be greater in women from ages 15 to 24 years and in men 20 to 24 years of age.[26] From 1975 to 1997, after implementing a national gonorrhea control program, the national rate of gonorrhea declined by 74%. However, an increase in rate was noted in 2010 to 2011.[26]

Risk factors Young adulthood, unmarried status, a previous history of gonorrhea, a history of STDs, multiple sex partners or new sex partners, illicit drug abuse, low education, and intermittent condom use are all risk factors.[26–28]

Clinical disease In women, the cervix is the most common site of infection. Women may be asymptomatic or present with mucopurulent vaginal discharge, abdominal pain, dyspareunia, dysuria, or intermenstrual bleeding. Gonorrhea in women can result in PID, and women may present with fever and abdominal/pelvic pain at that time. On pelvic examination, cervical motion tenderness, adnexal tenderness, or uterine tenderness may be present. Complications of PID include infertility, chronic pelvic pain, ectopic pregnancy, and perihepatitis.

Men infected with gonorrhea may present with dysuria or copious purulent or mucopurulent discharge.

Complications of gonorrhea in men are not common but can include epididymitis, periurethral abscess, disseminated gonococcal infection, seminal vesiculitis, and proctitis. Men with epididymitis may present with fever, swelling of the epididymis, or unilateral testicular pain. Proctitis is seen mainly in MSM.[29] Patients may present with rectal pain, tenesmus, constipation, rectal discharge, and rectal bleeding.

Diagnosis NAATs, culture, microscopy, and nucleic acid-base hybridization and amplification techniques can all be used for the detection of gonorrhea. A NAAT is the recommended test for detection of gonorrhea by the CDC. In women, an endocervical or vaginal swab is collected. This swab can be collected either by the patient themselves or by the clinician. In men, a urethral swab is collected. In both men and women a urine sample can be collected for gonorrhea. A culture is used for the detection of rectal and oropharyngeal gonorrhea infections. Culture is also useful when suspecting drug resistance.

Treatment The Gonococcal Isolate Surveillance Project is a surveillance system developed by the CDC in 1986 that monitors antimicrobial susceptibility trends of gonorrhea in the United States. Quinolones had been widely used in the treatment of gonorrhea since 1993. Since 2007, resistance to the quinolones has increased, and cephalosporins have become the treatment of choice.[24,30]

The recommended first-line treatment by the CDC for uncomplicated gonorrhea is ceftriaxone 250 mg intramuscularly (IM), plus either a single dose of azithromycin 1 g or doxycycline 100 mg twice a day for 7 days. Ceftriaxone alone is not recommended secondary to emerging resistance to cephalosporins.[31]

Alternative regimens Cefixime 400 mg single dose, plus azithromycin 1 g or doxycycline 100 mg twice a day for 7 days plus a test of cure in 1 week may be used if ceftriaxone is not available. Azithromycin 2 g plus a test of cure in 1 week is recommended if the patient has an allergy to cephalosporins. Test of cure with a culture or a NAAT is recommended. A confirmatory culture is performed if the NAAT is positive. If the culture is positive, then phenotypic antimicrobial susceptibility testing is recommended.[31] Azithromycin monotherapy is not recommended secondary to gastrointestinal adverse effects and an increase in the development of resistance by gonococci.

Outside the United States, spectinomycin 2 g IM is effective in patients who are unable to tolerate cephalosporins. Spectinomycin is not available in the United States.

Pregnancy Ceftriaxone 250 mg IM plus a single dose of azithromycin 1 g is recommended. An alternative regimen is azithromycin 2 g, single dose. A test of cure is recommended 3 to 4 weeks after initiating antibiotics.

Coinfection with *Chlamydia* Forty-six percent of men and women infected with gonorrhea have a coinfection with *Chlamydia*.[32] Ceftriaxone 250 mg IM, plus either a single dose of azithromycin 1 g or doxycycline 100 mg twice a day for 7 days, is recommended.

Partner management Patients infected with gonorrhea should refer their sex partners to a health care provider for treatment and evaluation. A patient's sex partner should be treated for both gonorrhea and *Chlamydia* if the infected patient's last sexual intercourse with the partner was 60 days or less before the onset of symptoms or the diagnosis with gonorrhea. Expedited partner therapy can be performed if necessary.[33] The person infected with gonorrhea must abstain from sexual intercourse until therapy for gonorrhea is completed and until the patient and the patient's sex partner become asymptomatic.[24]

Chlamydial infection

Cause and epidemiology *Chlamydia trachomatis* is an obligate intracellular, gram-negative bacterium. *Chlamydia* infection is the most common STD in the United States caused by a bacterium. Many patients are asymptomatic and thus most cases are not reported. In the United States, in the year 2011, 1,412,791 chlamydial infections were reported to the CDC.

Cases of *Chlamydia* were reported to be greater in women from ages 18 to 20 years and men from ages 20 to 24 years.[26] In sexually active females aged 14 to 19 years, it is estimated that 1 of 15 have *Chlamydia*.[34] In women, cases of *Chlamydia* were more than 2.5 times more common than in men, possibly because women tend to be screened more often than men.

Risk factors Young adulthood, multiple sex partners, intermittent use of condoms, cervical ectopy, a history of STD or HIV, low education, low socioeconomic class, and MSM are all risk factors.[34–37]

Clinical disease Many patients infected with *Chlamydia* are asymptomatic. Symptoms may occur weeks to months after being exposed to *Chlamydia*. In women, the cervix or the urethra are the most common sites of infection. Women may present with a mucopurulent vaginal discharge, dysuria, postcoital bleeding, intermenstrual vaginal bleeding. or urinary frequency. A complication of *Chlamydia* in women is PID, and women may present with abdominal and pelvic pain at that time. On pelvic examination, there is usually cervical motion tenderness and adnexal tenderness. Possible complications of PID are infertility, chronic pelvic pain, ectopic pregnancy,[38] and perihepatitis (Fitzhugh-Curtis syndrome). Complications of *Chlamydia* in pregnancy include preterm delivery and early rupture of membranes. The infection can also spread to the newborn and cause conjunctivitis or pneumonia.[38] Men infected with *Chlamydia* may present with dysuria or a watery or mucoid urethral discharge. Complications of *Chlamydia* in men are not common but can include epididymitis, proctitis, and reactive arthritis (Reiter's syndrome). Men with epididymitis may present with fever, swelling of the epididymis, and unilateral testicular pain. Proctitis is almost exclusively seen in MSM and may present with rectal pain, tenesmus, rectal discharge, and rectal bleeding. The triad of reactive arthritis includes arthritis, uveitis, and urethritis.

Diagnosis The CDC recommends screening for *Chlamydia* annually in sexually active women aged 25 years and younger. NAATs, culture, genetic probe, and antigen detection can all be used for the diagnosis of *Chlamydia*. NAATs are the most sensitive and specific tests for the detection of *Chlamydia*. In women, an endocervical or vaginal swab is collected either by the patient or by a clinician. In men, a urethral swab is collected. In both men and women, a urine sample can be collected for *Chlamydia*. NAATs are also used for the detection of rectal and oropharyngeal *Chlamydia trachomatis* infections.[24,39]

Treatment The recommended first-line treatments for *Chlamydia trachomatis* are azithromycin 1 g single dose or doxycycline 100 mg twice a day for 7 days. A meta-analysis of 12 randomized clinical trials for the treatment of *Chlamydia trachomatis* infection reported microbial cure rates of 97% with azithromycin and 98% with doxycycline.[40]

Alternative regimens Erythromycin base 500 mg 4 times a day for 7 days, erythromycin ethylsuccinate 800 mg orally 4 times a day for 7 days, levofloxacin 500 mg once daily for 7 days, or ofloxacin 300 mg twice a day for 7 days can all be used. Infected individuals should be tested for all other STDs, including HIV and hepatitis B and C.

Pregnancy Azithromycin 1 g single dose or amoxicillin 500 mg 3 times a day for 7 days is recommended. Erythromycin 500 mg 4 times a day for 7 days is an alternative regimen. A test of cure is recommended 3 to 4 weeks after initiating antibiotics in pregnancy.

Coinfection with gonorrhea Ceftriaxone 250 mg IM plus either a single dose of azithromycin 1 g or doxycycline 100 mg twice a day for 7 days is recommended for this coinfection or if coinfection is suspected.

Partner management The patient infected with *Chlamydia* should refer their sex partners to a health care provider for treatment and evaluation. The patient's sex partner should be treated for *Chlamydia* if the infected patient's last sexual intercourse with the partner was 60 days or less before the onset of symptoms or 60 days or less before the patient being diagnosed with *Chlamydia*. Expedited partner therapy may be used if necessary, but this varies by state.[33] The person infected with *Chlamydia* must abstain from sexual intercourse until therapy for *Chlamydia* is completed and until the patient and the patient's sex partner become asymptomatic.[24,39]

Trichomoniasis
Cause and epidemiology Trichomoniasis is caused by *Trichomonas vaginalis*, a flagellated protozoan. The disease is found worldwide, and 3.7 million people in the United States are affected by trichomoniasis. Women are more affected than men.

Risk factors A history of STDs, multiple sex partners or a new sex partner, intravenous (IV) drug abuse, and prostitution are risk factors.[24]

Clinical disease In women, the vulva, vagina, or urethra are the most common sites of infection. Women may be asymptomatic or present with frothy, clear, yellow or green purulent, thin, foul-smelling vaginal discharge, dysuria, dyspareunia, postcoital bleeding, and vulvar itching.

In women with HIV, trichomoniasis can result in PID.[41] Trichomoniasis may increase the risk of transmission of HIV,[42,43] tubal infertility,[44] the risk of cervical neoplasia,[45] and increase the risk for cuff cellulitis after abdominal hysterectomy.[46] Complications of trichomoniasis in pregnancy include preterm delivery, premature rupture of membranes, and low birth weight.[42,47] Men infected with trichomoniasis may be asymptomatic or present with dysuria or clear mucopurulent discharge. Complications of trichomoniasis in men can include epididymitis, prostatitis, infertility, and prostate cancer.

See http://www.trichomoniasis.org/Trichomonas_Vaginalis/Index.aspx for a picture of the organism.

Diagnosis Microscopy of vaginal discharge using a saline wet preparation in the office is usually performed for diagnosing trichomoniasis. This test has a sensitivity of 60% to 70%.[24,48] Tests cleared by the US Food and Drug Administration (FDA) with more than 83% sensitivity and more than 93% specificity include a test from OSOM Rapid Diagnostics, a division of Sekisui Diagnostics, and the Affirm VP III (BD Diagnostics, Franklin Lakes, NJ, USA) test. Results using OSOM and Affirm VP III are seen in 10 and 45 minutes, respectively. Another test, the APTIMA *T vaginalis,* a NAAT (Hologic/Gen Probe, San Diego, CA, USA), has a specificity of 87% to 100% and a sensitivity of 97% to 100%. Culture can also be performed with high sensitivity (95%) and specificity (>95%). In men, tests with high sensitivity include NAATs and transcription-mediated amplification.[24]

Treatment The recommended treatment of trichomoniasis is metronidazole 2 g orally in a single dose or tinidazole 2 g orally in a single dose. Patients should not drink alcohol 24 hours after completing treatment with metronidazole and 72 hours after completing treatment with tinidazole.

Alternative regimen Metronidazole 500 mg orally twice a day for 7 days.

Pregnancy The pregnant patient is treated if symptomatic. Metronidazole is recommended. If she is breastfeeding, the patient is advised not to breastfeed while on metronidazole and for 12 to 24 hours after the last dose. If on tinidazole, she is advised not to breastfeed while on the medicine and for 3 days after the last dose.

Partner management The sex partner should be treated and evaluated for STDs. Expedited partner therapy is possible.[33] Patients should not have sexual intercourse until they have completed treatment or the patient and patient's partner become asymptomatic.

Other organisms not covered in this article but which may be spread sexually and are causes of urethral or vaginal discharge are:

Ureaplasma spp
Mycoplasma spp
Gardnerella vaginalis

Diseases (or Organisms) Causing Genital Ulcers

Syphilis
Cause Syphilis is caused by the spirochete bacterium *Treponema pallidum*. Acquired infection is transmitted by direct contact with individuals with early syphilis. This disease is found only in human hosts. Transmission can also occur vertically from mother to baby.

Epidemiology Syphilis is a common worldwide STD. The number of syphilis cases in the United States peaked in 1990 before decreasing to all-time lows in 2000.[49] In 2001, the rates again began increasing annually before decreasing again in 2010. This increase is primarily because of increasing rates of infection in men. In 2011, 72% of primary and secondary (P&S) syphilis cases in 46 states and the District of Columbia that provided information about sex of sex partners were among MSM.[50] During 2010 to 2011, the rate of P&S syphilis increased 4.5% among Hispanics (from 4.4 to 4.6 cases per 100,000 population), 8.0% among American Indians/Alaska Natives (from 2.5 to 2.7 cases per 100,000 population), 9.5% among non-Hispanic whites (from 2.1 to 2.3 cases per 100,000 population), and 33.3% among Asian/Pacific Islanders (from 1.2 to 1.6 cases per 100,000 population). The rate decreased 6.6% among non-Hispanic blacks (from 16.6 to 15.5 cases per 100,000 population).[50]

Risk factors Most cases of syphilis in the United States are found in the MSM population. Other risk factors include HIV infection, using a combination of methamphetamine and sildenafil, and having acquired sexual partners through the Internet.[51] In 2002, 25% of cases of syphilis were in patients coinfected with HIV.[52] Syphilis itself is also a risk factor for acquiring HIV, similar to other ulcerative genital diseases. Other risk factors include promiscuity, the use of illicit drugs, poverty and uninsured status, and work as a sex worker.

Pathophysiology Transmission of *Treponema pallidum* occurs with direct contact with an infectious lesion during sex, but transmission can also occur by kissing or touching a person who has active lesions on their lips, oral cavity, breasts, or genitals.[53] It is estimated that transmission occurs in approximately one-third of patients exposed to lesions.[54]

Clinical disease Syphilis is often described as the great imitator, because many of the signs and symptoms are indistinguishable from other diseases. There are 4 different stages to this disease: primary, secondary, early latent, and late latent.

Primary syphilis presents as a chancre. This is a painless papule that subsequently erodes and becomes ulcerated. Lesions typically are located in the genital region; however, they can be located at any site of initial inoculation. These lesions are also associated with painless bilateral inguinal lymphadenopathy. The ulcers heal spontaneously in 4 to 6 weeks. Most patients are unaware of these lesions because there is no pain associated, thus increasing the risk of transmission to others.

Secondary syphilis occurs if treatment is not initiated at the primary stage. It can produce a wide range of symptoms. Typically, findings occur weeks to months after the initial infection. A key feature of this stage is development of a pale pink or reddish macular rash. The rash is typically diffuse and is present over the entire body, including the palms and soles. When the rash presents in moist areas of the body, the papules can enlarge to form gray-white lesions called condyloma lata. These lesions are highly infectious. Constitutional symptoms are also present during this stage, including fever, fatigue, weight loss, sore throat, and headache. Other complications including meningitis, hepatitis, nephropathy, arthritis, uveitis, and hepatitis can occur but are less common. See http://www.cdc.gov/std/syphilis/STDFact-Syphilis.htm for pictures and more information.

Early latent syphilis is the stage at which there is a normal physical examination in the presence of a positive treponemal antibody test. This stage is defined as a period of 1 year, after which the disease is termed late latent. Misclassification of latent syphilis is common and can have a negative impact on appropriate treatment duration or contact tracing.[55]

Late latent syphilis can develop in about 15% of people who have not been treated for syphilis, and can appear 10 to 20 years after infection was first acquired.[56] Typically, this stage of the disease is manifested by chronic end-organ complications, including neurosyphilis, cardiovascular syphilis, and gummatous syphilis. Neurosyphilis, infection of central nervous system (CNS), can occur at any time in the course of the disease. Early forms may involve the cerebrospinal fluid (CSF), meninges, and cerebral vasculature. Early infections can be asymptomatic, but have a CSF lymphocytosis, increased protein level and a positive Venereal Disease Research Laboratory (VDRL) test. Meningitis has abnormal cerebrospinal fluid (CSF) and causes headache, confusion, and stiff neck. Syphilis can also affect the eye or cause hearing loss. Arteritis can lead to an ischemic stroke. Late in the disease course, the infection involves the brain and spinal cord and is called general paresis and tabes dorsalis. These conditions are less common in the antibiotic era. General paresis causes forgetfulness and personality change. It may also cause hypotension, tremor, and dysarthria. Tabes dorsalis affects the posterior columns of the spinal cord. There are lancinating pains and sensory ataxia. The Argyll-Robertson pupil may be found plus absent reflexes in the legs and impaired vibratory and position sense. Lumbar puncture should always be considered with neurologic or ocular disease compatible with syphilis regardless of past history. Lumbar puncture should also be performed when HIV infection coexists with syphilis.

Syphilis in pregnancy Is serious, because there can be transplacental infection of the fetus. Eighty percent of women with syphilis are in the reproductive age group.[57] Universal screening in pregnancy is recommended by many international organizations. A nontreponemal test should be performed at the first prenatal visit and in the third trimester in all patients and at delivery in high-risk mothers. By treating any cases found immediately, most morbidity of syphilis in pregnancy can be eliminated. If pregnancy is diagnosed in a nontraditional setting (eg, prison, drug treatment center, emergency department), a syphilis test should be performed in case the woman does not seek prenatal care. A positive test should be confirmed with a treponemal antibody test (see later discussion) to eliminate false-positive results. Fetal infection does increase as pregnancy progresses but symptoms are most severe early in pregnancy. Manifestations include intrauterine growth restriction, stillbirth, preterm birth, neonatal death, and congenital anomalies. Congenital syphilis is usually caused by late or no prenatal care. The incidence in 2008 in the United States was 10.1 cases per 100,000 live-born infants.[58] Pregnant women should be treated with penicillin, as outlined later. Unless the patient has had a documented nonreactive serology in the past year, the case is considered latent, and 3 doses of benzathine penicillin are given 1 week apart. With penicillin allergy, the only proven option is desensitization to penicillin. Titers should be followed after treatment to assess resolution of infection. If infection is diagnosed after 20 weeks' gestation, ultrasonography can help diagnose fetal infection.

All infants born to mothers with syphilis should have serologic tests and a physical examination to detect congenital syphilis. An examination of the placenta and umbilical cord to test for antitreponemal antibodies can be performed. A description of the full workup and treatment is beyond the scope of this article, but the most common treatment is 10 days of penicillin G given IV. Please consult the CDC and the American Academy of Pediatrics for full information.[24,59] Physical examination findings can be subtle. Fever, hepatosplenomegaly, lymphadenopathy, edema, various rashes, jaundice, anemia, bony changes, and CSF abnormalities are the most common findings in neonates. Findings in late congenital syphilis include typical bony and facial features, hearing loss, Hutchinson's teeth, rhagades, keratitis, and corneal scarring.

Diagnosis The differential diagnosis of syphilis includes genital herpes, chancroid, scabies, genital warts, primary HIV infection, and noninfectious drug eruptions. History and physical examination findings alone often prove inaccurate. Nontreponemal and treponemal serologic tests are the mainstays of diagnosis. The nontreponemal tests are VDRL and rapid plasma reagin (RPR), which are used for initial screening. Treponemal specific tests are used to confirm the diagnosis of syphilis and rule out false-positive results. These tests include FTA-ABS (fluorescent treponemal antibody absorption) and MHA-TP (microhemagglutination assay for *T pallidum* antibodies). The nontreponemal tests become negative after treatment, whereas the specific treponemal tests remain positive. Dark-field microscopy, looking for the typical spirochetes, can be used to evaluate the chancre in primary syphilis.

Treatment Long-acting benzathine penicillin remains the mainstay of treatment of early syphilis. Bicillin L-A, 2.4 million units, given as a single IM dose is the recommended therapy. Be aware that Bicillin C-R, which contains equal amounts of procaine and benzathine penicillin, does not produce effective serum drug levels to effectively treat *Treponema pallidum*. Patients with latent syphilis of unknown duration should be treated with Bicillin L-A, 2.4 million units once weekly for 3 consecutive weeks. Complications of late latent syphilis have different treatment protocols. Neurosyphilis can be treated with 3 to 4 million units of penicillin G every 4 hours IV for 10 to 14 days as 1 option.

Additional treatment options for early syphilis include doxycycline 100 mg twice daily or tetracycline 500 mg 4 times daily for 14 days. Current evidence also shows efficacy with a single 2-g dose of oral azithromycin, although reports of macrolide resistance have begun to emerge. Ceftriaxone seems to have similar efficacy to penicillin in animal models, although the optimal dose and duration have yet to be determined.[24]

Chancroid
Synonym Soft sore.

Cause *Haemophilus ducreyi*, a gram-negative bacillus. It forms streptobacillary chains on Gram stain, often described as railroad tracks or a school of fish. It is difficult to culture without special media.

Epidemiology Infection occurs mainly in developing countries, although it occurs in North America and Europe and may be underdiagnosed in those regions. It is common in Africa and once was found in 60% of genital ulcers in South Africa.[60,61] It is also common in Southeast Asia and Latin America. It is associated with poverty and is often found in epidemics. The ulcers of chancroid have been found to increase the risk of HIV transmission.[62,63]

There were 24 reported cases in the United States in 2010; however, the disease becomes more prevalent if efforts are made to look for it.[64] With polymerase chain reaction (PCR) testing, it was found in 59% of genital ulcers in Jackson, MS.[65]

Risk factors More men are infected than women, especially uncircumcised men.[66] Use of cocaine and trading sex for drugs are also risk factors. Minority groups, heterosexuals, and female prostitutes are all at higher risk.

Pathophysiology The organism is highly infectious. It gains access through tiny abrasions that occur with sexual activity. The infection leads to an initial papule that develops into an ulcer, typically 1 to 2 cm in size. The ulcer forms an exudate and is highly contagious. Classically there are 3 zones: superficial with necrotic material, intermediate with edema, and a deep zone with lymphocytes and plasma cells. *Haemophilus ducreyi* may form a cytotoxin, which injures the epithelium and is toxic to fibroblasts and other cells, leading to the ulcer.[67] The infection causes painful lymphadenopathy in about half of cases and can form buboes.

Clinical disease The CDC defines a definite case when *Haemophilus ducreyi* is isolated from the lesion and a probable case when there are compatible clinical findings with a negative dark-field examination for treponemes, a negative serologic test for syphilis, and a negative culture for herpes (or a picture incompatible with herpes).[68]

Symptoms are the development of a painful genital papule that leads to an ulcer or more commonly multiple ulcers. The ulcer is soft rather than hard and shows exudate and irregular, ragged edges. It bleeds easily. The ulcer develops to about 1 to 2 cm in size and commonly involves the prepuce, corona, and glans of the penis on men and the labia, introitus, and perianal area in women. The incubation period is usually 3 to 10 days, but can be up to 35 days. There are painful inguinal lymph nodes in 50% of cases, most often unilateral, which can form buboes. The infection may cause extensive local tissue destruction, especially with HIV coinfection, but it does not disseminate. (See pictures at www.cdc.gov/std/training/clinicalslides/PowerPoint/chancroid.ppt).[69]

Diagnosis A purely clinical diagnosis is often made but this can be difficult. Gram stain of an ulcer swab can be performed, looking for gram-negative bacilli in typical parallel formation. This test has a low sensitivity.

Culture for the organism on special media is the gold standard, but is not widely available.[70] The specimen must be plated quickly for culture to be successful. PCR is now becoming more widely available and is more sensitive for diagnosis.[71] However, it is a more costly test in low-resource areas.

Treatment Local care should be given to the ulcer to keep it dry. Current antibiotic recommendations are either azithromycin 1 g once or ceftriaxone 250 mg IM once. Ciprofloxacin 500 mg twice a day for 3 days and erythromycin 500 mg 4 times a day for 7 days can also be used. In patients with HIV, it may be necessary to give longer courses of treatment. Drainage of buboes also aids healing. It is important to follow clinically to ensure healing, especially if the diagnosis was made on clinical grounds alone. Usually pain is better within 48 hours and the ulcer shows signs of healing within 72 hours. It is important to rule out syphilis. Syphilis and chancroid can coexist and both need to be treated. Any sex partners who have been exposed within 10 days must be treated even if they have no signs of disease.[24]

Herpes simplex virus
Synonym Genital herpes, cold sores, fever blisters.

Cause *Herpes simplex* virus (HSV) has 2 types: HSV-1 and HSV-2. Both types can lead to oral or genital herpes; however, HSV-1 is mainly oral and HSV-2 is mainly genital. HSV is classified as a human herpes virus (HHV). Other types of HHV include varicella-zoster virus, Epstein-Barr virus, cytomegalovirus, roseola virus, and Kaposi sarcoma–associated herpes virus.

Epidemiology HSV-1 and HSV-2 are common infections worldwide; at least 50 million persons have genital herpes in the United States alone.[24,72] Previous infection with HSV-1 also leads to a 3-fold increase in asymptomatic HSV-2 infection.[73] HSV-2 infection has also been established as risk factor for HIV-1 infection and transmission.[74]

Risk factors There are multiple risk factors for the development of genital herpes, including history of previous STD, early age of first sexual intercourse, and multiple sexual partners. In general, HSV-2 is more easily transmitted from men to women, thus making women more susceptible. Athletes who participate in sports in which there is direct close personal contact are also at risk.

Pathophysiology Infection is caused by exposure of a disrupted area of the mucosal surface to the virus. This exposure allows entry of the virus and subsequent replication in epithelial cells. The incubation period ranges from 2 to 30 days. Transmission from an individual can occur with or without active lesions as a result of shedding of the virus during asymptomatic periods. Regardless of the appearance of lesions, infection of the nerve endings can occur.

Clinical disease Genital herpes is caused by both HSV-1 and HSV-2 and is a chronic lifelong disease. There are 3 types of clinical manifestations of the disease: primary, nonprimary, and recurrent. A primary infection is diagnosed when a person is infected and there is no evidence of preexisting antibodies. Typically, patients present with painful, ulcerative, genital lesions. These lesions can also be associated with constitutional symptoms. Pictures can be found at http://www.cdc.gov/std/training/clinicalslides/slides-dl.htm. Nonprimary infections occur when there has previously been a type 1 or 2 infection and the subsequent infection is of the alternate type. Patients usually experience a less severe presentation of the disease compared with primary infections. Recurrent infection occurs when the original HSV type reactivates. Recurrence with HSV-1 typically occurs about 1 to 2 times a year. Without suppressive therapy, the median recurrence rate after the first episode of HSV-2 infection is about 4 times a year, with approximately 40% of patients having at least 6 recurrences and 20% having more than 10 recurrences in the first year.[75,76]

Herpes can be transmitted to the neonate, by direct contact of the fetus with infected vaginal secretions at the time of delivery. Although viral shedding can occur during an asymptomatic reactivation of disease, the most important determinate of neonatal infection is a primary maternal infection near the time of delivery. Any HSV primary infection should be treated in pregnancy. A woman with recurrences should receive suppressive therapy from 36 weeks' gestation on.[24] See the guidelines from the American College of Obstetricians and Gynecologists for more information on various scenarios of herpes in pregnancy.[77]

Diagnosis Differential diagnoses include syphilis, chancroid, lymphogranuloma venereum (LGV), scabies, and squamous cell carcinoma. Scraping of an infected lesion was previously used to diagnosis the disease either by Tzanck smear or cytology; however, this method is insensitive and lacks specificity and should be avoided. Viral cultures can be used with recognition that they have low sensitivity. HSV PCR, which has a higher sensitivity than a viral culture, is also obtained by scraping the ulcer. Type-specific serologic assays can also be used to differentiate HSV-1 or HSV-2 infections. If these tests yield a negative result, repeat testing in 6 to 12 weeks should occur.[78]

Treatment The goal of treatment is to shorten the duration of the clinical signs and symptoms of HSV infections. Initiation of oral antiviral therapy within 72 hours of lesion appearance may decrease duration and severity of illness by days to weeks.[79] The antiviral agents acyclovir, famciclovir, and valacyclovir seem to have similar efficacy for the treatment of primary genital herpes and for the suppression of recurrent infection.[80,81] The CDC recommends the following regimens:

- Primary infection: acyclovir 400 mg orally 3 times a day or 200 mg orally 5 times a day for 7 to 10 days, famciclovir 250 mg orally 3 times a day for 7 to 10 days, or valacyclovir 1 g orally twice a day for 7 to 10 days[24]
- Episodic therapy for recurrent HSV infections include: acyclovir 400 mg orally 3 times a day for 5 days, acyclovir 800 mg orally twice a day for 5 days, acyclovir 800 mg orally 3 times a day for 2 days, famciclovir 125 mg orally twice a day for 5 days, famciclovir 1 g orally twice a day for 1 day, famciclovir 500 mg orally once followed by 250 mg twice daily for 2 days, valacyclovir 500 mg orally twice a day for 3 days, or valacyclovir 1 g orally once a day for 5 days[24]
- In recurrent disease, suppressive therapy can reduce the frequency of genital herpes by 70% to 80%.[82] The following are recommended regimens for suppressive therapy: acyclovir 400 mg twice a day, famciclovir 250 mg orally twice a day, valacyclovir 500 mg or 1 g orally once a day[24]

Lymphogranuloma venereum (LGV)

Synonyms Lymphogranuloma inguinale, lymphopathia venereum, tropical bubo, Durand-Nicolas-Favre disease.

Cause LGV serovars of *Chlamydia trachomatis*, L1, L2, L3.

Epidemiology LGV has traditionally been considered a disease of the tropics with heterosexual transmission. It has never been a common disease, and is less common than other ulcerative STDs, such as herpes, chancroid, and syphilis.[83] Traditionally, LGV has been found most often in Africa, India, Southeast Asia, and the Caribbean.[84] Beginning in 2004, with an outbreak in the Netherlands, LGV has been found with an increasing incidence in North America, Europe, and Australia.[85] This outbreak has occurred almost entirely among MSM and most commonly involves proctitis rather than the more classic inguinal buboes.[86] The largest outbreaks have been reported in New York and the United Kingdom. The Western outbreak has been associated almost entirely with serovar L2 and often the subset of L2b.[87] There is a close association with HIV, although LGV is not considered an opportunistic infection but rather a coinfection.

Risk factors HIV is an independent risk factor,[88] and any coexisting ulcerative disease is also a risk factor. Other risk factors include other STDs, anal intercourse, travel abroad, and meeting sexual partners on the Internet.[89]

Pathophysiology The *Chlamydia* organism invades the genital area and spreads to local lymphatic tissue. This organism produces lymphangitis with necrosis and abscess formation of lymph nodes in the inguinal and femoral areas. This situation can lead to subsequent fibrosis.

Clinical disease The disease has classically 3 stages, which have been well described.

Stage I is the primary infection. A small genital ulcer or papule is found at the initial site of inoculation after an incubation period of 3 to 21 days. This infection also may be only mucosal inflammation. This initial lesion heals spontaneously in a matter of days and often goes unnoticed and is found in only 10% of patients. There are no significant symptoms of rectal disease at this stage.

Stage II is the secondary infection. After 2 to 6 weeks, the infection extends to the local inguinal and femoral nodes. Because the inguinal ligament bisects these groups of nodes, it often creates the groove sign, considered a classic sign of LGV. In a few cases, symptoms may be severe, with painful lymphangitis and systemic symptoms such as fever, headache and arthralgias. The nodes often form abscesses or buboes and may rupture spontaneously through the skin, or into the vagina or rectum.

In those with coexistent HIV infection, proctitis is the most common manifestation of disease at this stage. Symptoms include tenesmus, anal discharge, and bleeding. An inflammatory mass can form in the rectum and cause hemorrhage.

Eye infections have been reported with follicular conjunctivitis, keratitis, or iridocyclitis with local lymph node spread. Oral infections usually involve a painful lesion on the tongue, although other areas of the oral cavity can be infected. The cervical lymph nodes are involved.[90] After 3 to 4 months, the infection may resolve spontaneously, but often leads to the third stage.

Stage III is the late stage. The lymph nodes become scarred and fibrotic and obstruct lymphatic flow. This situation can lead to swelling or elephantiasis of the genital area. Also, anal fistulas may develop in the anogenital tract, with strictures and infertility resulting in the long-term.

(Pictures can be found at www.cdc.gov/std/training/clinicalslides/PowerPoint/lgv.ppt).

Diagnosis Clinical diagnosis is difficult, because the incidence is low, but in the MSM population with proctitis the index of suspicion should be high.

- The organism can be cultured from an ulcer or bubo but this is rarely performed because the false-negative rate is high and the culture is positive only about 30% of the time.
- Biopsy shows only nonspecific inflammation and cannot be relied on for diagnosis.
- Serologic tests (immunofluorescence or complement fixation) are the most common way to make the diagnosis, but they cannot distinguish *Chlamydia* serotypes and cannot distinguish between recent or past infections.
- NAATs and PCRs have been developed with excellent sensitivity and specificity. These are the recommended tests for rectal or oral lesions in which LGV is suspected. The tests are not widely available yet, but swabs can be sent to the local health department or to the CDC after consultation.[91,92]

Treatment When LGV is diagnosed, the recommended treatment is doxycycline 100 mg twice a day for 21 days. The alternative in pregnancy is erythromycin 500 mg 4 times a day for 21 days. Azithromycin 1 g weekly for 3 weeks has also been used successfully, but there is less evidence for this treatment. A test of cure is recommended at least 4 weeks after treatment.

Treatment of proctitis is the same; however, ceftriaxone 250 mg IM once is usually given as well.

Late-stage disease may require surgical drainage of abscesses and plastic surgery for the fibrosis and strictures.

Infected individuals should be tested for all other STDs, including HIV and hepatitis B and C.

Asymptomatic partners of those with documented LGV should receive the standard treatment of *Chlamydia*: doxycycline 100 mg twice a day for 7 days or azithromycin 1 g once.[24]

Granuloma inguinale
Synonyms Donovanosis, granuloma venereum.

Cause *Klebsiella granulomatis,* formerly *Calymmatobacterium granulomatis,* a gram-negative coccobacillus with a capsule and 2 end bulbs resembling a safety pin. These organisms are found in large macrophages and are called Donovan bodies.

Epidemiology This is an uncommon tropical disease found mainly in India, Papua New Guinea, South America, South Africa, the Caribbean, and Australia. It often occurs in epidemics. In 1986, 16% of genital ulcers in Durban, South Africa were caused by granuloma inguinale.[93] More recently, the percentage was about 4%.[94]

Risk factors tend to be poor hygiene and prostitution. The disease generally is found in impoverished and marginalized populations.

Pathophysiology The organism invades the skin of the genitalia to form an ulcer. It is thought that it can be transmitted by both sexual and nonsexual contact with the ulcer and can be transmitted to an infant during vaginal delivery.[95] It begins as a small papule and gradually enlarges into a painless ulcer with a raised border. Uncommonly, it can spread to the inguinal lymph nodes and cause pseudobuboes.

Clinical disease An invasive ulcer develops on the genitalia and gradually enlarges. The incubation period is 3 to 50 days, with most infections occurring after 30 to 40 days.[96] The initial ulcer is granulomatous, painless, and bleeds easily. Untreated, it enlarges gradually toward the groin and anus.

There are 4 types of ulcers: the classic ulcerogranulomatous form, a hypertrophic ulcer, a necrotic ulcer, and a sclerotic ulcer.[97]

Complications include secondary infection, scarring, and local genital elephantiasis. Squamous cell carcinoma can develop in the ulcers, although the old literature states that this occurs only 0.25% of the time. The organism can also rarely disseminate and infect other organs. It is also likely a risk factor in acquiring HIV.[96]

(See pictures at www.cdc.gov/std/training/clinicalslides/PowerPoint/Granuloma_inguinale.ppt).

Diagnosis Index of suspicion must be high in endemic areas, because other ulcerative genital diseases are more common. Culture is difficult and not readily available. A punch biopsy or a crush tissue preparation is the best way to show the diagnostic Donovan bodies. A smear made from the ulcer and stained with Giemsa can also be successful. A PCR test has been developed but is not in general use.

Treatment Many antibiotics have been successful. Most agencies and experts use either doxycycline (100 mg twice a day) or azithromycin (1 g weekly) for at least 3 weeks and sometimes longer if symptoms have not resolved at that point. An aminoglycoside (streptomycin or gentamicin) can be added if necessary. Other antibiotics that have been successful are ciprofloxacin 750 mg twice a day and trimethoprim/sulfamethoxazole double-strength twice a day both for 3 weeks. In pregnancy, erythromycin 500 mg 4 times a day for 3 weeks is recommended.

With concomitant HIV infection, treatment may need to be more prolonged.

In some areas lacking good diagnostic facilities, patients with genital ulcers should be treated for syphilis and chancroid as well as granuloma inguinale to cover the more common infections.

Plastic surgery is sometimes needed in neglected cases.

All contacts should be treated if they have had sexual relations with the patient within 60 days.

See **Table 1** for a comparison of the diseases causing genital ulcers.

Diseases of the Skin and Mucosa

HPV
Synonym HPV, genital warts, condyloma accuminata.

Cause HPV is a nonenveloped double-stranded DNA virus of the Papovaviridae family. There are more than 100 subtypes of HPV, of which specific ones infect the genital area. These subtypes are divided into low-risk and high-risk types based on the oncogenic potential. HPV-6 and HPV-11 cause approximately 90% of genital warts,[98] whereas the carcinogenic serotypes HPV-16 and HPV-18 cause approximately 70% of all cervical cancers worldwide.[99]

Epidemiology HPV is the most common STD, with a worldwide point prevalence of approximately 10%.[100] Approximately 6.2 million new HPV infections occur every year, and approximately 20 million individuals are currently infected in the United States.[101] It is also estimated that 75% to 80% of sexually active adults acquire a genital tract HPV infection before the age of 50 years.[102]

Risk factors The risk of HPV infection in women is directly related to the number of male sex partners and to the male partners' number of female sex partners.[103] Both vaginal and anal intercourse are major risk factors; however, penetrating intercourse is not required for transmission.[103,104] The strongest risk for the development of cancer is disease persistence.

Pathophysiology HPV is a nonenveloped, capsid virus with a life cycle that is integrally linked to the integrity of the host epithelium. Initial cellular infection occurs as a result of microscopic epithelial disruption.[105] Once these short-lived, infected cells desquamate, infectious HPV virions are released for the next round of infection. HPV infection can alter genital epithelial cell morphology as well as invade the immune system through a variety of mechanisms. These 2 events, although not clearly understood, are believed to increase the risk for HPV-associated cancers.

Clinical disease Asymptomatic genital HPV infection is common and usually self-limited; it is estimated that more than 50% of sexually active persons become infected at least once in their lifetime.[24] The body's immune system clears most HPV naturally within 2 years (about 90%), although some infections persist. Disease development is determined by HPV type. Genital warts are typically associated with types 6 and 11 and occur on the genital regions of both men and women. Cervical cancer is typically associated with types 16 and 18 and occurs after dysplastic changes on the cervix. Recurrent respiratory papillomatosis associated with types 6 and 11 is caused when warts grow in the pharynx or esophagus. Other cancers associated with types 16 and 18 that can occur, but are seen less frequently, include vulvar, vaginal, penile, anal, and oropharyngeal cancers. See http://www.cdc.gov/std/training/clinicalslides/slides-dl.htm for pictures of genital warts.

Diagnosis There is no recommendation for routine screening of the general population. In women aged 21 to 65 years, Pap smears should be obtained per current recommended intervals to screen for cellular changes related to HPV infection. In women older than 30 years, the recommendation is to screen with an HPV DNA test along with a Pap smear. Four tests have been approved by the FDA for use in the United States: the HC II High-Risk HPV test (Qiagen), HC II Low-Risk HPV test (Qiagen), Cervista HPV 16/18 test, and Cervista HPV High-Risk test (Hologics).[24]

Table 1
Characteristics and treatment of ulcerative STDs

	Herpes simplex	Syphilis	Chancroid	Lymphogranuloma Venereum	Granuloma Inguinale
Incubation	2–7 d	9–90 d	1–14 d	3–42 d	7–28 d but ≤6 mo
Lesion appearance	Superficial, moist vesicle	Papule becoming a 5-mm–15-mm sharply demarcated, elevated, nonpurulent ulcer	Papule becoming a ragged, undermined, purulent ulcer	Inconspicuous papule or pustule becoming a 2-mm–10-mm elevated ulcer	Papule becoming an elevated ulcer with a red base that bleeds easily
Number of lesions	Multiple	Usually 1	Usually multiple	Usually 1, may not be detected	Variable
Induration	None	Firm	Soft	Usually firm if found	Firm
Pain	Significant pain and tenderness	Pain uncommon	Pain common and tender	Variable	Pain uncommon
Inguinal adenopathy	Positive firm tender nodes	Firm, nontender nodes	Tender nodes may suppurate	Tender nodes, may suppurate	None but can form pseudobuboes
Treatment (see text for alternatives)	Acyclovir 400 mg tid for 7–10 d or famciclovir 250 mg tid × 7–10 d or valacyclovir 1 g bid × 7–10 d	Benzathine penicillin G 2.4 million units IM for primary disease	Azithromycin 1 g or ceftriaxone 250 mg IM	Doxycycline 100 mg bid for 3 wks	Doxycycline 100 mg bid or azithromycin 1 g weekly for at least 3 wks
Treat partners if exposed within	If symptomatic. Offer testing if asymptomatic	≥90 d	10 d	60 d	60 d

Adapted from Holmes KK, Sparling P, Stamm W, et al, editors. Sexually transmitted diseases. 4th edition. New York: McGraw-Hill; 2008.

Treatment Although there is no specific treatment of the virus itself, there are treatments for the serious diseases that HPV can cause, including genital warts, and cervical and other cancers.[106] Recommended regimens for external genital warts include:

1. Patient-applied: Podofilox 0.5% solution or gel, Imiquimod 5% cream, or Sinecatechins 15% ointment
2. Provider-administered: cryotherapy with liquid nitrogen or cryoprobe
3. Podophyllin resin 10% to 25% in a compound tincture of benzoin, trichloroacetic acid or bichloroacetic acid 80% to 90%
4. Surgical removal[24]

Efforts at prevention are the key to decreasing the prevalence of this disease. There are 2 HPV vaccines that are licensed in the United States: a bivalent vaccine (Cervarix) containing HPV types 16 and 18, and a quadrivalent vaccine (Gardasil), containing HPV types 6, 11, 16, and 18. Both vaccines offer protection against the HPV types that cause 70% of cervical cancers.[24]

Molluscum contagiosum
Cause A member of the poxvirus family.

Epidemiology This virus is present worldwide and has 4 distinct genotypes; however, genotype 1 is the predominant form and represents 90% of cases in the United States.[107] It has previously been thought of as a pediatric disease, but the number of adult cases has increased as a result of the AIDS epidemic.[108]

Risk factors It is a common childhood disease and not necessarily sexually transmitted. Healthy adolescents and adults can develop the disease, often caused by sexual transmission or in relation to participating in contact sports.[107] Atopic dermatitis may be a risk factor caused by the barrier breaks and immune cell dysfunction in atopic skin.[109] It is also associated with immune-deficient states.

Pathophysiology The virus invades the skin and replicates in the cell cytoplasm. It infects keratinocytes and mucosa, resulting in papular lesions. The lesions can occur on any part of the body and are often spread by autoinoculation from the original area of infection to other areas of the body. It is classified as an STD when the infection is located in the genital region of a sexually active individual. In children with anogenital lesions, it is most often the result of autoinoculation rather than sexual contact.[110] Infection can also be spread by sharing towels or bathing sponges.[107] The incubation period is estimated to be from 2 weeks to 6 months. It is a self-limited infection, with papules usually resolving spontaneously within 6 to 12 months, but they may persist for up to 4 years.[111]

Clinical disease The infection typically presents as 2-mm to 5-mm pearly papules with umbilicated centers. These areas may also have an underlying inflamed or eczematous appearance. They can occur anywhere on the body but spare the palms and soles. In immunosuppressed states, the lesions are larger and more diffuse. See http://www.cdc.gov/std/training/clinicalslides/slides-dl.htm for pictures of Molluscum.

Diagnosis Identification of lesions on the skin is usually sufficient to establish the diagnosis. Differential diagnoses include verruca, Penicillium marneffei, cryptococcosis, milia, basal cell carcinoma, keratoacanthoma, and condyloma accuminata. Skin biopsy can be useful if the cause of the lesion cannot be determined.

Henderson-Patterson bodies can be seen when hematoxylin-eosin stains are performed on histologic specimens. This procedure provides a definitive diagnosis.

Treatment In general, this disease is considered to be self-limited. The decision to treat is determined by the desired outcome by the clinician and patient. In general, the consensus is that sexually active individuals with *Molluscum* should be treated to avoid spread of the disease. In addition, immunocompromised patients may also benefit from early treatment.

First-line therapies include cryotherapy with liquid nitrogen applied to individual lesions for 6 to 10 seconds with a cotton-tipped applicator, curettage of individual lesions with a curette, cantharidin, a topical blistering agent that should only be applied by the clinician, or Podophyllotoxin, a commercially available topical solution or gel applied twice daily for 3 consecutive days each week for up to 4 weeks.

Second-line therapies that have been found to have limited efficacy, include Imiquimod 5% cream (applied 3 times weekly for up to 12 weeks), potassium hydroxide 5% to 10%, salicylic acid, or topical retinoids.

Ectoparasites

Pediculosis pubis
Synonym Crab lice.

Cause An infestation with the ectoparasite *Phthirus pubis.* The crab louse is 1 to 1.8 mm long, translucent, and shorter and broader than body and scalp lice. It has 4 of its 6 legs adapted with pincers to grasp hair shafts (picture at http://www.cdc. gov/parasites/lice/pubic/index.html). The parasite goes through the egg stage, which hatches in about a week, and then 3 nymphal stages before becoming an adult. The life span of the adult female is 3 to 4 weeks, during which time she lays about 30 eggs, called nits, that are attached firmly to hair shafts.

Epidemiology Pubic lice have been found worldwide, infesting about 2% to 10% of human populations and as far back in history as 10,000 years ago in the Old World.[112] Crab louse eggs have been found on a Chilean mummy from 2000 years ago in the New World.[113] This parasite infests only humans (not pets) and cannot survive more than 24 to 48 hours off the human host. It is generally transmitted by close sexual contact, although transmission by contact with infected fomites such as clothing, towels, or linens is possible.[114] The louse is not adapted to crawling on smooth surfaces, thus infection from a toilet seat is unlikely.[114] It is highly contagious, and about 95% of sexual contacts become infested.[115]

Risk factors include any risky sexual behavior, including prostitution. Teenagers and young adults are most often infected. In 1 large study in Spain performed at an STD clinic,[116] 1.8 women were infected to 1 male, with the yearly infection rate of 1.3% to 4.6%. In this study, there was a higher rate of infection in MSM than in heterosexual men.

Clinical disease The main symptom is itching in the pubic area. Although the genital area is the most common site, the lice can be found in any hairy area of the body (beard, chest) except the scalp. The eyelashes are another common site of involvement (*Pediculosis ciliaris*, see treatment in later discussion). At times, a bluish spot is noted at the site of the insect bite caused by a louse anticoagulant released during feeding. Inguinal lymphadenopathy occasionally occurs.

Pubic lice are not a vector for systemic disease, in contrast to body lice. Secondary local infection may occur as a result of scratching. (Pictures of pubic lice and scabies, another sexually transmitted ectoparasite, can be found at: www.cdc.gov/std/training/clinicalslides/PowerPoint/lice&scabies.ppt).

Diagnosis The diagnosis is made by finding lice or nits on hair shafts. Both lice and nits can be seen with the naked eye but a microscope helps to identify the species. It is important to check for other STIs if lice are found because there are often coexistent diseases.

Treatment The current recommendations are either:

- Permethrin 1% cream rinse applied to the area and washed off in 10 minutes or
- Pyrethrins with piperonyl butoxide applied to the affected areas and washed off after 10 minutes[24]

Alternatives include Malathion 0.5% applied to the affected area and washed off after 8 to 12 hours or Ivermectin 250 μg/kg by mouth repeated in 2 weeks. Ivermectin is not recommended in pregnant or lactating women or in children lighter than 15 kg.[24] No change in treatment is recommended with concomitant HIV infection.

Resistance to pediculicides is virtually nonexistent in pubic lice, but it has become a problem with head lice. It is possible that resistance could develop in the future.

Lice and nits are destroyed by heat, and any clothing should be washed in water at least 130° F for 30 minutes.[24] A hot iron is useful in folds and pleats. Sexual partners from the past month should be treated but nonsexual household contacts do not have to be treated if they do not show sins of infestation.[117]

It is difficult to use topical treatment of *Pediculosis cillaris*, and mechanical removal of lice and nits may be best after the application of ordinary petrolatum.[24] Ivermectin should be tried if mechanical removal is not possible, and the eyelashes have been removed in some cases.[118,119]

Scabies is not covered in this article but is spread with close contact including sexual contact.

Systemic Infections (Not Covered in this Article)

Hepatitis A, B, C, D
HIV
Cytomegalovirus
Human T-Cell Lymphotropic Virus
Group B *Streptococcus*

Gastrointestinal Pathogens Possibly Spread by Oral-Fecal Exposure During Sexual Acts (Not Covered in this Article)

Shigella
Campylobacter
Entamoeba
Giardia
Cryptosporidium
Enterobius
Strongyloides
Candida

See **Table 2** for the various STD syndromes and a summary of their diagnosis and treatment.

Table 2
Common presentations with likely organisms, tests, and treatments

Presentation	Organism(s)	Diagnostic Tests	Empirical Treatment
Male urethritis	Gonorrhea (GC), *Chlamydia*, *Mycoplasma*, *Ureaplasma*, *Trichomonas*, HSV	Gram stain of discharge, culture, NAAT of discharge or first voided urine	Ceftriaxone + doxycycline or azithromycin
Epididymitis	GC, *Chlamydia*	Same as above for any discharge	Same as above
Female urethritis or cystitis	GC, *Chlamydia*, HSV	Same as above	Same as above
Cervicitis	GC, *Chlamydia*, *Mycoplasma*	NAAT of discharge or first voided urine	Same as above if diagnosis confirmed
Vulvitis	Trichomoniasis, candidiasis	KOH and saline wet preparation of vaginal discharge	Metronidazole or antifungal treatment depending on diagnosis
PID	GC, *Chlamydia*, *Gardnerella*, *Mycoplasma*, group B *Streptococcus*, anaerobes	NAAT of cervical discharge	Outpatient: ceftriaxone + doxycycline + metronidazole or ofloxacin Hospital: either cefotetan or cefoxitin + doxycycline or clindamycin + gentamycin
Genital ulcer	HSV I and II, syphilis, chancroid, LGV, granuloma inguinale	Viral culture of ulcer, RPR, ulcer smear for dark-field or Gram stain examination, NAAT or serology for LGV	Antiviral treatment of herpes plus penicillin
Proctitis	*Chlamydia*, LGV, GC, HSV, syphilis	NAAT, RPR, culture	Ceftriaxone 250 mg IM + doxycycline 100 mg bid × 7 d
Proctocolitis or enteritis	*Campylobacter*, shigellosis, amebiasis, giardiasis	Stool examination and culture	Depends on diagnosis
Acute arthritis	GC, *Chlamydia*, hepatitis B	Test for STDs as above or serologic test for hepatitis	Depends on diagnosis
Genital warts	HPV	Physical examination	Podophyllin or destructive measures
Squamous cell carcinoma and dysplasia of cervix	HPV	PCR or hybrid capture assay on cervical specimen	Colposcopy and depends on diagnosis

Adapted from Kasper DL, Fauci AS. Harrison's Infectious Diseases. New York: McGraw-Hill; 2010. p. 285.

PREVENTION OF STDS

The basic principles of prevention of STDs are: education and counseling of patients and providers, rapid early diagnosis and treatment, partner notification and treatment, condom use, and vaccination. Social factors are important as mentioned earlier, and having better access to care is critical in meeting prevention goals.

Patient education involves primary prevention for those sexually active and secondary prevention for those who already have an STD. Decreasing the number of sexual partners, avoiding high-risk partners (such as prostitutes), being aware of the symptoms of STDs and the need for rapid treatment, avoidance of sex if symptoms are present, knowledge of the spread of STDs including HIV infection, and the proper use of condoms are all important educational points.

Education begins with being willing to discuss sexual issues with patients. All patients, including adolescents, should have a sexual history taken and those at risk given counseling. Good evidence has shown that behavioral counseling interventions with multiple sessions conducted both in STD clinics and in primary care can reduce the STD incidence in at-risk adult and adolescent populations.[120] Even low-intensity interventions with 2 sessions have been shown to have some effect.[121] The education of adolescents is particularly important and also presents its own challenges. A study from Nigeria showed that using peers to help in the educational process was acceptable and successful in increasing reproductive health knowledge among adolescents.[122]

Condoms, when used correctly and consistently, have been shown to reduce the incidence of most STDs, except the ectoparasites. The most common type is the latex condom, which is effective but cannot be used by anyone with a latex allergy. They are also not compatible with oil-based lubricants or medications. There are also condoms made from synthetic materials such as polyurethane. These condoms are also effective and are compatible with all lubricants but they are more expensive. Condoms made from natural membranes are less effective, because they have small pores that allow the passage of viruses. This type of condom is not recommended. Condom effectiveness depends on patient motivation, skill, and knowledge of use. A condom placed on the penis before any genital contact greatly reduces the spread of any pathogen to or from the penile urethra. Those diseases causing skin or mucosal ulceration are also reduced, but if the involved area is not entirely covered, transmission can still occur.[24] The World Health Organization reached a consensus on 5 key messages for condom instructions:

a. Use a new condom for each act of sexual intercourse
b. Place the condom on the tip of the erect penis with the rolled side out before any genital contact
c. Unroll the condom all the way to the base of the penis
d. Immediately after ejaculation, hold the rim of the condom and withdraw the penis while still erect
e. Throw the condom away safely[123]

Vaccinations are available for HPV and hepatitis A and B. The hepatitis A vaccine is recommended for all children older than 1 year, travelers to countries where hepatitis A is endemic, and high-risk groups such as MSM, IDU, patients with an STD, and patients seeking care at a clinic because of concerns about an STD. The hepatitis B vaccine is recommended for all children, beginning at birth. It is also recommended for MSM, IDU, patients with HIV/AIDS, and Asian/Pacific islanders, who are also a high-risk group. Patients seeking care for an STD or possible STD should also be offered the hepatitis B vaccine, if not already immune. MSM and IDU should be tested for chronic hepatitis B infection because it is common in these populations. Between 15% and 25% of new cases of hepatitis B occur in the MSM group. Lack of vaccination represents a missed opportunity to prevent this serious disease.[122]

There are 2 vaccines available for the prevention of HPV, as mentioned earlier: HPV-2 against the oncogenic serotypes 16 and 18 and HPV-4 with activity against types 16 and 18 as well as the nononcogenic types 6 and 11 that cause genital warts. Either vaccine can be given to all girls between the ages of 9 and 26 years. The HPV-4 vaccine is also recommended for men in this same age group.

Antiviral medication is useful for preventing the spread of genital herpes. Valacyclovir, at 500 mg once daily, has been shown to reduce virus transmission in patients with genital herpes. This finding is true whether there are active lesions or not. Using condoms and rapidly treating outbreaks are also essential.

A new preventive treatment of HIV was approved by the FDA in July 2012. Pre-exposure prophylaxis with a combination of tenofovir disoproxil fumerate and emtricitabine has been shown to be effective in preventing HIV if taken regularly before sexual activity. It is being recommended for very-high-risk groups only at this time. More information is available in other articles elsewhere in this issue on HIV and hepatitis.

Male circumcision has been shown to lower the risk of STD acquisition in men in various studies. Most of this work has been carried out with HIV transmission, including 3 randomized trials in Africa. Circumcision reduced the rate of female to male transmission of HIV by 50% to 60%.[124] These results are in heterosexual men, and it is not known if the same results would be found in the MSM population. Circumcision does not seem to reduce HIV transmission from men to women. However, female partners of circumcised men did report lower rates of genital ulcers and a reduced risk of Trichomonas and bacterial vaginosis in 1 study.[125]

Reporting and partner notification are important tools to stop the spread of STDs in a community. Gonorrhea, syphilis, Chlamydia, chancroid, and AIDS are reportable in all states. When partners are tested, up to half are found to be infected, even though they are often asymptomatic. In some cases, it may be necessary to give the treatment course to the infected patient to pass along to their contact, a practice known as expedited partner therapy. This is not the ideal practice and may not be legal in some states, but it is often the best way to get treatment to a partner.[33]

REFERENCES

1. Workowski KA, Levine WC, Wasserheit JN. U.S. Centers for Disease Control and Prevention Guidelines for the Treatment of Sexually Transmitted Diseases: an opportunity to unify clinical and public health practice. Ann Intern Med 2002; 137:255–62.
2. CDC. STD Trends in the US 2010: National data for Chlamydia, gonorrhea and syphilis. Atlanta (GA): US Department of Health and Human Services; 2011. Available at: http://www.cdc.gov/std/stats10/trends.htm. Accessed September 3, 2012.
3. Decker MR, Miller E, McCauley HL, et al. Sex trade among young women attending family-planning clinics in Northern California. Int J Gynaecol Obstet 2012;117(2):173–7.
4. Maheux B, Haley N, Rivard M, et al. STD risk assessment and risk reduction counseling by recently trained family physicians. Acad Med 1995;70(8):726–8.
5. Seubert DE, Thompson IM, Gonik B. Partner notification of sexually transmitted disease in an obstetric and gynecology setting. Obstet Gynecol 1999;94: 399–402.

6. Weisbord JS, Koumans EH, Toomey KE, et al. Sexually transmitted diseases during pregnancy: screening, diagnostic and treatment practices among prenatal care providers in Georgia. South Med J 2001;94(1):47–53.

7. Gonzalez JS, Hendrikson ES, Collins EM, et al. Latinos and HIV/AIDS: examining factors related to disparity and identifying opportunities for psychosocial intervention research. AIDS Behav 2009;13:582–602.

8. DeNavas-Walt C, Proctor BD, Smith JC. U.S. Census Bureau, current population reports, P60–238, income, poverty and health insurance coverage in the United States: 2009. Washington, DC: US Government Printing Office; 2010.

9. Wiehe SE, Rosenman MB, Wang J, et al. Chlamydia screening among young women: individual- and provider-level differences in testing. Pediatrics 2011; 127(2):e336–44.

10. CDC. Special Focus Profiles: STDs in racial and ethnic minorities. STD Surveillance. 2010. Available at: http://www.cdc.gov/std/stats10/minorities.htm. Accessed September 3, 2012.

11. Forhan SE, Gottlieb SL, Sternberg MR, et al. Prevalence of sexually transmitted infections among female adolescents aged 14-19 in the United States. Pediatrics 2009;124:1505.

12. Tripp J, Viner R. Sexual health, contraception and teenage pregnancy. BMJ 2005;330:590–3.

13. Weinstock H, Berman S, Cates W. Sexually transmitted diseases among American youth: incidence and prevalence estimates, 2000. Perspect Sex Reprod Health 2004;36(1):6–10.

14. Tu W, Batteiger BE, Wiehe S, et al. Time from first intercourse to first sexually transmitted infection diagnosis among adolescent women. Arch Pediatr Adolesc Med 2009;163:1106.

15. Burstein GR, Gaydos CA, Diener-West M, et al. Incident Chlamydia trachomatis infections among inner-city adolescent females. JAMA 1998;280:521.

16. Fortenberry JD. Adolescent substance use and sexually transmitted disease risk: a review. J Adolesc Health 1995;16:304.

17. Niccolai LM, Ethier KA, Kershaw TS, et al. New sex partner acquisition and sexually transmitted disease risk among adolescent females. J Adolesc Health 2004;34:216.

18. Thrall JS, McCloskey L, Ettner SL, et al. Confidentiality and adolescents' use of providers for health information and for pelvic examinations. Arch Pediatr Adolesc Med 2000;154:885.

19. Jena AB, Goldman DP, Kamdar A, et al. Sexually transmitted diseases among users of erectile dysfunction drugs: analysis of claims data. Ann Intern Med 2010;153:1–7.

20. Harned MS, Panatlone DW, Ward-Ciesielski EF, et al. The prevalence and correlates of sexual risk behaviors and sexually transmitted infections in outpatients with borderline personality disorder. J Nerv Ment Dis 2011;199:832–8.

21. Low N, Broutet N, Adu-Sarkodie Y, et al. Global control of sexually transmitted infections. Lancet 2006;368:2001.

22. CDC. Sexually transmitted disease surveillance, 2008. Atlanta (GA): US Department of Health and Human Services; 2009.

23. Peterman TA, Tian LH, Metcalf CA, et al. High incidence of new sexually transmitted infections in the year following a sexually transmitted infection: a case for rescreening. Ann Intern Med 2006;145:564.

24. Centers for Disease Control and Prevention. Sexually transmitted diseases treatment guidelines, 2010. MMWR 2010;59(No. RR-12):1–109.

25. Centers for Disease Control and Prevention. Sexually transmitted disease, gonorrhea, fact sheet. Atlanta (GA): CDC; 2013. Available at: http://www.cdc.gov/std/gonorrhea/STDFact-gonorrhea.htm. Accessed June 21, 2013.
26. Centers for Disease Control and Prevention. Sexually transmitted disease surveillance 2011. Atlanta (GA): US Department of Health and Human Services; 2011.
27. Klausner JD, Barrett DC, Dithmer D. Risk factors for repeated gonococcal infections: San Francisco, 1990-1992. J Infect Dis 1998;177:1766.
28. Hook EW 3rd, Reichart CA, Upchurch DM, et al. Comparative behavioral epidemiology of gonococcal and chlamydial infections among patients attending a Baltimore, Maryland, sexually transmitted disease clinic. Am J Epidemiol 1992;136:662.
29. Handsfield HH, Sparling PF. Neisseria gonorrhoeae. In: Mandell GL, Bennett JE, Dolin R, editors. Principles and practice of infectious diseases. 4th edition. New York: Churchill Livingstone; 1995. p. 1909.
30. Centers for Disease Control and Prevention (CDC). Update to CDC's sexually transmitted diseases treatment guidelines, 2006: fluoroquinolones no longer recommended for treatment of gonococcal infections. MMWR 2007;56:332.
31. Centers for Disease Control and Prevention. Update to CDC's sexually transmitted diseases treatment guidelines, 2010: oral cephalosporins no longer a recommended treatment for gonococcal infections. MMWR 2012;61:590.
32. Datta SD, Sternberg M, Johnson RE, et al. Gonorrhea and chlamydia in the United States among persons 14 to 39 years of age, 1999 to 2002. Ann Intern Med 2007;147:89.
33. Centers for Disease Control and Prevention. Expedited partner therapy in the management of sexually transmitted diseases. Atlanta (GA): US Department of Health and Human Services; 2006. Available at: http://www.cdc.gov/std/treatment/EPTFinalReport2006.pdf. Accessed September 3, 2012.
34. Centers for Disease Control and Prevention. Sexually transmitted disease, chlamydia, fact sheet. Atlanta (GA): CDC; 2013. Available at: http://www.cdc.gov/std/chlamydia/stdfact-chlamydia.htm. Accessed June 21, 2013.
35. Warszawski J, Meyer L, Weber P. Criteria for selective screening of cervical *Chlamydia trachomatis* infection in women attending private gynecology practices. Eur J Obstet Gynecol Reprod Biol 1999;86:5.
36. Gaydos CA, Howell MR, Pare B, et al. *Chlamydia trachomatis* infections in female military recruits. N Engl J Med 1998;339:739.
37. Phillips RS, Hanff PA, Holmes MD, et al. *Chlamydia trachomatis* cervical infection in women seeking routine gynecologic care: criteria for selective testing. Am J Med 1989;86:515.
38. Centers for Disease Control and Prevention. *Chlamydia trachomatis* genital infection–United States, 1995. MMWR Morb Mortal Wkly Rep 1997;46(9):193–8.
39. Geisler WM. Diagnosis and management of uncomplicated *Chlamydia trachomatis* infections in adolescents and adults: summary of evidence reviewed for the 2010 Centers for Disease Control and Prevention Sexually Transmitted Diseases Treatment Guidelines. Clin Infect Dis 2011;53(Suppl 3):S92.
40. Lau CY, Qureshi AK. Azithromycin versus doxycycline for genital chlamydial infections: a meta-analysis of randomized clinical trials. Sex Transm Dis 2002;29:497–502.
41. Moodley P, Wilkinson D, Connolly C, et al. *Trichomonas vaginalis* is associated with pelvic inflammatory disease in women infected with human immunodeficiency virus. Clin Infect Dis 2002;34:519.

42. Centers for Disease Control and Prevention. Sexually transmitted disease, tricho-moniasis fact sheet. Atlanta (GA): CDC; 2012. Available at: http://www.cdc.gov/std/trichomonas/STDFact-Trichomoniasis.htm. Accessed June 21, 2013.

43. Laga M, Manoka A, Kivuvu M, et al. Non-ulcerative sexually transmitted diseases as risk factors for HIV-1 transmission in women: results from a cohort study. AIDS 1993;7:95.

44. Grodstein F, Goldman MB, Cramer DW. Relation of tubal infertility to history of sexually transmitted diseases. Am J Epidemiol 1993;137(5):577.

45. Zhang ZF, Begg CB. Is Trichomonas vaginalis a cause of cervical neoplasia? Results from a combined analysis of 24 studies. Int J Epidemiol 1994;23:682.

46. Soper DE, Bump RC, Hurt WG. Bacterial vaginosis and trichomoniasis vaginitis are risk factors for cuff cellulitis after abdominal hysterectomy. Am J Obstet Gynecol 1990;163:1016.

47. Cotch MF, Pastorek JG 2nd, Nugent RP, et al. Trichomonas vaginalis associated with low birth weight and preterm delivery. The Vaginal Infections and Prematurity Study Group. Sex Transm Dis 1997;24:353.

48. Krieger JN, Tam MR, Stevens CE, et al. Diagnosis of trichomoniasis. Comparison of conventional wet-mount examination with cytologic studies, cultures, and monoclonal antibody staining of direct specimens. JAMA 1988;259:1223.

49. Centers for Disease Control and Prevention. Primary and secondary syphilis–United States, 1998. MMWR Morb Mortal Wkly Rep 1999;48:873.

50. Centers for Disease Control and Prevention. 2011 Sexually transmitted disease surveillance- syphilis. Available at: http://www.cdc.gov/std/Syphilis2011/default.htm. Accessed February 28, 2013.

51. Wong W, Chaw K, Kent CK, et al. Risk factors for early syphilis among gay and bisexual men seen in an STD clinic in San Francisco, 2002-2003. Sex Transm Dis 2005;32:458.

52. Centers for Disease Control and Prevention. Congenital syphilis–United States, 2002. MMWR Morb Mortal Wkly Rep 2003;53:716.

53. Centers for Disease Control and Prevention. Transmission of primary and secondary syphilis by oral sex–Chicago, Illinois, 1998-2002. MMWR Morb Mortal Wkly Rep 2004;53:966.

54. Hook EW, Marra CM. Acquired syphilis in adults. N Engl J Med 1992;326:1060.

55. Peterman TA, Kahn RH, Ciesielski CA, et al. Misclassification of the stages of syphilis: implications for surveillance. Sex Transm Dis 2005;32:144.

56. Centers for Disease Control and Prevention. Sexually transmitted diseases – syphilis-CDC fact sheet. Available at: http://www.cdc.gov/std/syphilis/STDFact-Syphilis-detailed.htm. Accessed February 28, 2013.

57. Centers for Disease Control and Prevention. 2008 Sexually Transmitted Disease Surveillance. Table 33: Primary and secondary syphilis reported cases and rates per 100,000 population by age group and sex: United States, 2004-2008. Available at: http://www.cdc.gov/std/stats08/tables/33.htm. Accessed February 28, 2013

58. Centers for Disease Control and Prevention. Congenital syphilis–United States, 2003-2008. MMWR Morb Mortal Wkly Rep 2010;59:413.

59. American Academy of Pediatrics. Syphilis. In: Pickering LK, editor. Red Book: 2012 Report of the Committee on Infectious Diseases, vol. 29. Elk Grove Village (IL): American Academy of Pediatrics; 2012. p. 690.

60. Lai W, Chen CY, Morse SA, et al. Increasing relative prevalence of HSV-2 infection among men with genital ulcers from a mining community in South Africa. Sex Transm Infect 2003;79:202.

61. O'Farrell N. Increasing prevalence of genital herpes in developing countries: implications for heterosexual HIV transmission and STI control programs. Sex Transm Infect 1999;75:377.

62. Plummer FA, Simonson JN, Cameron DW, et al. Co-factors in male to female transmission of HIV. J Infect Dis 1991;163:233.

63. Gelfanova V, Humphreys TL, Spinola SM. Characterization of *Haemophilus ducreyi*-specific T-cell lines from lesions of experimentally infected human subjects. Infect Immun 2001;69:4224.

64. Dillon SM, Cummings M, Rajagopalan S, et al. Prospective analysis of genital ulcer disease in Brooklyn, New York. Clin Infect Dis 1997;24:945.

65. Mertz KJ, Weiss JB, Webb RM, et al. An investigation of genital ulcers in Jackson, Mississippi with use of a multiplex polymerase chain reaction assay: high prevalence of chancroid and human immunodeficiency virus infection. J Infect Dis 1998;178:1060.

66. Hart G. Venereal disease in a war environment: incidence and management. Med J Aust 1975;1:808.

67. Cope LD, Lumbley S, Latimer JL, et al. A diffusible cytotoxin of *Haemophilus ducreyi*. Proc Natl Acad Sci U S A 1997;94:4056.

68. Wharton M, Chorba TL, Vogt RL, et al. Case definitions for public health surveillance. MMWR Morb Mortal Wkly Rep 1990;39:1.

69. Mabey D, Richens J. Sexually transmitted infections. In: Cook GC, Zumla A, editors. Manson's tropical diseases. Edinburgh (United Kingdom): Elsevier Science; 2003. p. 444.

70. Riedner G, Todd J, Rusizoka M, et al. Possible reasons for an increase in the proportion of genital ulcers due to herpes simplex virus from a cohort of female bar workers in Tanzania. Sex Transm Infect 2007;83:91.

71. DiCarlo RP, Martin DH. The clinical diagnosis of genital ulcer disease in men. Clin Infect Dis 1997;25:292.

72. Xu F, Sternberg MR, Kottiri BJ, et al. Trends in herpes simplex virus type 1 and type 2 seroprevalence in the United States. JAMA 2006;296:964.

73. Langenberg AG, Corey L, Ashley RL, et al. A prospective study of new infections with herpes simplex virus type 1 and type 2. Chiron HSV Vaccine Study Group. N Engl J Med 1999;341:1432.

74. Freeman E, Weiss HA, Glynn JR, et al. Herpes simplex virus 2 infections increase HIV acquisition in men and women: systematic review and meta-analysis of longitudinal studies. AIDS 2006;20:73–83.

75. Gupta R, Warren T, Wald A. Genital herpes. Lancet 2007;370:2127.

76. Corey L, Adams HG, Brown ZA, et al. Genital herpes simplex virus infections: clinical manifestations, course, and complications. Ann Intern Med 1983;98:958.

77. American College of Obstetricians and Gynecologists. Gynecological herpes simplex virus infections. ACOG Practice Bulletin No. 57. Obstet Gynecol 2004;104:1111–7.

78. Guerry SL, Bauer HM, Klausner JD, et al. Recommendations for the selective use of herpes simplex virus type 2 serological tests. Clin Infect Dis 2005;40:38–45.

79. Cernik C, Gallina K, Brodell RT. The treatment of herpes simplex infections: an evidence-based review. Arch Intern Med 2008;168:1137.

80. Perry CM, Wagstaff AJ. Famciclovir. A review of its pharmacological properties and therapeutic efficacy in herpesvirus infections. Drugs 1995;50:396.

81. Perry CM, Faulds D. Valacyclovir. A review of its antiviral activity, pharmacokinetic properties and therapeutic efficacy in herpesvirus infections. Drugs 1996;52:754.

82. Diaz-Mitoma F, Sibbald RG, Shafran SD, et al. Oral famciclovir for the suppression of recurrent genital herpes: a randomized controlled trial. Collaborative Famciclovir Genital Herpes Research Group. JAMA 1998;280:887–92.
83. Behets FM, Andriamiadana J, Randrianasolo D, et al. Chancroid, primary syphilis, genital herpes and lymphogranuloma venereum in Antananarivo, Madagascar. J Infect Dis 1999;180:1382.
84. Scieux C, Barnes R, Bianchi A, et al. Lymphogranuloma venereum: 27 cases in Paris. J Infect Dis 1989;160:662.
85. Blank S, Schillinger JA, Harbatkin D. Lymphogranuloma venereum in the industrialized world. Lancet 2005;365:1607.
86. White JA. Manifestations and management of lymphogranuloma venereum. Curr Opin Infect Dis 2009;22:57.
87. Martin-Iguacel R, Libre JM, Nielson H, et al. Lymphogranuloma venereum proctocolitis: a silent endemic disease in men who have sex with men in industrialized countries. Eur J Clin Microbiol Infect Dis 2010;29:917.
88. Van der Bij AK, Spaargaren J, Morré SA, et al. Diagnostic and clinical implications of anorectal lymphogranuloma venereum in men who have sex with men: a retrospective case-control study. Clin Infect Dis 2006;42:186.
89. Ward H, Martin I, Macdonald N, et al. Lymphogranuloma venereum in the United Kingdom. Clin Infect Dis 2007;44:26.
90. Bedi R, Scully C. Tropical oral health. In: Cook GC, Zumla A, editors. Manson's tropical diseases. Edinburgh (United Kingdom): Elsevier Science; 2003. p. 521.
91. Hampton T. Lymphogranuloma venereum targeted: those at risk identified; diagnostic test developed. JAMA 2006;295:2592.
92. Bachmann LH, Johnson RE, Cheng H, et al. Nucleic acid amplification tests for diagnosis of Neisseria gonorrhoeae and Chlamydia trachomatis rectal infections. J Clin Microbiol 2010;48:1827.
93. O'Farrell N, Hoosen AA, Coetzee K, et al. Genital ulcer disease in women in Durban, South Africa. Genitourin Med 1991;67:327.
94. Kharsamy AB, Mohabeer Y, Goga R, et al. Aetiology of genital ulcer disease and HIV infection among men attending a STD clinic. 13th Meeting of the International Society for Sexually Transmitted Diseases Research, Abstract 533. Denver, July 11-14, 1999.
95. Govender D, Naidoo K, Chetty R. Granuloma inguinale (donovanosis). An unusual cause of otitis media and mastoiditis in children. Am J Clin Pathol 1997;108:510.
96. O'Farrell N. Donovanosis. Sex Transm Infect 2002;78:452.
97. O'Farrell N, Moi H. European Guidelines for the management of donovanosis. Int J STD AIDS 2010;21(9):609.
98. Beutner KR. Nongenital human papillomavirus infections. Clin Lab Med 2000;20:423.
99. deSanjose S, Quint WG, Alemany L, et al. Human papillomavirus genotype attribution in invasive cervical cancer: a retrospective cross-sectional worldwide study. Lancet Oncol 2010;11:1048.
100. de Sanjose S, Diaz M, Castellsague X, et al. Worldwide prevalence and genotype distribution of cervical human papillomavirus DNA in women with normal cytology: a meta-analysis. Lancet Infect Dis 2007;7:453.
101. Center for Disease Control and Prevention. Genital HPV infection–CDC fact sheet. Atlanta (GA): CDC; 2004.
102. Center for Disease Control and Prevention, Workowski KA, Berman SM. Sexually transmitted disease treatment guidelines, 2006. MMWR Recomm Rep 2006;55:1.
103. Ho GY, Bierman R, Beardsley L, et al. Natural history of cervicovaginal papillomavirus infection in young women. N Engl J Med 1998;338:423.

104. Winer RL, Lee SK, Hughes JP, et al. Genital human papillomavirus infection: incidence and risk factors in a cohort of female university students. Am J Epidemiol 2003;157:218.
105. Doorbar J. Molecular biology of human papillomavirus infection and cervical cancer. Clin Sci (Lond) 2006;110:525.
106. Center for Disease Control and Prevention. Incidence, prevalence, and cost of sexually transmitted infections in the United States, February 2013. Available at: http://www.cdc.gov/std/stats/STI-Estimates-Fact-Sheet-Feb-2013.pdf. Accessed February 28, 2013
107. Dohil MA, Lin P, Lee J, et al. The epidemiology of *Molluscum contagiosum* in children. J Am Acad Dermatol 2006;54:47.
108. Koopman RJ, van Merrienboer FC, Vreden SG, et al. *Molluscum contagiosum*: a marker for advanced HIV infection. Br J Dermatol 1992;126:528.
109. Kakourou T, Zacharides A, Anastasiou T, et al. *Molluscum contagiosum* in Greek children: a case series. Int J Dermatol 2005;44:221–3.
110. Braue A, Ross G, Varigos G, et al. Epidemiology and impact of childhood *Molluscum contagiosum*: a case series and critical review of the literature. Pediatr Dermatol 2005;22:287.
111. Center for Disease Control and Prevention. Clinical information: *Molluscum contagiosum*. Available at: http://www.cdc.gov/ncidod/dvrd/molluscum/clinical_overview.htm. Accessed February 28, 2013.
112. Anderson AL, Chaney E. Pubic Lice (*Phthirus pubis*): history, biology and treatment vs. knowledge and beliefs of US college students. Int J Environ Res Public Health 2009;6(2):592.
113. Rick FM, Rocha GC, Dittmar K, et al. Crab louse infestation in pre-Columbian America. J Parasitol 2002;88(6):1266.
114. Galiczynski EM, Elston DM. What's eating you? Pubic lice (*Phthirus pubis*). Cutis 2008;81:109.
115. Letau LA. Nosocomial transmission and infection control aspects of parasitic and ectoparasitic diseases. Part III. Ectoparasites/summary and conclusions. Infect Control Hosp Epidemiol 1991;12:179.
116. Varela JA, Otero L, Espinosa E, et al. *Phthirus pubis* in a sexually transmitted diseases unit. Sex Transm Dis 2003;30(4):292.
117. Stone SP, Goldfarb JN, Bacelieri RE. Scabies, other mites and pediculosis. In: Wolf K, Goldsmith LA, Katz SI, et al, editors. Fitzpatrick's dermatology in general medicine. New York: McGraw-Hill; 2008. p. 2029.
118. Burkhart CN, Burkhart CG. Oral ivermectin therapy for *Phthiriasis palpebrum*. Arch Ophthalmol 2000;118:134.
119. Ikeda N, Nomoto H, Hayasaka S, et al. *Phthirus pubis* infestation of the eyelashes and scalp hairs in a girl. Pediatr Dermatol 2003;20:356.
120. Lin JS, Whitlock E, O'Connor E, et al. Behavioral counseling to prevent sexually transmitted infections: a systematic review for the U.S. preventive services task force. Ann Intern Med 2008;149:497–508.
121. Dilley JW, Woods WJ, Loeb L, et al. Brief cognitive counseling with HIV testing to reduce sexual risk among men who have sex with men: results from a randomized controlled trial using paraprofessional counselors. J Acquir Immune Defic Syndr 2007;44:569.
122. Okanlawon FA, Asuzu MC. Effect of peer education intervention on secondary school adolescents' reproductive health knowledge in Saki, Nigeria. Afr J Med Med Sci 2011;40(4):353–60.

123. World Health Organization & The Department of Reproductive Health and Research, Johns Hopkins Bloomberg School of Public Health/Center for Communication Programs, INFO Project. Family planning: a global handbook for providers. Baltimore (MD); Geneva (Switzerland): CCP and WHO; 2007.

124. Gostin LO, Hankins CA. Male circumcision as an HIV prevention strategy in Sub-Saharan Africa: sociolegal barriers. JAMA 2008;300:2539.

125. Gray RH, Kigozi G, Serwadda D, et al. The effects of male circumcision on female partners' genital tract symptoms and vaginal infections in a randomized trial in Rakai, Uganda. Am J Obstet Gynecol 2009;200:42.e1.

Management of Human Immunodeficiency Virus in Primary Care

Jarrett K. Sell, MD

KEYWORDS

- Human immunodeficiency virus • Antiretroviral • Opportunistic infections
- Pre-exposure prophylaxis

KEY POINTS

- Improved routine op-out screening can help identify the 20% to 25% of persons living with human immunodeficiency virus (HIV) in the United States who remain undiagnosed.
- All patients with HIV, regardless of CD4 cell count, should be considered for antiretroviral treatment.
- Understanding of opportunistic infection prophylaxis, proper vaccination, and comorbid risk factor modification can improve life expectancy for many patients living with chronic stable HIV infection.
- Expanded recommendations for treatment of HIV infected persons and prophylaxis will likely significantly increase the number of persons in the United States who receive anti-retroviral treatment.
- Primary care providers have the opportunity to be more actively involved in the screening, prevention, and management of HIV.

INTRODUCTION

Since the identification of AIDS in 1981, the human immunodeficiency virus (HIV) has accounted for an estimated 30 million deaths, and more than 34 million people are infected with HIV worldwide. Effort has been made to improve education and access to treatment. As a result, new HIV infections declined by 17% worldwide from 2001 to 2009 according to the World Health Organization. However, despite a reduction in new HIV infections, the total number of persons living with HIV continues to increase as a result of an improved life expectancy with treatment.

At the start of the AIDS epidemic in the early 1980s, primary care physicians were on the front line helping to define HIV and manage the initially untreatable course of advanced AIDS. With the advent of highly active antiretroviral therapy in the

Penn State Hershey Department of Family and Community Medicine, Penn State Milton S. Hershey Medical Center, 500 University Drive, Hershey, PA 17033, USA
E-mail address: jsell@hmc.psu.edu

Prim Care Clin Office Pract 40 (2013) 589–617
http://dx.doi.org/10.1016/j.pop.2013.05.002
0095-4543/13/$ – see front matter © 2013 Elsevier Inc. All rights reserved.

mid-1990s, many persons infected with HIV transferred to the care of infectious disease specialists, who had the expertise to manage the complicated regimens and side effects of this therapy. During this time, many primary care physicians deferred HIV management to specialists, who assumed much of the HIV and primary care needs for HIV-infected persons.

Now that more HIV patients have normal CD4 counts and low viral loads on simpler antiviral regimens, primary care physicians have the opportunity to return to taking a more active role in meeting the needs of HIV-infected persons who are often, at this stage, similar to noninfected persons. Primary care providers are well trained in management of chronic diseases, such as lipid disorders, depression, and cardiovascular disease, which have become the primary mortality risk for stable patients with HIV.

Because of the high prevalence of persons currently living in the United States with HIV, primary care providers increasingly have the opportunity to be directly involved in HIV screening, prevention, and chronic care of those with HIV. Because the prevalence of HIV infection in the general US population is 0.5%,[1] the typical primary care physician averages approximately 10 HIV-infected persons in their practice. Current trends also show a higher incidence in Hispanics and African Americans in the United States, with an increasing proportion of heterosexual transmission (**Table 1**).

Screening

Despite advances in treatment, the availability of reliable screening, and generous financial aid for medical care, approximately 20% to 25% of persons infected with HIV in the United States have not been tested and are unaware of their status. Primary care providers serve a vital role in the diagnosis and prevention of HIV infection by being knowledgeable about current screening recommendations and methods. There are cost-effective and reliable testing options that are appropriate for use in screening (**Box 1**).

Improved screening rates for HIV have the benefit of early diagnosis and limiting the spread of the virus. With earlier diagnosis, patients have the option to start with antiretroviral therapy earlier, which has been shown to reduce mortality.[2] Patients who are tested and diagnosed with an HIV infection have the opportunity to limit high-risk behaviors and affect transmission to uninfected individuals. A meta-analysis[3] has shown that, compared with controls who are not already HIV positive, individuals recently diagnosed with HIV infection reduce the frequency of unprotected anal or vaginal intercourse by 68%.

In the 20% to 25% of HIV-infected individuals who remain undiagnosed, the opposite is true. Those who are unaware that they are HIV positive account for 54% of new sexual transmissions of HIV each year.[4] Delayed diagnosis also accounts for a

Table 1
New HIV infections in the United States based on age, race/ethnicity, and transmission in 2010

Age (y)	%	Race/Ethnicity	%	Transmission	%
13–29	36	Black	46	MSM	61
30–39	25	Latino	20	Heterosexual	27
40–49	24	White	29	IVDU	8
50+	15	Other	4	MSM/IVDU	3

Abbreviations: IVDU, intravenous drug use; MSM, men who have sex with men.
Data from Centers for Disease Control and Prevention. HIV surveillance report: diagnoses of HIV infection and AIDS in the United States and dependent areas. 2010. Available at: http://www.cdc.gov/hiv/pdf/statistics_surveillance_report_vol_22.pdf. Accessed January, 2013.

Box 1
HIV screening rationale
• Reliable, affordable screening test available
• People aware of HIV status reduce high-risk behaviors, resulting in less transmission
• Antiretroviral therapy less effective if started later
• HIV-infected persons who are unaware of their status account for a disproportionate number of new cases of sexually transmitted HIV

disproportionate amount of deaths from AIDS. Of persons who have been recently diagnosed, 36.4% go on to develop AIDS in the following year,[5] which shows the large number of infected persons who are unaware of their status for a prolonged period.

In 2006, in response to low rates of HIV screening and a plateau in the number of patients who remained undiagnosed, the US Centers for Disease Control and Prevention (CDC) updated their recommendations and called for all persons 13 to 64 years of age to be screened at least once for HIV. Barriers to screening found in **Box 2** prompted the need to change the screening strategy to change patient and physician behavior.

Risk-based screening of only patients who are symptomatic or have risk factors alone has been shown to miss many persons who are infected. Approximately 25% of patients with HIV infection report no risk factors.[6] Risk-based screening assessments may also not accurately take into account the risk behaviors of sexual partners. Therefore, the 2006 CDC guidelines recommend opt-out screening. In opt-out screening, screening can be recommended in a less judgmental fashion that does not follow risk assessment and can allow HIV screening to be added to other acceptable screening tests.

An example of offering HIV testing in opt-out screening: "As a part of routine care, we test everyone for HIV, unless they refuse, just like we test cholesterol, blood sugar levels and other health conditions."

Other medical organizations, including the US Preventive Services Task Force in its 2012 draft recommendations, support the 2006 CDC guidelines for universal opt-out screening for HIV (**Table 2**), and most state laws are consistent with the CDC. Repeat or additional screening can then be performed in high-risk groups (**Box 3**).

DIAGNOSIS
Primary HIV Infection

Primary HIV infection commonly causes a mononucleosislike illness (fever, lethargy, myalgias, rash, lymphadenopathy, pharyngitis, and headache) within 28 days of

Box 2
Barriers to HIV testing
1. Time
2. Complicated or lengthy consent process
3. Perception that patients are low risk
4. Reimbursement costs
5. Lack of training to counsel or interpret results
6. Poor patient acceptance

Table 2 Screening recommendations for HIV	
Organization	**Recommendation**
CDC	Routinely screen all patients aged 13–64 y at least once, as well as all pregnant women (2006)
USPSTF	Routinely screen all patients aged 15–65 y at least once, as well as all pregnant women (2012 Draft Recommendation)
AAFP	Strongly recommends that physicians screen for HIV in all adolescents and adults at increased risk for HIV infections (2005) Updated recommendation: Recommends that clinicians screen adolescents and adults ages 18 to 65 years for HIV infection. Younger adolescents and older adults who are at increased risk should also be screened (2013)
ACP	Recommends that clinicians adopt routine screening for HIV and encourage patients to be tested (2009)
ACOG	Recommends routine screening for women aged 19–64 y and target screening for women with risk factors outside that age range (2008)
AAP	Recommends that pediatricians offer routine HIV screening, beginning at ages 16 to 18 years old in communities where prevalence is >0.1% (2011)

Abbreviations: AAFP, American Academy of Family Practice; AAP, American Academy of Pediatrics; ACOG, American College of Obstetrics and Gynecology; ACP, American College of Physicians; USPSTF, United States Preventive Services Task Force.

infection but is underdiagnosed because of the nonspecific nature of these symptoms. HIV viremia is often present within 4 to 11 days of initial transmission,[7] but other laboratory testing is often nonspecific with leukopenia, thrombocytopenia, and increased transaminase levels. Initial HIV RNA levels (**Box 4**) are often greater than 100,000 copies/mm^3 and then decrease to a steady state 6 months after infection. However, HIV antibodies often are not present during primary HIV infection and are not typically detectable with current assays until 3 to 6 weeks after initial transmission. The laboratory diagnosis of primary HIV infection is therefore defined by a high HIV RNA level or a positive p24 antigen test with a negative (or indeterminate) HIV antibody assay (**Table 3**).

Chronic HIV Infection

If primary HIV infection is not suspected, HIV antibody testing alone is sufficient for initial testing. Fifty percent of HIV-infected persons have a positive antibody test by 4 weeks, and 100% have a positive test at 6 months after initial transmission.

Box 3 Repeat testing for high-risk groups
• Intravenous drug users and their sex partners
• Persons who exchange sex for money/drugs
• Sex partners of HIV-positive persons
• Persons who have had more than 1 sex partner since their last HIV test
• Persons being treated for active tuberculosis (TB)
• Persons undergoing testing for sexually transmitted infection

Box 4
Indications for HIV RNA testing

- Diagnosis of suspected primary HIV infection
- Initial evaluation of newly diagnosed chronic HIV infection
- 2 to 8 weeks after starting a new antiretroviral regimen, then repeat every 4 to 8 weeks until less than 200 copies/mm^3, then every 3 to 6 months
- Indeterminate HIV antibody

Table 3
Testing for suspected acute (primary) HIV infection

HIV Antibody	HIV RNA	Diagnosis
−	+	Acute HIV[a]
−	−	No HIV
+	+	Chronic HIV or late acute HIV
+	−	Repeat test (laboratory error or long-term nonprogressor)

[a] Expect HIV RNA level >100,000 copies/mm^3 with acute HIV infection.

Enzyme-linked immunosorbent assay (ELISA) testing is used as an initial antibody screening test with Western blot confirmation. A positive Western blot result includes identification of at least 2 bands (p24, gp41, gp160/120). An indeterminate Western blot result can occur in 4% to 20% of reactive ELISAs because of a single p24 band or weak other bands and requires HIV RNA testing to confirm the diagnosis (**Table 4**). Antibody testing can be initially performed at home, in the office, or in many other nonclinical settings that can expand testing opportunities. Whole blood, plasma, or oral mucosal samples can be used for testing, and in July, 2012 OraQuick was approved by the US Food and Drug Administration (FDA) for home testing of oral secretions. The OraQuick test has a 1/5000 false-positive rate and 1/12 false-negative rate. Positive home or rapid testing requires standard serum testing for confirmation. Visit http://hivtest.cdc.gov to find a testing site near you.

Table 4
Testing for suspected chronic HIV infection

HIV Antibody	HIV RNA	Diagnosis
+	Not needed	Chronic HIV
−	Not needed	No HIV (no further testing needed)
Indeterminate	+	Acute HIV with seroconversion in progress[a]
Indeterminate	−	HIV infection unlikely (repeat antibody testing in 3 mo)

[a] Repeat HIV RNA to confirm result and repeat antibody testing at 1, 3, and 6 months until seroconversion is evident.

INITIAL MANAGEMENT

Initial evaluation of persons with HIV infection should include a comprehensive physical examination and discussion about past and future high-risk behaviors. Particular focus should be placed on sexual practices, drug use, previous sexually transmitted infections, previous residences (for consideration of fungal disease exposure), history of TB infection or exposure, and animal contact. HIV-infected persons are at greater risk for several infectious complications that can be effectively prevented or treated as an integral part of their chronic disease management. Initial laboratory testing (**Table 5**) can help guide treatment and prevention. It is important to know the severity or stage of HIV infection (**Box 5**) currently and historically.

Immunizations

Safe administration of appropriate vaccines is an integral part of preventive care in HIV-infected persons. Recommended vaccinations are summarized in **Table 6**. Unique challenges in HIV-infected persons include the optimal timing of vaccinations during the course of the HIV infection. In general, vaccine response and subsequent immunity is improved if vaccines are provided earlier in the course of HIV infection, when patients have higher initial CD4 counts.[9–11] Live vaccines should be avoided with advanced immunosuppression (CD4 count <200 cells/mm^3).

Comorbidities

HIV-infected persons have higher rates of noninfectious comorbidities (**Box 6**) than their uninfected peers. This higher risk can be attributable to antiretroviral therapy, HIV infection itself, lifestyle, or social factors. An understanding of these risks can help primary care physicians, who are often familiar with these conditions, decrease morbidity and mortality for their HIV-infected patients.

OPPORTUNISTIC INFECTIONS
Prophylaxis

In general, the more widespread use of effective antiretroviral therapy has resulted in a significant decline in opportunistic infections in HIV-infected persons over the past decade. Total rates of opportunist infections have decreased during 1994 to 1997, 1998 to 2002, and 2003 to 2007 to rates (per 1000 person-years) of 89.0, 25.2 and 13.3, respectively. During 2003 to 2007, the most common opportunistic infections (per 1000 person-years) were: esophageal candidiasis (5.2), PCP (3.9), cervical cancer (3.5), MAC (2.5), and CMV disease (1.8). A third of opportunistic infections were diagnosed at CD4 counts greater than 200 cells/mm^3.[12] An overview of prophylaxis of common opportunistic infections in HIV-infected persons is found in **Table 7**.

Select Opportunistic Infections

Cryptococcal meningitis
Cryptococcal meningitis can occur with CD4 counts less than 100 cells/mm^3 and is the most common life-threatening fungal infection among persons infected with HIV. Cryptococcal meningitis affected 5% to 8% of HIV-infected persons before the onset of widespread use of antiretrovirals.[13] Diagnosis should be suspected in patients with a fever and headache and CD4 count less than 100 cells/mm^3. The presentation may be more subtle and subacute than in patients with acute bacterial meningitis.

Table 5
Initial laboratory testing for HIV-infected persons

Laboratory Test	Comments
CBC with platelets and differential	Rules out baseline cytopenias and is needed to calculate CD4 count
CD4 count with percentage	Used to determine need for antiretroviral therapy and opportunist infection prophylaxis. Predicts prognosis. Can be variable, especially during acute infection
Chemistry panel	Rules out renal dysfunction, hepatic dysfunction, diabetes
Lipid panel	Rules out baseline lipid disorders. HIV infection and many antiretroviral drugs may in increase risk of dyslipidemia
Urinalysis	Assess renal function initially and specifically with nephrotoxic drugs (tenofovir, indinavir)
HIV RNA level	Used to monitor response to antiretroviral therapy and assess prognosis
HIV resistance testing	Important for future treatment, even if therapy is to be delayed. Must have an increased HIV RNA level to perform this test
Syphilis serology (RPR or VDRL)	Higher risk of syphilis in persons infected with HIV
Hepatitis C serology (anti-hepatitis C virus Ab)	Order hepatitis C virus genotype and viral load, if Ab test is positive, for confirmation
Hepatitis B serology (HBsAb, HBcAb, HBsAg)	Immunize with hepatitis B vaccine if not immune or infected
Hepatitis A serology (anti-HAV Ab)	Immunize with hepatitis A vaccine if not immune or infected
Toxoplasmosis IgG	Determines need for prophylaxis or prevention. Repeat testing if CD4 <100 cells/mm^3
CMV IgG	Determines patients who should receive CMV-negative or leukocyte-depleted blood for transfusions. Should be tested only in those who are low risk (not in MSM nor IVDU, who are assumed positive)
VZV IgG	Consider vaccination if seronegative and CD4 count >200 cells/mm^3
G6PD screen	Important to prevent hemolysis with oxidative drugs (dapsone, primaquine, and sulfonamides)
HLA B*5701 screen	Before use of abacavir
Coreceptor tropism assay	Before initiation of a CCR5 antagonist
Chlamydia/gonorrhea screen	Screen initially and then periodically based on reported behaviors, symptoms, prevalence
Pap smear	Women should have Pap testing twice during the first year after diagnosis and then annually afterward if normal. Consider anal Pap smears for MSM. Role of HPV DNA testing not defined in HIV
Tuberculin test (PPD or IGRA)	>5 mm for PPD consider positive. Routine anergy skin testing not recommended
Chest radiograph	Consider for symptomatic patients or those with a positive PPD
Testosterone	Consider for patients with fatigue, weight loss, decreased libido, depression, erectile dysfunction, or reduced bone density

Abbreviations: Ab, antibody; Ag, antigen; CBC, complete blood count; G6PD, glucose-6-phosphate dehydrogenase; HBc, Hepatitis B core; HBs, Hepatitis B surface; IGRA, interferon γ release assay; IVDU, intravenous drug users; MSM, men who have sex with men; PPD, purified protein derivative; RPR, rapid plasma reagin; VDRL, venereal disease research laboratory.

Box 5
Stages of HIV infection

Acute Primary HIV Infection

- 1 to 4 weeks after transmission
- Symptomatic in 50% to 90%
- Fever (86%), lethargy (74%), myalgias (59%), rash (57%), headache (55%), pharyngitis (52%), adenopathy (44%)[8]

Asymptomatic HIV Infection

- Average of 8 to 10 years
- Gradual decline of CD4 levels with stable HIV RNA levels

Early Symptomatic HIV Infection

- AIDS-related complex
- Thrush, vaginal candidiasis, herpes zoster, oral hairy leukoplakia, peripheral neuropathy, diarrhea, weight loss

AIDS

- CD4 count less than 200
- CD4 cell % of total lymphocytes less than 14%
- AIDS-defining opportunistic infections:
  - Pneumocystis pneumonia (PCP), cryptococcal meningitis, recurrent bacterial pneumonia, *Candida* esophagitis, central nervous system toxoplasmosis, TB, non-Hodgkin lymphoma, disseminated coccidiomycosis/histoplasmosis, Kaposi sarcoma

Advanced HIV

- CD4 count less than 50
- Cytomegalovirus (CMV) disease, *Mycobacterium avium* complex (MAC)

Table 6
Recommended vaccines for HIV-infected persons

Vaccine	Comments
Hepatitis A	Recommended for hepatitis A virus nonimmune persons who are at risk
Hepatitis B	Recommended for all hepatitis B virus nonimmune or noninfected persons
Human papillomavirus	Recommended for females and males aged 9–26 y
Influenza (inactivated)	Recommended annually. Avoid live attenuated intranasal vaccine
Measles, mumps, and rubella[a]	Recommended in nonimmune persons with CD4 count >200 cells/mm^3
Meningococcal	Recommended if at risk (per routine recommendations for non–HIV-infected persons)
Pneumococcal	Recommended. Revaccinate once 5 y after first dose
Tetanus, diphtheria, and pertussis (Tdap/Td)	Recommended. Adults should receive Tdap once, then continue Td every 10 y
Varicella[a]	Consider in nonimmune persons if CD4 count >200 cells/mm^3 (give 2 doses 3 mo apart)
Zoster[a]	Insufficient data in HIV-infected persons. Contraindicated if CD4 <200 cells/mm^3

[a] Live vaccines.

Data from Centers for Disease Control and Prevention. Advisory Committee on Immunization Practices. Recommended adult immunization schedule United States. MMWR Morb Mortal Wkly Rep 2012;61(04):1–7.

Box 6
Common complications of HIV infection or treatment (with suspected causes)

Metabolic: dyslipidemia (HIV, protease inhibitors [PIs] > nonnucleoside reverse transcriptase inhibitors [NNRTIs]), diabetes mellitus (PIs)

Coronary artery disease (PIs + HIV)

Lipodystrophy (PIs)

Peripheral neuropathy (HIV, didanosine [ddI], stavudine [d4T])

Lactic acidosis (nucleoside reverse transcriptase inhibitors [NRTIs])

Hepatotoxicity (NNRTIs + PIs)

Renal disease: nephropathy, nephrolithiasis

Bone: osteoporosis, bone marrow toxicity (AZT)

Malignancy: anal carcinoma, cervical carcinoma, lymphoma

Psychiatric: depression, anxiety, addiction

Hypogonadism

Tobacco abuse

PCP

PCP is caused by the fungus *Pneumocystis jiroveci* (formerly *Pneumocystis carinii*) and, without preventive treatment (**Box 7**) or widespread antiretroviral use, would affect approximately 80% of HIV-infected persons.[14] Historically, it has been the most common AIDS-defining opportunistic infection, but its incidence has declined with prophylaxis (**Box 8**) and effective antiretroviral therapy.[12] First-line treatment of PCP is trimethoprim-sulfamethoxazole (TMP-SMX). Although side effects and allergic reactions can be common, low-dose use or desensitization can be options to improve tolerability. Alternative options are listed in see **Box 8**. Testing for

Table 7
Overview of prophylaxis of common opportunistic infections in HIV-infected persons

Organism	Indication for Prophylaxis	Preferred Treatment
Hepatitis A	Susceptible patients	Hepatitis A vaccine
Hepatitis B	All patients	Hepatitis B vaccine
Influenza	All patients	Annual influenza vaccine
PCP	CD4 count <200 cells/mm^3	TMP-SMZ
TB	PPD >5 mm or contact with active TB	INH
Toxoplasma	IgG Ab (+) and CD4 <100 cells/mm^3	TMP-SMX
MAC	CD4 <50 cells/mm^3	Azithromycin (Pfizer, New York, NY, USA)
Streptococcus pneumoniae	CD4 >200 cells/mm^3	Pneumococcal vaccine
VZV	CD4 >200 cells/mm^3 and Ab negative	Varicella vaccine

Abbreviations: Ab, antibody; INH, isoniazid; MAC, *mycobacterium avium* complex; PCP, pneumocystis pneumonia; PPD, purified protein derivative; TB, tuberculosis; TMP-SMX, trimethoprim-sulfamethoxazole; VZV, varicella zoster virus.

Box 7
Indications for PCP prophylaxis

- CD4 count less than 200 cells/mm^3
- CD4 count less than 14% cells/mm^3
- History of oral candidiasis
- History of AIDS-defining illness
- CD4 count greater than 200 to 250 cells/mm^3 if monitoring CD4 count every 1 to 3 months is not possible

Data from Kaplan JE, Benson C, Holmes KK, et al. Guidelines for prevention and treatment of opportunistic infections in HIV-infected adults and adolescents: recommendations from CDC, the National Institutes of Health, and the HIV Medicine Association of the Infectious Diseases Society of America. MMWR Recomm Rep 2009;58(RR-4):1–207.

---

glucose-6-phosphate dehydrogenase (G6PD) deficiency should be considered in persons, especially of Mediterranean, Indian, or southeast Asian descent, for whom treatment with dapsone, primaquine, or sulfonamides is considered. TMP-SMX is also effective for prophylaxis against *Toxoplasma* encephalitis. Therefore, additional prophylaxis for toxoplasmosis should be considered if TMP-SMX is not used. PCP prophylaxis can be discontinued when a patient maintains a CD4 count greater than 200 cells/mm^3 for at least 3 months.

Toxoplasma
Toxoplasma encephalitis, which is caused by the protozoan parasite *Toxoplasma gondii*, most commonly occurs at CD4 counts of less than 100 cells/mm^3. Most

---

Box 8
Recommended Treatment Options for Primary and Secondary Prophylaxis of PCP

Preferred choice:
- TMP-SMX DS daily
- TMP-SMX SS daily

Alternatives:
- TMP-SMX DS 3 times/wk
- Dapsone (Jacobus Pharmaceutical Co, Inc, Princeton, NJ, USA) 100 mg daily or 50 mg twice a day
- Dapsone 50 mg every day + pyrimethamine 50 mg every week + leucovorin 25 mg every week
- Aerosolized pentamidine 300 mg every month
- Atovaquone 1500 mg daily
- Atovaquone 1500 mg daily + pyrimethamine 25 mg daily + leucovorin 10 mg daily

Abbreviations: DS, double strength; SS, single strength; TMP-SMX, trimethoprim-sulfamethozazole.
Data from Kaplan JE, Benson C, Holmes KK, et al. Guidelines for prevention and treatment of opportunistic infections in HIV-infected adults and adolescents: recommendations from CDC, the National Institutes of Health, and the HIV Medicine Association of the Infectious Diseases Society of America. MMWR Recomm Rep 2009;58(RR-4):1–207.

---

humans are infected from ingesting undercooked lamb, beef, pork, or venison or cat feces and are typically initially asymptomatic. In the era before widespread antiretroviral use, the lifetime risk of *Toxoplasma* encephalitis in patients with AIDS who were seropositive for *Toxoplasma* was 10% to 50%.[15] TMP-SMX is the preferred drug for *Toxoplasma* encephalitis prophylaxis, with alternative regimens that consist of dapsone plus pyrimethamine plus leucovorin, or atovaquone with or without pyrimethamine and leucovorin. *Toxoplasma* encephalitis prophylaxis should be started at CD4 count less than 100 cells/mm^3 and can be discontinued in patients who have a CD4 count greater than 200 cells/mm^3 for at least 3 months.[13]

MAC

MAC is a group of nontuberculous mycobacterium which includes *Mycobacterium avium* and *Mycobacterium intracellulare*, which are both human pathogens and are typically found in soil, water, and several animals. Humans can become hosts via the gastrointestinal tract or the lungs. In the era before widespread antiretroviral use, 15% to 40% of HIV-infected patients developed disseminated MAC,[16] which is primarily caused by *M avium*.[13] Disseminated MAC remains a common opportunistic infection in HIV-infected persons with advanced immunosuppression and a CD4 count of less than 50 cells/mm^3 at a rate of 2.5 per 1000 patient years from 2003 to 2007.[12] Symptoms of MAC infection may include: weight loss, fever, night sweats, fatigue, diarrhea, and anemia. Routine screening for MAC is not recommended because of low sensitivity, nor are specific measures to prevent exposures, because MAC is ubiquitous in the environment. However, blood culture testing is recommended before initiation of prophylaxis. Azithromycin is often the preferred treatment choice because of fewer drug-drug interactions than with clarithromycin and rifabutin (**Box 9**). Prophylaxis may be discontinued if CD4 counts remain higher than 100 cells/mm3 for at least 3 months.

TB

TB continues to be a significant global infection in HIV-infected and noninfected persons. In the United States, 4% of the general population has latent TB,[13] and persons who are infected with HIV have a higher rate of conversion of latent to active TB independent of CD4 count. It is recommended that all persons initially diagnosed with HIV,

---

Box 9
Recommended treatment options for prophylaxis of MAC

Preferred choices:

- Azithromycin 1200 mg every week
- Clarithromycin (Abbott Laboratories, Abbott Park, IL, USA) 500 mg twice a day
- Azithromycin 600 mg 2 times/wk

Alternatives:

- Rifabutin 300 mg daily[a,b]

   [a] Rule out active TB before starting rirabutin to avoid TB resistance.
   [b] CYP3A inducer, therefore should be used with caution to avoid drug-drug interactions.
   Data from Kaplan JE, Benson C, Holmes KK, et al. Guidelines for prevention and treatment of opportunistic infections in HIV-infected adults and adolescents: recommendations from CDC, the National Institutes of Health, and the HIV Medicine Association of the Infectious Diseases Society of America. MMWR Recomm Rep 2009;58(RR-4):1–207.

Box 10
Indications for tuberculosis (TB) testing

- Initial diagnosis of HIV
- Yearly for high-risk individuals (active drug users, incarcerated persons)
- Clinical symptoms of TB
- Patients with a history of a low CD4 count (<200 cells/mm^3) who respond to antiretroviral therapy and have CD4 count >200 cells/mm^3

---

those with symptoms, and those who have known or high-risk exposure be tested for TB using the tuberculin skin test or interferon γ release assay (**Box 10**). A positive tuberculin skin test in an HIV-infected person is defined as more than 5 mm of induration when evaluated 48 to 72 hours after the test was performed. Anergy testing with empiric isoniazid treatment of anergic HIV-infected persons has not been shown to reduce the rate of active TB, progression of HIV disease, or death.[17] Therefore, routine anergy testing is not recommended.

All HIV-infected persons who have latent disease should receive treatment (**Box 11**), because their rate of conversion to active TB is greater than in non-HIV-infected persons.[18] Treatment of latent TB in HIV-infected persons reduces the risk of progression to active TB by approximately 60%.[19] Isoniazid is the preferred treatment of latent TB and can be given without significant interaction with antiretroviral medications. However, patients treated with isoniazid should be monitored closely for hepatitis, which can occur more commonly with increased age, alcohol consumption, and pregnancy. For patients who cannot tolerate isoniazid or are exposed to isoniazid-resistant TB, rifampin and rifabutin are alternatives **Box 12**.

ANTIRETROVIRAL TREATMENT
Treatment Initiation

Treatment of HIV with antiretroviral therapy is primarily based on CD4 cell count and clinical status. Efficacy, cost, side effects, and patient preference must also be taken into account. In the United States, recommendations regarding the optimal time to initiate antiretroviral therapy have evolved over the past 2 decades to take into account available treatment options and data regarding risks and benefits (**Table 8**).

Initial data to guide treatment of asymptomatic patients came from MACS (the Multicenter AIDS Cohort Study),[20,21] which looked at the natural course of untreated patients with HIV infection and progression to AIDS before treatment was made available. This study showed that untreated patients with a CD4 count of 201 to 350 cells/mm^3 had a 3-year risk for developing AIDS of 38.5%, and patients with a CD4 count of more than 350 cells/mm^3 had a 14.3% risk. Since the 1990s, much discussion and

---

Box 11
Indications for treatment of latent tuberculosis (TB) in HIV

- Positive diagnostic test for TB without previous treatment of active or latent TB
- Negative diagnostic test for TB but close contact with a person with active pulmonary TB
- History of untreated or inadequately treated healed TB (old fibrotic lesions on chest radiograph) regardless of diagnostic test results

---

Box 12
Recommended treatment of latent TB in HIV

Preferred choices:

- Isoniazid 300 mg daily for 9 months[a]
- 900 mg via Directly Observed Therapy (DOT) twice weekly for 9 months[a]

Alternatives:

- Rifampin 600 mg daily for 4 months
- Rifabutin for 4 months[b]

  [a] Consider pyridoxine 25 mg daily.
  [b] Dose dependent on concomitant antitetroviral therapy because of drug-drug interactions.

Table 8
Benefits versus risks of early antiretroviral therapy

Benefits	Risks
Reduced AIDS-related mortality	Drug toxicity
Reduced non–AIDS-related mortality	Cost
Reduced transmission	Antiretroviral resistance
Reduced opportunistic infections	Compliance
Restoration or preservation of immunologic function	

---

research have focused on early versus deferred initiation of antiretroviral therapy for asymptomatic patients with HIV. Key thresholds for initial initiation of therapy include CD4 counts of greater than 200 cells/mm^3, 350 cells/mm^3, or 500 cells/mm^3. In relative terms, the initial CD4 count has greater prognostic value than the HIV RNA viral level and therefore is one of the primary factors used to determine when to start treatment (**Box 13**).

Several observational and randomized controlled (**Table 9**) studies have shown greater reduction of mortality, opportunistic infections, and non-AIDS morbidity and

---

Box 13
When to initiate antiretroviral treatment (strength of recommendation taxonomy)

- Based on CD4 count:
  - <less than 350 (AI)
  - 350 to 500 (AII)
  - greater than 500 (BIII)
- Specific conditions regardless of CD4:
  - Pregnancy (AI)
  - History of AIDS-defining illness (AII)
  - Hepatitis B coinfection (AII)
  - Age younger than 50 years (BIII)

Table 9
Select studies on optimal CD4 count for initiation of antiretroviral therapy in HIV

Study Title	Study Design	Population Studied	Results
Antiretroviral Therapy (ART) Cohort Collaboration[22]	Observational cohort	12,574 antiretroviral-naive adult patients in Europe and United States who started antiretroviral therapy with at least 3 drugs	Less mortality and AIDS progression if ART started with CD4 >200 HIV RNA levels did not predict mortality
British Columbia Cohort[23]	Observational cohort	1219 antiretroviral-naive patients starting triple drug antiretroviral therapy in British Columbia	Lower risk of death and AIDS progression with CD4 >200 Risk of death and progression to AIDS was greatest for HIV RNA levels >100,000
Johns Hopkins Cohort[24]	Observational cohort	1173 antiretroviral-naive patients treated with antiretroviral therapy in United States	More rapid 3-y progression if CD4 <200 even if viral suppression was obtained No difference in 3-y progression when comparing CD4 201–350 vs >350
Swiss Cohort[25]	Observational cohort	283 Antiretroviral-naive patients in Europe	5 times decreased 3-y progression with start of ART at CD4 >350 Benefits offset by high rates of adverse events
North American AIDS Cohort Collaborative Collaboration on Research and Design (NA-ACCORD)[2]	Observational cohort	17,517 asymptomatic, antiretroviral-naive patients in the United States and Canada comparing early vs deferred therapy	69% increased risk of death for patients who deferred ART compared with starting at CD4 351–500 94% increased risk of death with deferred therapy compared with starting at CD4 >500
CIPRA-HT-001[26]	Randomized controlled	816 antiretroviral-naive patients in Haiti. Randomized to start ART at CD4 200–350 vs CD4 <200 or AIDS-defining condition	Lower risk of death and TB with initiation of ART at CD4 = 200–350
Strategies for Management of Antiretroviral Therapy (SMART)[27]	Randomized controlled	5472 initial patients with CD4 counts >350	Continuous initiation of ART at CD4 >350 compared with <250 may reduce opportunistic disease and serious non-AIDS events
HPTN 052[28]	Randomized controlled	1763 serodiscordant antiretroviral-naive couples in 9 countries with CD4 counts 350–550. Randomized to initiate ART immediately (early) or after CD4 count was <250 or HIV symptoms (late)	Early initiation of ART reduced rates of sexual transmission 96% and clinical events

Abbreviations: ART, antiretroviral therapy; HPTN, health prevention trials network.

mortality with earlier introduction of antiretroviral therapy. This evidence, when combined with the reduced toxicity and complexity of drug regimens, has led to a progressively more aggressive recommended approach to the treatment of HIV patients in the United States. As a result, guidelines in March, 2012 from the Department of Health and Human Services (DHHS) recommend treating all HIV-infected patients.

Treatment Options

After the discovery of zidovudine, the first available antiretroviral, in the late 1980s, there was an explosion of therapeutic options for HIV management in the mid to late 1990s. Recent advances have led to more effective and less complicated drug regimens with fewer side effects. Medications approved for the treatment and prevention of HIV infection are targeted to several steps in the life cycle of the HIV RNA virus as it enters and replicates in CD4 host cells. Five groups of antiretrovirals are approved for treatment. They include: (1) nucleoside and nucleotide reverse transcriptase inhibitors (NRTIs and NtRTIs), (2) non-nucleoside reverse transcriptase inhibitors (NNRTIs), (3) protease inhibitors (PIs), (4) entry inhibitors (CCR5 coreceptor antagonists and fusion inhibitors), and (5) integrase strand transfer inhibitors (INSTI) (**Tables 10** and **11**).

Current guidelines for treatment of HIV in the United States are provided primarily by the DHHS (**Boxes 14** and **15**) and the International AIDS Society-USA (IAS-USA) (**Box 16**). All regimens consist of at least 3 antiretrovirals used in combination to help reduce resistance and improve efficacy. Initial treatment of patients in the United States who have never taken antiretrovirals in the past is the focus of this discussion. Current initial treatment regimens comprise a backbone or base of an NRTI pair (containing lamivudine (3TC) or emtricitabine (FTC) as one of the agents) plus either an NNRTI or a ritonavir-boosted PI. Most PIs are used in combination with low-dose ritonavir.

Initiation of antiretroviral therapy or switching a regimen requires close laboratory monitoring to assess efficacy and tolerability of each regimen (**Table 12**). The baseline HIV RNA level should be rechecked 2 to 8 weeks after starting a new regimen, with an expected decrease in HIV RNA within 4 weeks of at least 1.0 log compared with the baseline. The HIV RNA level should then be rechecked every 4 to 8 weeks until the HIV RNA level becomes undetectable (<20–70 copies/mL depending on the assay). Most patients are able to reach an undetectable HIV RNA level in 12 to 24 weeks. A delayed or poor response to antiretroviral therapy may be caused by resistance, baseline increased HIV RNA levels, therapy adherence, drug interactions, or drug absorption. After the HIV RNA level becomes undetectable, levels can be checked every 3 to 4 months. Select patients who have shown adherence and tolerability to a specific regimen with undetectable HIV RNA levels for 2 years and are clinically and immunologically stable may check HIV RNA levels every 6 months.

The HIV RNA response is more clinically relevant after the initiation of antiretroviral therapy than following the CD4 response, which can be inconsistent and variable. CD4 count changes often lag behind HIV RNA levels, with an expected increase in CD4 count of 50 to 100 cells/mm^3 each year with successful treatment response. Generally, patients should have their CD4 count checked every 3 to 4 months, and those who have a stable increased CD4 count should be checked every 6 to 12 months. Approximately two-thirds of patients are able to achieve a CD4 count greater than 500 cells/mm^3 after 5 years.[29] A poor, or discordant, CD4 response in the setting of adequate viral suppression does not indicate treatment failure and is seen in less than 10% of patients. In the setting of a discordant CD4 response, bone marrow suppression from marrow suppressive drugs (ie, zidovudine, TMP-SMX, interferon,

Table 10
Available Individual Antiretrovirals for Treatment of HIV

Generic Name	Brand Name	Dosing	Comments
NRTI/NtRTI:			
Abacavir (ABC)	Ziagen (GlaxoSmithKline, Middlesex, United Kingdom)	Every day or twice a day, with or without food	Caution in patients with coronary artery diease or pretreatment HIV RNA >100,00 copies/mL Avoid use if positive for HLA B*5701
Didanosine (ddI)	Videx (Bristol Myers-Squibb, New York, NY, USA)	Every day; 0.5 h before or 2 h after meal	
Emtricitabine (FTC)	Emtriva (Gilead Sciences, Foster City, CA, USA)	Every day, with or without food	
Lamivudine (3TC)	Epivir (GlaxoSmithKline, Middlesex, United Kingdom)	Every day or twice a day, with or without food	
Stavudine (d4T)	Zerit (Bristol Myers-Squibb, New York, NY, USA)	Twice a day, with or without food	
Tenofovir (TDF)	Viread (Gilead Sciences, Foster City, CA, USA)	Every day, with or without food	
Zidovudine (AZT, ZDV)	Retrovir (GlaxoSmithKline, Middlesex, United Kingdom)	Twice a day or 3 times a day, with or without food	
NNTRI:			
Delavirdine (DLV)	Rescriptor (Pfizer, New York, NY, USA)	Three times a day, with or without food	
Efavirenz (EFV)	Sustiva (Bristol Myers-Squibb, New York, NY, USA)	Every day, every bedtime on an empty stomach	
Etravirine (ETR)	Intelence (Tibotec, Inc [Janssen Therapeutics], Titusville, NJ, USA)	Twice a day, after a meal	
Nevirapine (NVP)	Viramune (Boehringer Ingelheim, Ridgefield, CT, USA)	Every day for 14 d, then twice a day, with or without food	
Rilpivirine (RPV)	Edurant (Tibotec, Inc [Janssen Therapeutics], Titusville, NJ, USA)	Every day, with food	Avoid use with PPIs

PI:

Atazanavir (ATV)	Reyataz (Bristol-Myers Squibb, New York NY, USA)	Every day, with food	Caution with histamine 2 antagonists and PPIs
Darunavir (DRV)	Prezista (Tibotec, Inc [Janssen Therapeutics], Titusville, NJ, USA)	Every day or twice a day, with food	
Fosamprenavir (FPV)	Lexiva (GlaxoSmithKline, Middlesex, United Kingdom)	Every day or twice a day, unboosted: without food. Boosted w/RTV: with food	
Indinavir (IDV)	Crixivan (Merck, Whitehouse Station, NJ, USA)	Twice a day or 3 times a day. Unboosted: 1 h before meal or 2 h after. Boosted w/RTV: take with or without food	
Lopinavir + Ritonavir (LPV/r)	Kaletra (Abbott Laboratories, Abbott Park, IL, USA)	Every day or twice a day, with or without food	
Nelfinavir (NFV)	Viracept (Agouron Pharmaceuticals, San Diego, CA, USA)	Twice a day or 3 times a day, with food	
Ritonavir (RTV)	Norvir (Abbott Laboratories, Abbott Park, IL, USA)	With other PIs, with food	
Saquinavir (SQV)	Invirase (Hoffmann-La Roche, Basel, Switzerland)	Twice a day, with meal or within 2 h after meal	
Tipranavir (TPV)	Aptivus (Boehringer Ingelheim, Ridgefield, CT, USA)	Twice a day, with food	

INSTI:

Raltegravir (RAL)	Isentress (Merck & Co., Inc, Whitehouse Station, NJ, USA)	Twice a day, with or without food	
Elvitegravir (EVG)	A component of Stribild	Every day, with food	

Entry Inhibitors:

Fusion inhibitor: Enfuvirtide (ENF, T-20)	Fuzeon (Hoffmann-La Roche & Trimeris, Durham, NC, USA)	Twice a day, subcutaneously	
CCR5 Antagonist: Maraviroc (MVC)	Selzentry (Pfizer, New York, NY, USA)	Twice a day, with or without food	

Abbreviation: PPIs, proton pump inhibitors.
Drugs in bold type are preferred agents.

Table 11
Available antiretroviral combinations for treatment of HIV

Generic Name	Brand Name	Dosing	Comments
NRTI Combinations:			
Abacavir + lamivudine	Epzicom (GlaxoSmithKline, Middlesex, United Kingdom)	Every day	
Tenofovir + emtricitabine	Truvada (Gilead Sciences, Foster City, CA, USA)	Every day	
Zidovudine + lamivudine	Combivir (GlaxoSmithKline, Middlesex, United Kingdom)	Twice a day	
Zidovudine + lamivudine + abacavir	Trizivir (GlaxoSmithKline, Middlesex, United Kingdom)	Twice a day	
Single-Tablet Combinations:			
Tenofovir + emtricitabine + efavirenz	Atripla (Bristol-Myers Squibb, New York, NY, USA and Gilead Sciences, Foster City, CA, USA)	Every day, empty stomach	
Tenofovir + emtricitabine + rilpivirine	Complera (Gilead Sciences, Foster City, CA, USA)	Every day, with food	
Tenofovir + emtricitabine + cobicistat + elvitegravir	Stribild (Gilead Sciences, Foster City, CA, USA)	Every day, with food	For CrCl >70 mL/min

Abbreviation: CrCL, creatinine clearance.

pyrimethamine, sulfadiazine, ganciclovir, valganciclovir, and etoposide) and other causes (ie, lymphoma, disseminated histoplasmosis) should be excluded.

Antiretroviral Side Effects and Drug Interactions

Selection of appropriate antiretrovirals and management of other medical conditions must take into account side effects (**Table 13**) and drug interactions. All NNRTIs and

---

Box 14
DHHS guidelines: preferred regimens for treatment-naive patients (March, 2012)

NNRTI-Based Regimen:

Efavirenz (EFV) + tenofovir (TDF) + emtricitabine (FTC)

PI-Based Regimen:

Atazanavir (ATV) + ritonavir (RTV) + tenofovir (TDF) + emtricitabine (FTC)

INSTI-Based Regimen:

Raltegravir (RAL) + tenofovir (TDF) + emtricitabine (FTC)

Preferred Regimen for Pregnant Women:

Lopinavir (LPV) + ritonavir (RTV) + zidovudine (ZDV) + lamivudine (3TC)

Comments:

- Avoid use of efavirenz (EFV) during first trimester of pregnancy or in women who may become pregnant
- Use tenofovir (TDF) with caution in patients with renal insufficiency
- Avoid use of atazanavir (ATV) + ritonavir (RTV) in patients using greater than 20 mg of omeprazole

---

Box 15
DHHS guidelines: alternative regimens for treatment-nave patients (March, 2012)

NNRTI-Based Regimen:

Efavirenz (EFV) + abacavir (ABC) + lamivudine (3TC)

Rilpivirine (RPV) + tenofovir (TDF) + emtricitabine (FTC)

Rilpivirine (RPV) + abacavir (ABC) + lamivudine (3TC)

PI-Based Regimen:

Atazanavir (ATV) + ritonavir (RTV) + abacavir (ABC) + lamivudine (3TC)

Darunavir (DRV) + ritonavir (RTV) + abacavir (ABC) + lamivudine (3TC)

Fosamprenavir (FPV) + ritonavir (RTV) + abacavir (ABC) + lamivudine (3TC)

Fosamprenavir (FPV) + ritonavir (RTV) + tenofovir (TDF) + emtricitabine (FTC)

Lopinavir (LPV) + ritonavir (RTV) + abacavir (ABC) + lamivudine (3TC)

Lopinavir (LPV) + ritonavir (RTV) + tenofovir (TDF) + emtricitabine (FTC)

INSTI-Based Regimen:

Elvitegravir + cobicistat + tenofovir + emtricitabine

Raltegravir + abacavir (ABC) + lamivudine (3TC)

PIs are metabolized in the liver by cytochrome P450 (CYP) 3A isoenzymes, leading to risk of virologic failure or adverse effects if they interact with other drugs that induce or inhibit these enzymes. Azole antifungals, rifamycins, benzodiazepines, hepatitis C virus PIs, 3-hydroxy-3-methylglutaryl-coenzyme A reductase inhibitors (statins), and methadone are examples of drugs that metabolized by CYP enzymes and therefore can interact with antiretrovirals. See **Box 17** for a list of common drug-drug interactions with antiretroviral medications. A more comprehensive list of drug interactions and side effects can be found at http://aidsinfo.nih.gov/guidelines in Tables 13, 14 and 15a-15e.[35]

Antiretroviral Treatment Failure and Resistance

Antiretroviral treatment failure can be caused by multiple factors and be categorized as: virologic failure (inability to suppress viral level or rebound), immunologic failure

---

Box 16
IAS-USA guidelines: preferred regimens for treatment-naive patients (July, 2012)

NNRTI-Based Regimen:

Efavirenz (EFV) + tenofovir (TDF) + emtricitabine (FTC)

Efavirenz (EFV) + abacavir (ABC) + lamivudine (3TC)

PI-Based Regimen:

Darunavir (DRV) + ritonavir (RTV) + tenofovir (TDF) + emtricitabine (FTC)

Atazanavir (ATV) + ritonavir (RTV) + tenofovir (TDF) + emtricitabine (FTC)

Atazanavir (ATV) + ritonavir (RTV) + abacavir (ABC) + lamivudine (3TC)

INSTI-Based Regimen:

Raltegravir (RAL) + tenofovir (TDF) + emtricitabine (FTC)

Table 12
Recommended laboratory monitoring for initial and maintenance antiretroviral therapy

Laboratory	Start	2–8 wk	Every 3–6 mo	Every 6 mo	Every 12 mo
Basic chemistry	+	+	+		
Alanine aminotransferase, aspartate aminotransferase, bilirubin	+	+	+		
Complete blood count	+	+ (if on zidovudine)	+		
Lipids	+	+ (consider)		+ (if last check abnormal)	+ (if last check normal)
Fasting glucose	+			+ (if last check abnormal)	+ (if last check normal)
Urinalysis	+			+ (if on tenofovir)	
Pregnancy test	+				

Data from DHHS. Panel on Antiretroviral Guidelines for Adults and Adolescents. Guidelines for the use of antiretroviral agents in HIV-1-infected adults and adolescents. Department of Health and Human Services. Available at: http://aidsinfo.nih.gov/contentfiles/lvguidelines/AdultandAdolescentGL.pdf. Accessed January, 2013. and Aberg JA, Kaplan JE, Libman H, et al. Primary care guidelines for the management of persons infected with human immunodeficiency virus: 2009 update by the HIV medicine Association of the Infectious Diseases Society of America. Clin Infect Dis 2009;49:651–81.

(continued CD4 decline), and clinical failure (disease progression). The most common cause of treatment failure is poor medication adherence.[36] Poor adherence is a significant issue in HIV treatment, which can increase the risk of resistance and complicate future therapy. North American and European studies show that newly infected persons have 6% to 16% resistance to at least 1 antiretroviral and 3% to 5% resistance to multiple classes of antiretrovirals.[37] Resistance occurred in 7% to 24% of persons with acute or early HIV infection in San Francisco during 2002 to 2009.[38] Resistance testing can be performed via genotype (generally preferred) or phenotype testing and can help guide current as well as future therapy (**Box 18**).

Table 13
Common side effects of antiretroviral classes

All PIs	All NNRTIs	All NRTIs
Hyperlipidemia Lipodystrophy Hepatotoxicity Gastrointestinal intolerance Including bleeding risk for hemophiliacs Glucose intolerance	Rash, including Stevens-Johnson syndrome Hepatotoxicity (especially NVP) Lipid disorders	Lactic acidosis and hepatic steatosis (highest risk with d4T, then ddI and ZDV, lower with TDF, ABC, 3TC, and FTC) Lipodystrophy (higher risk with d4T)

Abbreviations: ABC, abacavir; ddI, didanosine; d4t, stavudine; FTC, emtricitabine; NVP, nevirapine; 3TC, lamivudine; TDF, tenofovir; ZDV, zidovudine.

Box 17
Common drug-drug interactions with antiretroviral medications

Known Drug Interactions:

- Statins and PIs
- Erectile dysfunction agents and PIs
- Methadone and select PIs or NNRTIs
- Fluticasone and PIs

Probable Drug Interactions:

- Antidepressants and PIs or NNRTIs
- Oral contraceptives and PIs
- Warfarin and PIs or NNRTIs
- Dihydropyridine calcium channel blockers and PIs
- Proton pump inhibitors or histamine 2 blockers and atazanavir
- Certain antifungal agents and PIs or NNRTIs
- Certain anticonvulsants and PIs or NNRTIs
- Certain benzodiazepines

Possible Drug Interactions:

- Herbal products and PIs or NNRTIs
- Oral hypoglycemics and PIs or NNRTIs
- Antipsychotics and PIs or NNRTIs

PREVENTION
Occupational Postexposure Prophylaxis

Many primary care providers are involved in the care of workers who have accidental occupational exposure, particularly in the health care field. The risk of seroconversion after percutaneous and mucous membrane exposure to blood infected with HIV is 0.3% and 0.09%, respectively,[39] which is less than the risk of acquiring hepatitis B or C. Characteristics of exposure that have been shown to increase risk are shown in **Box 19** and may help to guide the decision to start postexposure prophylaxis (PEP). Initial studies with zidovudine (Retrovir, GlaxoSmithKline, Middlesex, United Kingdom) for PEP show a decreased risk of HIV transmission of 80%.[40]

Box 18
Indications for resistance testing

- After initial diagnosis, even if therapy is not initiated
- Before initiation of antiretroviral therapy
- If HIV RNA level is detectable 24 weeks after initiation of therapy and is no longer declining
- HIV RNA level initially declines and then starts to increase
- HIV RNA levels increase after sustained suppression

Box 19
Increased risk of HIV transmission with

- Higher volume of blood
- Visible blood on the needle or device before the injury
- Needlesticks involving a needle that had been used in an artery or vein
- Deep tissue injury
- Higher viral load of the source patient
- Terminally ill source patient
- Hollow-bore needles

Data from Cardo DM, Culver DH, Ciesielski CA, et al. A case-control study of HIV seroconversion in health care workers after percutaneous exposure. Centers for Disease Control and Prevention Needlestick Surveillance Group. N Engl J Med 1997;337(21):1485–90.

The 2005 US Public Health Service guideline for the management of occupational exposures is summarized in **Boxes 20** and **21**,[41] and expert consultation can be found through the National Clinicians Post-exposure Prophylaxis Hotline (PEPline) (see listed resources). PEP is believed to most effective if initiated less than 48 hours after exposure, but there is not a defined cutoff at which PEP cannot be considered. Several regimens (listed in **Box 21**) can be considered based on risk of exposure, HIV resistance and symptoms of the source patient, and the exposed person's unique health conditions. The basic 2-drug regimen is sufficient for lower-risk exposures, and a third drug is added for higher-risk exposures.

Nonoccupational Postexposure Prophylaxis

Nonoccupational exposure prophylaxis (NPEP) encompasses the treatment of persons who have known contact with blood or other body fluids from known HIV-infected persons and is guided by recommendations from the DHHS recommendations from 2005.[42] Exposure can occur in HIV-discordant couples with a broken condom, rape, and many other accidental situations. Antiviral treatment can be considered in cases of substantial exposure risk (**Fig. 1**) and if treatment is initiated within 72 hours of contact. Data to support NPEP are based on several small observational studies[43–45] and experience with occupational postexposure treatment.

Box 20
General considerations for PEP

- Initiate PEP as soon as possible after exposure
- Continue PEP for 28 days
- Perform HIV antibody testing initially, 6 weeks, 3 months, and 6 months after exposure
- Encourage exposed persons to avoid secondary transmission

Data from Panlilio AL, Cardo DM, Grohskopf LA, et al. U.S. Public Health Service. Updated U.S. Public Health Service guidelines for the management of occupational exposures to HIV and recommendations for postexposure prophylaxis. MMWR Recomm Rep 2005;54(RR-9):1–17.

Box 21
Recommendations for PEP from the 2005 US Public Health Service guideline

Preferred Basic Regimens:

- Zidovudine + lamivudine
- Zidovudine + emtricitabine
- Tenofovir + emtricitabine
- Tenofovir + lamivudine

Alternative Basic Regimens:

- Stavudine + lamivudine
- Stavudine + emtricitabine
- Didanosine + lamivudine
- Didanosine + emtricitabine

Preferred Expanded Regimen = Basic Regimen + the following

- Lopinavir-ritonavir

Alternative Expanded Regimen = Basic Regimen + 1 of the following

- Atazanavir
- Atazanavir + ritonavir
- Fosamprenavir
- Fosamprenavir + norvir
- Indinavir + ritonavir
- Saquinavir + ritonavir
- Nelfinavir
- Efavirenz

Data from Panlilio AL, Cardo DM, Grohskopf LA, et al. U.S. Public Health Service. Updated U.S. Public Health Service guidelines for the management of occupational exposures to HIV and recommendations for postexposure prophylaxis. MMWR Recomm Rep 2005;54(RR-9):1–17.

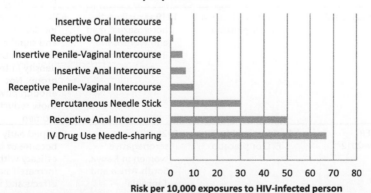

Fig. 1. Estimated transmission risk of HIV acquisition with exposure to an HIV-infected person, assuming no condom use.

Pre-Exposure Prophylaxis

Pre-exposure prophylaxis (PrEP) encompasses the preventive treatment of high-risk persons who are currently HIV-uninfected but at high future risk. This group may include those who routinely engage in high-risk sex or those who are in a serodiscordant relationship, in which 1 partner is infected with and the other is un-infected. Several recent studies (**Table 14**) have shown mixed results, and con-troversy remains concerning the best way to prevent HIV transmission in these high-risk groups. Lack of long-term safety data, potential side effects (headaches, abdominal pain, weight loss, decreased bone density, nephrotoxicity), drug resis-tance, and cost (estimated to be at least $10,000/y in the United States) remain significant concerns with PrEP. PrEP does not completely eliminate risk and cannot be taken as a morning-after pill. Behavior disinhibition has not been seen in trials to date.

Table 14
Select studies of PrEP in HIV

Study Title–Year	Study Design	Population Studied	Results
iPrEx Study–2010[30]	Randomized to TDF-FTC or placebo	2499 HIV-seronegative MSM in South America, United States, Thailand, and South Africa	44% reduction in incidence of HIV in treated group
VOICE (MTN-003) Study–Ongoing[31]	Randomized to oral TDF, oral TDF-FTC, oral placebo, vaginal TDF, or vaginal placebo	5000 HIV-negative women in Africa	Oral TDF and vaginal TDF study arms were stopped because of lack of efficacy. TDF-FTC is still being studied
Partners PrEP Study–2012[32]	Randomized to TDF, TDF, TDF-FTC or placebo	4758 serodiscordant heterosexual couples in Kenya and Uganda	67% and 75% reduction in incidence of HIV in TDF and TDF-FTC groups respectively
TDF2 Study–2012[33]	Randomized to TDF-FTC or placebo	1219 sexually active heterosexual men and women in Botswana	62% reduction in incidence of HIV and significant decline in bone density in treated group. Not enough power to show reduction in women
FEM-PrEP Study–2012[34]	Randomized to TDF-FTC or placebo	2120 HIV-seronegative women in Kenya, South Africa and Tanzania	Stopped early because of lack of efficacy with increased side effects and low drug adherence

Abbreviations: FTC, emtricitabine; MSM, men who have sex with men; TDF, tenofovir.

Box 22
Summary of PrEP CDC guidelines

- Tenofovir-emtricitabine (Truvada) daily indefinitely, based on risk
- HIV testing before treatment and every 2 to 3 months
- Screen for hepatitis B and sexually transmitted infections (every 3–6 months)
- Follow renal function before treatment and then annually
- Counsel regarding risk reduction and adherence

Based on recent studies, the CDC in August, 2012 published guidelines (see **Box 22**) for clinicians considering the use of PrEP for the prevention of HIV infection in heterosexually active adults,[46] which followed the 2011 guidelines for men who have sex with men.[47] In July, 2012 the FDA approved tenofovir-emtricitabine (Truvada) for PrEP, which may greatly increase the number of persons in the United States who are treated with antiretrovirals. This trend will likely increase the number of primary care physicians who prescribe antiretrovirals, or see patients on antiretrovirals, as the number of eligible patients increases. PrEP with antiretrovirals can be considered in addition to other prevention strategies (**Box 23**).

PREGNANCY

The CDC, the American College of Obstetricians and Gynecologists, and the American Academy of Pediatrics all recommend screening pregnancy women using the opt-out strategy. Women at high risk for HIV infection should be offered repeat screening in the third trimester. Use of antiretroviral therapy during pregnancy has resulted in significant reduction of vertical or maternal-fetal transmission and is an essential component in the reduction of children who are infected with HIV.

Perinatal treatment has been able to reduce transmission rates from 25% to 30% without treatment to 2% or lower with combined antiretroviral therapy.[48] It is recommended that all HIV-positive women receive treatment during pregnancy, with early initiation. Benefits of earlier introduction can be weighed against potential teratogenic risks during the first trimester. Treatment goals are similar to those in nonpregnant women with the use of a minimum of 3 antiretroviral agents, most commonly 2 NNRTIs plus a PI. Pregnancy guidelines differ from treatment of nonpregnant

---

Box 23
HIV prevention methods

- Barrier methods (condoms)
- Counseling
- HIV screening/testing
- Treatment of HIV-infected individuals
- PrEP

Table 15
Recommended Antiretroviral Treatment during Pregnancy

Antiretroviral Class	Recommended	Alternative	Use in Special Circumstances	Insuffcient Data to Recommend
NRTI/NtRTI	Zidovudine Lamivudine	Emtricitabine Abacavir Tenofovir	Didanosine Stavudine	
NNRTI	Nevirapine[b]		Efavirenz	Etravirine Rilpivirine
PIs[a]	Atazanavir Lopinavir Ritonavir	Darunavir Saquinavir	Indinavir Nelfinavir	Fosamprenavir Tipranavir
Entry inhibitors				Entuvirtide Maraviroc
Integrase inhibitors			Raltegravir	

[a] Most PIs are boosted with low-dose ritonavir.
[b] Avoid use of nevirapine in treatment-naive women with CD4 counts >250 cells/mm³ because of risk of hepatotoxicity and fatal rash.
 Data from Recommendations for use of antiretroviral drugs in pregnant HIV-1-infected women for maternal health and interventions to reduce perinatal HIV transmission. 2012. Available at: http://aidsinfo.nih.gov/guidelines. Accessed January, 2013.

guidelines in recommending zidovudine, which has a long history of success in pregnancy, and using efavirenz, which is potentially teratogenic, only in special circumstances (**Table 15**). Drug selection during pregnancy is guided by selection of agents to avoid toxicity to the mother and developing fetus. Intrapartum intravenous zidovudine can then be considered for women with HIV RNA levels greater than 300 copies/mL or unknown levels, and infants born to HIV-infected mothers should be continued on zidovudine for a minimum of 6 weeks for prophylaxis. Additional information regarding HIV management can be found in the resources listed in **Box 24**.

Box 24
Select additional HIV resources

- Primary Care Guidelines for the Management of Persons Infected with HIV: 2009 Update by the HIV Medical Association of the IDSA[49]
- AIDSinfo: DHHS (http://aidsinfo.nih.gov)
- HIV InSite (http://hivinsite.ucsf.edu)
- AIDS Education and Training Centers (http://www.aidsetc.org)
- IAS-USA (http://www.iasusa.org)
- American Academy of HIV Medicine (http://www.aahivm.org)
- HIV Medicine Association (http://www.hivma.org)
- National Clinicians' Post-Exposure Prophylaxis Hotline (PEPline) (1-888- HIV-4911)
- National Perinatal HIV Hotline (1-888-448–8765)
- CDC Web site for HIV testing sites (http://hivtest.cdc.gov)

REFERENCES

1. Hall HI, Song R, Rhodes P, et al. Estimation of HIV incidence in the United States. JAMA 2008;300:520–9.
2. Kitahata MM, Gange SJ, Abraham AG, et al. Effect of early versus deferred antiretroviral therapy for HIV on survival. N Engl J Med 2009;360(18):1815–26.
3. Marks G, Crepaz N, Senterfitt JW, et al. Meta-analysis of high-risk sexual behavior in persons aware and unaware they are infected with HIV in the United States: implications for HIV prevention programs. J Acquir Immune Defic Syndr 2005; 39:446–53.
4. Marks G, Crepaz N, Senterfitt JW, et al. Estimating sexual transmission of HIV from persons aware and unaware that they are infected with the virus in the US. AIDS 2005;20:1447–50.
5. Shouse R, Kajese T, Hall H, et al. Late HIV testing–34 states, 1996-2005. MMWR Morb Mortal Wkly Rep 2009;58(24):661–5.
6. Peterman TA, Todd KA, Mupanduk I. Opportunities for targeting publicly funded human immunodeficiency virus counseling and testing. J Acquir Immune Defic Syndr 1996;12:69–74.
7. Niu MT, Stein DS, Schnittman SM. Primary human immunodeficiency virus type 1 infection: review of pathogenesis and early treatment intervention in humans and animal retrovirus infections. J Infect Dis 1993;168(6):1490–501.
8. Vanhems P, Hughes J, Collier AC, et al. Comparison of clinical features, CD4 and CD8 responses among patients with acute HIV-1 infection from Geneva, Seattle and Sydney. AIDS 2000;14(4):375–81.
9. Kroon FP, Van Dissel JT, De Jong JC, et al. Antibody response to influenza, tetanus and pneumococcal vaccines in HIV-seropositive individuals in relation to the number of CD4+ lymphocytes. AIDS 1994;8(4):469–76.
10. Rodriguez-Barradas MC, Alexandraki I, Nazir T, et al. Response of human immunodeficiency virus-infected patients receiving highly active antiretroviral therapy to vaccination with 23-valent pneumococcal polysaccharide vaccine. Clin Infect Dis 2003;37(3):438–47.
11. Lange CG, Lederman MM, Medvik K, et al. Nadir CD4+ T-cell count and numbers of CD28+ CD4+ T-cells predict functional responses to immunizations in chronic HIV-1 infection. AIDS 2003;17(14):2015–23.
12. Buchacz K, Baker RK, Palella FJ Jr, et al, HOPS Investigators. AIDS-defining opportunistic illnesses in US patients, 1994-2007: a cohort study. AIDS 2010; 24(10):1549–59.
13. Kaplan JE, Benson C, Holmes KK, et al. Guidelines for prevention and treatment of opportunistic infections in HIV-infected adults and adolescents: recommendations from CDC, the National Institutes of Health, and the HIV Medicine Association of the Infectious Diseases Society of America. MMWR Recomm Rep 2009; 58(RR-4):1–207.
14. Fishman JA. Prevention of infection due to *Pneumocystis carinii*. Antimicrob Agents Chemother 1998;42:995–1004.
15. Richards FO Jr, Kovacs JA, Luft BJ. Preventing toxoplasmic encephalitis in persons infected with human immunodeficiency virus. Clin Infect Dis 1995;21(Suppl 1):S49–56.
16. Masur H. Recommendations on prophylaxis and therapy for disseminated *Mycobacterium avium* complex disease in patients infected with the human immunodeficiency virus. Public Health Service Task Force on Prophylaxis and Therapy for Mycobacterium avium Complex. N Engl J Med 1993;320:898–904.

17. Gordin FM, Matts JP, Miller C, et al. A controlled trial of isoniazid in persons with anergy and human immunodeficiency virus infection who are at high risk for tuberculosis. N Engl J Med 1997;337:315–20.
18. Markowitz N, Hansen NI, Hopewell PC, et al. Incidence of tuberculosis in the United States among HIV-infected persons. The pulmonary complications of HIV Study Group. Ann Intern Med 1997;126:123–32.
19. Bucher HC, Griffith LE, Guyatt GH, et al. Isoniazid prophylaxis for tuberculosis in HIV infection: a meta-analysis of randomized controlled trials. AIDS 1999;13:501–7.
20. Mellors JW, Rinaldo CR Jr, Gupta P, et al. Prognosis in HIV-1 infection predicted by the quantity of virus in plasma. Science 1996;272:1167–70.
21. Mellors JW, Munoz A, Giorgi JV, et al. Plasma viral load and CD4+ lymphocytes as prognostic markers of HIV-1 infection. Ann Intern Med 1997;126:946–54.
22. Egger M, May M, Chene G, et al. Prognosis of HIV-1-infected patients starting highly active antiretroviral therapy: a collaborative analysis of prospective studies. Lancet 2002;360:119–29.
23. Hogg RS, Yip B, Chan KJ, et al. Rates of disease progression by baseline CD4 cell count and viral load after initiating triple-drug therapy. JAMA 2001;286: 2568–77.
24. Sterling TR, Chaisson RE, Keruly J, et al. Improved outcomes with earlier initiation of highly active antiretroviral therapy among human immunodeficiency virus-infected patients who achieve durable virologic suppression: longer follow-up of an observational cohort study. J Infect Dis 2003;188:1659–65.
25. Opravil M, Ledergerber B, Furrer H, et al. Clinical efficacy of early initiation of HAART in patients with asymptomatic HIV infection and CD4 cell count > 350 x 10(6)/l. AIDS 2002;16:1371–81.
26. Severe P, Juste MA, Ambroise A, et al. Early versus standard antiretroviral therapy for HIV-infected adults in Haiti. N Engl J Med 2010;363:257–65.
27. Emery S, Neuhaus JA, Phillips AN, et al. Major clinical outcomes in antiretroviral therapy (ART)-naive participants and in those not receiving ART at baseline in the SMART study. Strategies for Management of Antiretroviral Therapy (SMART) Study Group. J Infect Dis 2008;197:1133–44.
28. Cohen MS, Chen YQ, McCauley M. Prevention of HIV-1 infection with early antiretroviral therapy. N Engl J Med 2011;365(6):493–505.
29. Egger M, Hirschel B, Francioli P, et al. Impact of new antiretroviral combination therapies in HIV infected patients in Switzerland: prospective multicentre study. Swiss HIV cohort study. BMJ 1997;315(7117):1194–9.
30. Grant RM, Lama JR, Anderson PL, et al. Preexposure chemoprophylaxis for HIV prevention in men who have sex with men. N Engl J Med 2010;363:2587–99.
31. Microbicide Trials Network. [Online]. Available at: http://www.mtnstopshiv.org/studies/70. Accessed January, 2013.
32. Baeten JM, Donnell D, Ndase P, et al. Antiretroviral prophylaxis for HIV prevention in heterosexual men and women. N Engl J Med 2012;367(5):399–410.
33. Thigpen M, Kebaabetswe PM, Paxton L, et al. Antiretroviral preexposure prophylaxis for heterosexual HIV transmission in Botswana. N Engl J Med 2012;367(5): 423–34.
34. Van Damme L, Corneli A, Ahmed K, et al. Preexposure prophylaxis for HIV infection among African women. N Engl J Med 2012;367(5):411–22.
35. Available at: http://aidsinfo.nih.gov/guidelines. Accessed January, 2013.
36. Harrigan PR, Hogg RS, Dong WW, et al. Predictors of HIV drug-resistance mutations in a large antiretroviral-naive cohort initiating triple antiretroviral therapy. J Infect Dis 2005;191(3):339–47.

37. Panel on Antiretroviral Guidelines for Adults and Adolescents. Guidelines for the use of antiretroviral agents in HIV-1-infected adults and adolescents. Department of Health and Human Services 2011;1–166.

38. Jain V, Liegler T, Vittinghoff E, et al. Transmitted drug resistance in persons with acute/early HIV-1 in San Francisco, 2002-2009. PLoS One 2010;5(12):e15510.

39. Bell DM. Occupational risk of human immunodeficiency virus infection in health-care workers: an overview. Am J Med 1997;102(5B):9–15.

40. Cardo DM, Culver DH, Ciesielski CA, et al. A case-control study of HIV seroconversion in health care workers after percutaneous exposure. Centers for Disease Control and Prevention Needlestick Surveillance Group. N Engl J Med 1997; 337(21):1485–90.

41. Panlilio AL, Cardo DM, Grohskopf LA, et al, US Public Health Service. Updated US public health service guidelines for the management of occupational exposures to HIV and recommendations for postexposure prophylaxis. MMWR Recomm Rep 2005;54(RR-9):1–17.

42. Smith DK, Grohskopf LA, Black RJ, et al. Antiretroviral postexposure prophylaxis after sexual, injection-drug use, or other nonoccupational exposure to HIV in the United States: recommendations from the US Department of Health and Human Services. MMWR Recomm Rep 2005;54(RR-2):1–20.

43. Schechter M, Do Lago RF, Mendelsohn AB, et al. Behavioral impact, acceptability, and HIV incidence among homosexual men with access to postexposure chemoprophylaxis for HIV. J Acquir Immune Defic Syndr 2004;35(5):519–25.

44. Martin JN, Roland ME, Neilands TB, et al. Use of postexposure prophylaxis against HIV infection following sexual exposure does not lead to increases in high-risk behavior. Clin Infect Dis 2005;41(10):1507–13.

45. Kahn JO, Martin JN, Roland ME, et al. Feasibility of postexposure prophylaxis (PEP) against human immunodeficiency virus infection after sexual or injection drug use exposure: the San Francisco PEP study. J Infect Dis 2001;183(5): 707–14.

46. Centers for Disease Control and Prevention (CDC). Interim guidance for clinicians considering the use of preexposure prophylaxis for the prevention of HIV infection in heterosexually active adults. MMWR Morb Mortal Wkly Rep 2012;61(31):586–9.

47. Centers for Disease Control and Prevention (CDC). Interim guidance: preexposure prophylaxis for the prevention of HIV infection in men who have sex with men. MMWR Morb Mortal Wkly Rep 2011;60(3):65–8.

48. Public Health Service Task Force recommendations for use of antiretroviral drugs in pregnant HIV-1-infected women for maternal health and interventions to reduce perinatal HIV-1 transmission in the United States. November 17, 2005. Available at: http://aidsinfo.nih.gov/ContentFiles/PerinatalGL07062006051.pdf. Accessed January, 2013.

49. Aberg JA, Kaplan JE, Libman H, et al. Primary care guidelines for the management of persons infected with human immunodeficiency virus: 2009 update by the HIV Medicine Association of the Infectious Diseases Society of America. Clin Infect Dis 2009;49:651–81.

Tick-borne Infections in the United States

George G.A. Pujalte, MD, CAQSM[a,b,*], Joel V. Chua, MD[c,d]

KEYWORDS

- Ticks • Babesiosis • Tularemia • Ehrlichiosis • Lyme • Tick-borne • Spirochetes

KEY POINTS

- Avoiding high-risk habitats during periods of peak tick activity is the first line of defense.
- Other prevention strategies include (1) bed nets, (2) tick repellents, (3) permethrin for clothing, (4) N,N-diethyl-m-toluamide (DEET) for skin, (5) wearing long pants and tucking pant legs into socks, and (6) use of Citrodiol.
- 24 to 48 hours of attachment to the host are required before infection occurs; diseases can be prevented by early tick removal.
- Removal of the tick can be done by vertical traction onto tick body as it is grasped gently, best done with angled, medium-tipped, and blunt forceps.
- *Ixodes scapularis* nymphs can be killed by deltamethrin at forest-lawn interfaces of residential properties.
- Vegetation management is a method of controlling ticks, including controlled burns, brush removal, mowing, and placing a border between tick-infested forested habitats and adjacent lawns.
- Removal of leaf litter from forest floor exposes ticks to desiccation.

INTRODUCTION

Tick-borne infections usually present initially in primary care clinics and are the consequence of humans' close interaction with nature. These infections are easily treatable, but may result in considerable morbidity and mortality; therefore, an accurate and early clinical diagnosis is imperative. In diagnosing tick-borne infections, a thorough epidemiologic and travel history is pertinent. Because these diseases are

Funding Sources: Nil.
Conflict of Interest: Nil.
[a] Department of Family and Community Medicine, Penn State Milton S. Hershey Medical Center, 500 University Drive, Hershey, PA 17033, USA; [b] Department of Orthopaedics and Rehabilitation, Penn State Milton S. Hershey Medical Center, Hershey, PA, USA; [c] Infusion Solutions of Delaware, 200 Banning Street, Suite 260, Dover, DE, USA; [d] Department of Medicine, Kent General Hospital - Bayhealth Medical Center, 640 South State Street, Dover, DE, USA
* Corresponding author. Department of Family and Community Medicine, Penn State Milton S. Hershey Medical Center, 500 University Drive, Hershey, PA 17033.
E-mail address: gpujalte@hmc.psu.edu

related to a specific tick vector, its geographic reach is limited to where that certain tick can be found (**Table 1**). Location is therefore the key to stratifying the likelihood of a certain vector-associated infection's occurrence. The pathogens that cause tick-borne infections are viruses, obligate intracellular organisms (*Rickettsia*, *Ehrlichia*, and *Anaplasma*), spirochete bacteria (*Borrelia* [Lyme disease]), or parasites (*Babesia*).[1,2]

There are instances when a patient may come to the doctor's office carrying a tick, either attached to the body or previously removed. Recognizing the specific tick by its size, color, stripes, and pattern may be a challenge, but is helpful in delineating potential pathogens that it may carry (**Table 2**). Not all ticks carry diseases.

Although tick-borne infections are also seen in Europe and Africa, this article is limited to tick-borne infections seen in the United States.

Although tick-borne infections generally present with protean constitutional symptoms such as fever, chills, arthralgia, and body malaise, there are certain features unique to some of these infections. For example, *Borrelia burgdorferi* (the causal agent for Lyme disease) causes the classic targetlike rash known as erythema migrans (**Table 3**).

Table 4 summarizes the medications commonly used for the various conditions discussed in this article.

TICK-BORNE RELAPSING FEVER
Presentation

Fever is intermittent and high. It is usually greater than 40°C. Delirium may be present. A week from the tick bite usually passes before signs and symptoms appear. Nausea, vomiting, arthralgias, fever, chills, night sweats, and generalized malaise are usually apparent. On examination, meningeal signs and splenomegaly may be apparent. Splenic rupture, myocarditis, pneumonitis, cranial nerve palsy, coma, iridocyclitis, hemoptysis, and epistaxis may also be present.[1,2]

Pathogen

Borrelia hermsii, a spirochete, is the causative agent for tick-borne relapsing fever. The chief vectors are ticks of the *Ornithodoros* genus. Hares, rabbits, squirrels, chipmunks, mice, and rats may serve as reservoir hosts. Mountainous areas west of the Mississippi River have the most cases in the United States. Occurrence of the disease is sporadic and may be in familial clusters.[16]

Diagnosis

During a febrile episode, cerebrospinal fluid, bone marrow, or blood may have detectable spirochetes. Thrombocytopenia with or without leukocytosis may also be noted.[1]

Management

Doxycycline is the treatment of choice. Erythromycin is a viable alternative.[17] If given during the late febrile stage, a Jarisch-Herxheimer reaction, characterized by seizures, rigors, sweating, fever, headache, and generalized malaise, may occur with treatment. Giving acetaminophen 2 hours before and after antibiotic administration may lessen the severity of the reaction. Nonsteroidal antiinflammatory drugs or steroid administration do not ameliorate the reaction's cardiopulmonary disturbances.

Table 1
Geographic distribution of tick-borne illnesses

Patient Seen In or With Recent Travel To	Illness	Associated Reservoirs and/or Tick/s	Organism/s
Mountainous areas, west of the Mississippi	Relapsing fever	Hares, rabbits, and rodents carrying genus Ornithodoros ticks	Genus *Borrelia* spirochete
Rocky Mountain region, in the Colorado mountains (in campers, between March and September)	Colorado tick fever	*Dermacentor andersoni*: the wood tick	RNA orbivirus
Northeastern United States	Babesiosis	*Ixodes scapularis*: the deer tick and/or the black-legged tick	*Babesia divergens* and/or *Babesia microti*
Southeastern United States	Tularemia	*Dermacentor variabilis*: the dog tick. Reservoirs are ground squirrels, rabbits, hares, voles, muskrats, water rats, and other rodents	*Francisella tularensis*
Western United States		*D andersoni*: the wood tick. Same reservoirs as listed earlier	
Southeastern and south-central United States; rural areas in all states (except Hawaii)		*Amblyomma americanum*: the lone star tick. Same reservoirs as listed earlier	
Northeastern and upper Midwestern United States, northern California	Human granulocytotropic anaplasmosis	*I scapularis*: the deer tick and/or the black-legged tick. Reservoirs are rodents, deer, ruminants, horses	*Anaplasma phagocytophilum*
Southeastern United States	Human monocytotropic ehrlichiosis	*D variabilis*: the dog tick. Reservoirs are white-tailed deer, coyotes, dogs	*Ehrlichia chaffeensis*
South-central United States		*A americanum*: the lone star tick. Same reservoirs as listed earlier	
All states, except Montana; most in the Great Lakes area and the northeast	Lyme disease	The white-footed mouse: *I scapularis*, the deer tick, and/or the black-legged tick. Reservoir is the white-footed mouse	*Borrelia burgdorferi*
Southern and eastern states	Rocky Mountain spotted fever	*D variabilis*: the dog tick	*Rickettsia rickettsii*
All states except Alaska, Hawaii, and Maine; only found in the Western Hemisphere		*D andersoni*: the wood tick	

Data from Refs.[1–7]

Table 2
The ticks

Illness	Associated Tick	Size of Tick	Distinguishing Features	Illustration
Tick-borne relapsing fever	Genus *Ornithodoros*	About 3–4 mm long, 2 mm wide, 1 mm thick	Oval shape, mouth parts show ventrally, gray color, no dorsal shield	Fig. 1A
Colorado tick fever	*D andersoni*: the wood tick	About 3–4 mm long, 2 mm wide, 1 mm thick	Teardrop shaped; short mouth parts; females with white shield, brown abdomen, and partial shields; males brown with white markings, full shields; 11 festoons	Fig. 1B
Babesiosis, human granulocytotropic anaplasmosis, and Lyme disease	*I scapularis*: the deer tick and/or black-legged tick	About 2 mm long, 1 mm wide, 0.5 mm thick	Teardrop shaped; long mouth; females with black partial shield and brick-red abdomen; males with black full shield and lighter red abdomen	Fig. 1C
Tularemia, human monocytotropic ehrlichiosis, and Rocky Mountain spotted fever	*D variabilis*: the dog tick	About 3–4 mm long, 2 mm wide, 1 mm thick	Teardrop shaped; short mouth parts; females with white shield, brown abdomen, and partial shields; males brown with white markings, full shields; 11 festoons	Fig. 1D
	D andersoni: the wood tick	About 3–4 mm long, 2 mm wide, 1 mm thick	Teardrop shaped; short mouth parts; females with white shield, brown abdomen, and partial shields; males brown with white markings, full shields; 11 festoons	Fig. 1E
	A americanum: the lone star tick	About 2 mm long, 1 mm wide, 0.5 mm thick; female is about 4–5 mm long, 3 mm wide, 2 mm thick	Rounded; longest mouth parts; females red-brown with white spot star, partial shield; males red-brown with full shield	Fig. 1F

Data from Refs.[1–7]

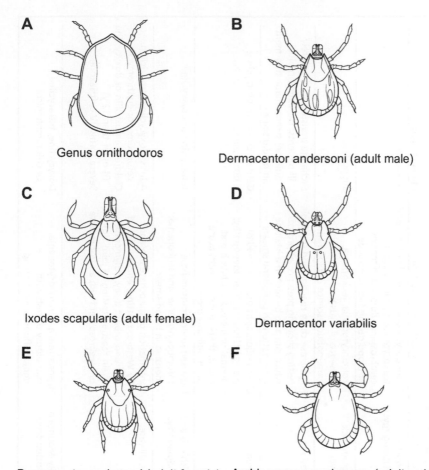

Genus ornithodoros

Dermacentor andersoni (adult male)

Ixodes scapularis (adult female)

Dermacentor variabilis

Dermacentor andersoni (adult female)   Amblyomma americanum (adult male)

Fig. 1. The tick vectors.

COLORADO TICK FEVER
Presentation

Within 1 week (usually 3–6 days) after the tick bite, the patient usually begins having flulike symptoms. Sore throat is the presentation in one-third of patients.[18] Saddleback fever is the pathognomonic feature. This biphasic fever initially lasts for about 3 days, followed by a period of defervescence for 1 to 3 days, and concludes with the reappearance of the fever for another few days. Colorado tick fever may be associated with conjunctivitis, rash, and meningitis.[16]

Pathogen

The wood tick *Dermacentor andersoni* transmits the RNA orbivirus that causes Colorado tick fever. The Rocky Mountain region has the most cases every year. The annual incidence is probably higher than most reported numbers because the initial presentation is generally benign.[19] Severe complications may occur in patients who have had a splenectomy or those who are immunocompromised.

Table 3
Presentation key or unique aspects to consider

Key and/or Unique Aspect/s of Presentation	Tick-borne Illness to Consider	What to Look for in Work-up	Management
Cranial nerve palsy, epistaxis, iridocyclitis, hemoptysis, splenomegaly, meningeal signs (even coma), signs and symptoms of splenic rupture, myocarditis, and/or pneumonitis	Tick-borne relapsing fever	Thrombocytopenia, normal or increased leukocyte count, spirochetes in cerebrospinal fluid, bone marrow, or blood during febrile episode	Doxycycline
Saddleback fever	Colorado tick fever	Thrombocytopenia, leukopenia, presence of virus noted through immunofluorescence in blood smears	Supportive
Renal failure, hemoglobinuria, jaundice (fever with hemolytic anemia)	Babesiosis	Polymerase chain reaction and serologic testing showing presence of protozoa, which can also be seen in a Maltese cross pattern in peripheral smears	Exchange transfusion in severely ill patients; clindamycin plus quinine; symptomatic treatment in mild disease
Pericarditis, acute respiratory distress syndrome, pneumonia, and pleural effusion; skin ulcers with associated lymphadenopathy	Tularemia	Chest radiographs showing triad of pleural effusions, hilar adenopathy; normal or increased white blood count; titers consistent with acute or chronic infection	Gentamicin or streptomycin ± doxycycline
Petechial, maculopapular, or macular rash	Ehrlichiosis and anaplasmosis	Increased serum transaminase, thrombocytopenia, and leukopenia; morulae in blood smear	Tetracycline or doxycycline
Stage 1 (early localized): lymphadenopathy, arthralgias, fatigue, erythema migrans rash Stage 2 (early disseminated): central nervous system symptoms, secondary cutaneous annular lesions Stage 3 (late chronic): myocardial and neurologic abnormalities, keratitis, dermatitis, and central nervous system impairment	Lyme disease	Confirmation of spirochete presence by Western blotting, enzyme-linked immunosorbent assay, polymerase chain reaction testing of joint fluid or cerebrospinal fluid, and/or culture	Adults: doxycycline, amoxicillin, cefuroxime, or erythromycin Children: amoxicillin or doxycycline (if older than 12 y) Severe forms: IV ceftriaxone
Abdominal petechial rash also affecting pads and soles of feet, pleuritic chest pain	Rocky Mountain spotted fever	Hyponatremia, thrombocytopenia, skin biopsy of rash with immunofluorescent staining	Doxycycline, tetracycline, or chloramphenicol

Abbreviation: IV, intravenous.
Data from Refs.[1–7]

Table 4
Medications for tick-borne illnesses

Tick-borne Illness	Options for Medications, with Doses and Duration of Treatment
Tick-borne relapsing fever[8]	Doxycycline[a] 100 mg po BID for 5–10 d Or Erythromycin: 500 mg or 12.5 mg/kg PO for 5–10 d (an effective alternative when tetracyclines are contraindicated) Or Ceftriaxone: 2 g IV per day for 10–14 d (preferred for patients with central nervous system involvement)
Colorado tick fever[9]	No specific treatment. Antipyretics for symptomatic relief.
Babesiosis[10,11]	Atovaquone: 750 mg PO BID for 7–10 d Plus Azithromycin: 500–1000 mg on the first day, then 250–1000 mg PO daily for the following days, or 600 mg PO 3 times per day for a total of 7–10 d or until parasitemia is cleared Or Clindamycin: 300–600 mg IV 4 times per day, or 1.2 g IV 2 times per day, or 600 mg orally 3 times per day Plus Quinine: 650 mg PO 3 times per day for 1 wk or until parasitemia is cleared
Tularemia[12]	Preferred choices for adults: Streptomycin: 1 g IM or IV 2 times per day for 10–14 d Or Gentamicin: 5 mg/kg IM or IV per day for 10–14 d Or Doxycycline[a]: 100 mg IV or PO 2 times per day for 14–21 d Or Chloramphenicol: 15 mg/kg IV 4 times per day for 14–21 d Or Ciprofloxacin: 400 mg IV or (750 mg PO) 2 times per day for 14–21 d Preferred choices for children: Streptomycin: 15 mg/kg IM or IV 2 times per day (should not exceed 2 g/d) for 10–14 d Or Gentamicin: 2.5 mg/kg IM or IV 3 times per day for 10–14 d Or Doxycycline[a]: if weight ≥45 kg, 100 mg IV 2 times per day. If weight <45 kg, 2.2 mg/kg IV 2 times per day for 14–21 d Or Chloramphenicol: 15 mg/kg IV 4 times per day for 14–21 d Or Ciprofloxacin: 15 mg/kg IV 2 times per day for 14–21 d Preferred choices for pregnant women: Gentamicin: 5 mg/kg IM or IV once per day for 10–14 d Or Streptomycin: 1 g IM or IV 2 times per day for 10–14 d
Human ehrlichiosis and anaplasmosis[13]	Doxycycline[a]: 100 mg PO 2 times per day, minimum of 3 d after defervescence to maximum of 14–21 d (avoid in pregnancy)

(continued on next page)

Table 4 (continued)	
Tick-borne Illness	**Options for Medications, with Doses and Duration of Treatment**
Lyme disease[14]	Preferred choices for adults: Amoxicillin: 500 mg 3 times per day for 14 d Or Doxycycline[a]: 100 mg 2 times per day for 14 d Or Cefuroxime axetil: 500 mg 2 times per day for 14 d Or Ceftriaxone: 2 gm IV 1 time per day for 14–28 d (If with meningitis, encephalitis, carditis, and/or arthritis) Preferred choice for children 8 y of age or older: Amoxicillin: 50 mg/kg per day in 3 divided doses (maximum, 500 mg per dose) for 14 d Preferred choice for children less than 8 y old: Amoxicillin: 4 mg/kg per day in 2 divided doses (maximum, 100 mg per dose) for 14 d Cefuroxime axetil: 30 mg/kg per day in 2 divided doses (maximum, 500 mg per dose) for 14 d
Rocky Mountain spotted fever[15]	Doxycycline[a]: 100 mg every 12 h for 7 d or for 2–3 d after fever has defervesced

Abbreviations: BID, twice a day; IM, intramuscularly; PO, by mouth.
[a] Avoid doxycycline for patients younger than 8 years old because of risk of tooth discoloration.

Diagnosis

Immunofluorescence reveals the presence of the virus in blood smears. Thrombocytopenia and leukopenia may be present as well.[1]

Management

Supportive treatment is usually all that is needed, and specific medications are not required; there is no specific antiviral medication available. Other tick-borne diseases may have been covered empirically already with doxycycline or tetracycline by the time the diagnosis is elucidated.[1]

BABESIOSIS
Presentation

One to 4 weeks after inoculation, flulike symptoms develop, just like in other tick-borne diseases. Patients may have headaches, myalgias, sweating, and fever. In asplenic patients, babesiosis may present with renal failure, jaundice, hemoglobinuria, hemolytic anemia, and high fever, resembling falciparum malaria. In young, healthy adults or children, babesia infection can be subclinical and self-limiting.[1,2]

Pathogen

Protozoans *Babesia microti* and *Babesia divergens* cause babesiosis. As such, babesiosis is the only tick-borne disease caused by protozoans in the United States. Various species of the *Ixodes* tick serve as the vector. The northeastern United States have the most cases.[1,2,7]

Diagnosis

History and a physical examination aid the most in diagnosis. Exposure history is appropriate. Fever is evident. Hemolytic anemia may be present. The Maltese cross, a characteristic tetrad, may be evident in blood smears, an indication of the presence of the causative protozoans. Polymerase chain reaction and serologic tests are also available.[1]

Management

Symptomatic treatment is all that is required for mild disease. Patients should be treated with quinine with clindamycin if they present with rising parasitemia, progressive anemia, and persistent high fevers. Atovaquone with azithromycin is an excellent alternative regimen.[20] Children may be treated with the same medications at reduced doses. Severely ill patients with high parasitemia have benefited from exchange transfusions.[1,2,20]

TULAREMIA
Presentation

Human tularemia infection depends on the route of entry of the bacterium.[6] Various syndromes have been described to encapsulate the clinical manifestations of tularemia based on the mode of infection: typhoidal (ingestion of contaminated water); pulmonary (inhalation of aerosolized bacteria); oropharyngeal/gastrointestinal (ingestion of infected meat); oculoglandular (conjunctiva exposure); and, the most common, ulceroglandular (direct skin inoculation) syndrome.[16] Myalgias, fatigue, malaise, headache, chills, and fever rapidly ensue 3 to 6 days after inoculation. One-third of patients present with coughing. Pericarditis, acute respiratory distress syndrome, pneumonia, pleural effusions, sore throat, and skin ulcers may be noted as well.[21] Vomiting and nausea may also occur. Except in typhoidal or glandular tularemia, the infected site, which could be the roof of the mouth, an eye, an arm, or a finger, may present with an inflamed papule within 24 to 48 hours of inoculation. An ulcer crater with colorless exudates results after the papule ulcerates and becomes pustular. Draining suppuration may be noted in regions of lymphadenopathy. Posterior auricular or cervical nodes are commonly affected in children. The femoral and inguinal nodes are more likely to be affected in adults.[1]

Pathogen

The bacterium that causes tularemia, or rabbit fever, is called *Francisella tularensis*. In the western United States, the tick vector is *D andersoni*, whereas in the southeastern and south-central states the tick vectors are *Dermacentor variabilis* and *Amblyomma americanum*. Contamination, inhalation, inoculation, and ingestion are the main ways of transmitting the bacteria. Infected rabbits that are skinned by their hunters may have lesions from which the bacteria pass, this time through microlesions on the hunters' skin. This is the main route of transmission in the winter. Horse flies, deer flies, and ticks are the vectors of transmission in the summer. Infection may also ensue from consuming contaminated water or undercooked infected meat, although this is uncommon.[1,2,6,21,22]

Diagnosis

A primary pustular lesion on an extremity, the characteristic symptoms outlined earlier, and exposure to ticks, wild rodents, or rabbits should lead a medical provider to suspect tularemia, particularly if in the context of correct geographic setting by history or location. The organism can be highly infectious and so it is dangerous to try to isolate the organism from sputum, lymph nodes, or skin lesions, although this would be diagnostic. The potential of the pathogen being used as a biological weapon brings this reality to the fore. Culture media or infected tissues should be handled with extreme caution. The diagnosis may be confirmed by acute and convalescent titers. White blood cell count may be normal or increased. Pulmonary tularemia is more likely to present with abnormal chest radiographic finding, such as a triad of pleural effusions, hilar adenopathy, and oval opacities, compared with other tick-borne diseases.[22–24]

Management

Confirmatory laboratory test results need not be back before treatment is begun. Streptomycin and gentamicin are both bactericidal against *F tularensis* and are therefore the drugs of choice.[6,22] The dose of gentamicin needs to be reduced if renal disease is present. Fluoroquinolones such as levofloxacin and ciprofloxacin have been used to treat this infection.[6] Although they may not prevent node suppuration or relapses, tetracyclines or chloramphenicol may also be used.[25]

EHRLICHIOSIS AND ANAPLASMOSIS
Presentation

The clinical presentation of both human monocytotropic ehrlichiosis (HME) and human granulocytotropic anaplasmosis (HGA) are similar. Fever (97% in HME, and 94%–100% in HGA), myalgia, headache (81% in HME, and 61%–85% in HGA), malaise, cough, and chills[26] comprise the influenza like syndrome that marks both infections. Although only about one-tenth to one-third of cases exhibit rashes, if present the rash appears as a petechial, macular, or maculopapular lesion on the upper extremities and trunk. Rarely (less than 5%), the palms and soles may also have the rash. It may be difficult to clinically distinguish ehrlichiosis from Rocky Mountain spotted fever.[1]

Pathogen

Anaplasma phagocytophilum (formerly classified and named *Ehrlichia equi* or *Ehrlichia phagocytophila*) is a small, gram-negative bacterium that primarily infects granulocytes, and therefore is called HGA. In contrast, *Ehrlichia chaffeensis* targets monocytes and causes HME. They are distinct epidemiologically but are clinically indistinguishable.[27] Human anaplasmosis is predominantly seen in the northeastern and Midwestern United States during the months of May, June, and July. It is during this time of year that the primary vector, the ixodid ticks (American deer ticks) are most active, and when human contact with its reservoir host is at its peak. Coinfection with Lyme disease and babesiosis is common because of a shared vector: *Ixodes scapularis*.[1,2,11] HME is seen mostly in the southeastern to south-central United States. Although it can be seen year-round, HME cases mostly occur between the months of April and September, with a peak in July. Its primary vectors are the American dog tick (*D variabilis*) and the lone star tick (*Amblyomma americanum*).[1,2,11]

Diagnosis

Increased serum transaminases, thrombocytopenia, and leukopenia are commonly seen in patients with either ehrlichiosis or anaplasmosis. A patient presenting with acute-onset fever with leukopenia, thrombocytopenia, and increased serum transaminases coupled with a recent history of tick bite in an endemic area should trigger empiric treatment with doxycycline, until HME or HGA has been ruled out. Specific serologies may initially be negative and a convalescent phase serologic titer may need to be repeated in 2 to 4 weeks.[26–28] Seroconversion during convalescence is the principal method of diagnosing human ehrlichiosis and anaplasmosis. The diagnosis necessitates documentation of a single serum antibody titer greater than or equal to 1:128, or a 4-fold increase or decrease in antibody titer with a minimum peak of 1:64.[1,2,26] Identification of morulae within the cytoplasm of monocytes, macrophages, and neutrophils via microscopic examination using a blood smear may help in the diagnosis, but may require a trained eye to detect.

Management

Confirmation with laboratory tests should not be awaited before treatment of ehrlichiosis and anaplasmosis is begun, as with other tick-borne diseases. The treatment of choice is doxycycline.[28] Tetracycline is a good alternative. Although there may be a small risk of aplastic anemia with its use, and it may not be readily available in some centers, chloramphenicol is an alternative treatment. Antibiotics should be given for 5 to 7 days until there is evidence of clinical improvement and after fever subsides, and then continued for at least 3 days more.[28] Severe cases may require longer treatment courses.

LYME DISEASE
Presentation

Lyme disease typically presents in 3 stages. Seven to 10 days after the tick bite, stage 1 (early localized Lyme disease) occurs, in which 75% of patients develop the typical rash, called erythema migrans, at the site of the tick bite. This rash is a red, expanding, annular papule or macule with central clearing up to 50 cm in diameter. Regional lymphadenopathy, coughing, headaches, arthralgias, fatigue, and low-grade fevers may ensue as part of an influenzalike syndrome that characterizes this stage.[1,2,7,29]

A few weeks after the initial infection, stage 2 (early disseminated Lyme disease) may occur. Later stages of Lyme disease (stage 2 and late/chronic Lyme disease) only occur if the infection is left untreated at stage 1. Central nervous system symptoms, adenopathy, fever, and multiple secondary cutaneous annular lesions characterize stage 2. The patient may also have pharyngitis and coughing.[1,2,7,29]

Keratitis, dermatitis, central nervous system impairment, and chronic arthritis characterize stage 1 (late chronic Lyme disease). Cardiomegaly, pericarditis, atrioventricular block, radiculopathies, Bell palsy, and meningoencephalitis may also occur at this stage.[14]

Pathogen

Lyme disease is the most common vector-borne infectious disease in the United States.[29] It is caused by the spirochete *B burgdorferi*. *I scapularis*, or the black-legged tick, is the main vector in the United States (see **Table 2**). The female tick often attaches herself to the white-tailed deer during winter, and so it is also known as the deer tick. Small mammals such as the white-footed mouse serve as natural reservoirs for *B burgdorferi*. Tick nymphs or larvae become infected when they feed on such mammals. The nymphs then usually infect humans, although adult ticks may also do this. The risk of transmission of *B burgdorferi* only becomes substantial if the infected nymph remains attached for 36 hours or longer. Adult ticks must remain attached for more than 48 hours.[30–33] Fleas, flies, or mosquitoes cannot transmit Lyme disease. Lyme disease cannot be transmitted by blood products.[34]

Diagnosis

In an endemic area, patients presenting with typical erythema migrans require no laboratory confirmation, because only about 30% have positive Lyme serologies during this early phase.[35] The enzyme-linked immunosorbent assay (ELISA) test is about

72% specific and 89% sensitive. The Lyme Western blot test is used to confirm a positive ELISA test. The Lyme Western blot immunoglobulin (Ig) G is almost 100% positive (ie, more than 5 bands positive of the 10 total IgG bands) if the test is done in patients with an active infection for longer than 1 month, as in the case of late Lyme disease.[35] Therefore, in patients who have been ill for more than 4 weeks, a positive Western blot IgM test by itself (negative IgG test) is most likely a false-positive. Lyme DNA polymerase chain reaction assays allow specific diagnosis of this infection using sterile fluids such as the synovial fluid and cerebrospinal fluid in diagnosing Lyme arthritis and neuroborreliosis, respectively.[25] It takes weeks for cultures from most body fluids and tissues to turn positive for B burgdorferi, which limits their usefulness.

Management

If a tick was attached for less than 36 hours, the risk of infection with B burgdorferi is minimal to nonexistent. There is no need for routine antibiotic prophylaxis in such cases.[14,34] In the typical practice setting, the likelihood of infection is less than 3.5%. One 200-mg dose of doxycycline is cost-effective only if the likelihood of infection is more than that, according to a cost-effectiveness analysis.[35,36] Antibiotic treatment is curative in most cases if symptoms develop. Doxycycline is the recommended antibiotic if the patient is older than 12 years. For patients 12 years old and younger, amoxicillin is the recommended antibiotic. For patients who cannot take tetracyclines or are allergic to penicillin, cefuroxime is a viable alternative. For uncomplicated cases, treatment usually ranges from 14 to 21 days. Intravenous antibiotics, with a switch to oral therapy once the patient is no longer in high-degree atrioventricular block, may be needed in severe or late disease, particularly in patients with cardiovascular or neurologic manifestations. At least 30 days of treatment should be administered in these advanced cases. Retreatment may be necessary, because treatment failures may occur in late disease.[37]

ROCKY MOUNTAIN SPOTTED FEVER
Pathogen

Rocky Mountain spotted fever is the most common rickettsial disease in the United States and is caused by Rickettsia rickettsii.[11] About 2000 cases of Rocky Mountain spotted fever are reported every year in the United States, thus making it the most frequently reported rickettsial disease.[38] All states except Alaska, Hawaii, and Maine have reported cases, and the disease is limited to the Western Hemisphere. Infections may occur year-round in the southern United States, although the disease is more common in the coastal Atlantic states from April to September.[25] The most common vector in the southern and eastern United States is the dog tick, D variabilis. In the western United States, the wood tick, D andersoni, is the principal vector. Person-to-person transmission does not seem to occur. Children 5 to 9 years of age are the most commonly afflicted with Rocky Mountain spotted fever.[39]

Presentation

Between 50% and 70% of patients with tick-borne disease recall getting bitten by a tick.[25,39] Rocky Mountain spotted fever symptoms usually begin 5 to 7 days after inoculation. Vomiting, nausea, frontal headaches, fever, leg muscle pain, back pain, and generalized malaise are common symptoms. Abdominal pain, pleuritic chest pain, sore throat, and nonproductive cough are other symptoms. An exanthem appearing within the first few days of symptoms, associated with chills, fever, and a sudden headache, comprise the classic presenting symptoms. The forearms, ankles, wrists, palms, and soles present with the initial lesions. Pressure applied onto the lesions, which are macular and pink, causes them to fade. The rash becomes maculopapular and then petechial as it extends onto the face, neck, trunk, buttocks, and axilla. Large areas of ulceration and ecchymosis may result as the lesions coalesce. Neurologic compromise may occur, along with circulatory and respiratory failure.[40] Poor outcomes and complications usually occur in patients with glucose-6-phosphate dehydrogenase deficiency.[15]

Diagnosis

History and a physical examination may be all that is needed to diagnose Rocky Mountain spotted fever. Rocky Mountain spotted fever should be a consideration in patients presenting with headaches and fever in endemic areas during peak months of tick exposure. Immunofluorescent staining for Rickettsia after skin biopsy of a rash, if present, is highly specific, although sensitivity may be only slightly more than 60%. Hyponatremia and thrombocytopenia may be noted, although laboratory testing is of limited usefulness.[15] Within the convalescence period, latex agglutination titers and increase of specific ELISA may be useful.[1]

Management

Immediate treatment is imperative when hyponatremia, thrombocytopenia, and the rash are noted. A minimum of 7 days of treatment with chloramphenicol, doxycycline, or tetracycline is needed for Rocky Mountain spotted fever.[28] There is a lack of evidence that Rocky Mountain spotted fever responds to fluoroquinolones, although there are reports that these may also be effective.[41] Early treatment is crucial in order to effect optimal response to antibiotics. From epidemiologic and clinical findings, appropriate antibiotic treatment should be initiated immediately when Rocky Mountain spotted fever is suspected. Laboratory confirmation need not be obtained before treatment is instituted.[42]

TICK-BORNE ILLNESS PREVENTION STRATEGIES

Avoiding high-risk habitats during periods of peak tick activity is the first line of defense against tick bites.[3]

Using bed nets when sleeping on the ground or camping, using tick repellents containing permethrin for clothing and N,N-diethyl-m-toluamide (DEET) for the skin, wearing long pants, tucking pant legs into socks, and avoiding tick-infested areas, especially during the summer months, are some measures that may prevent tick exposure. The effectiveness of a product called Citriodiol, available on the market and derived from lemon-scented eucalyptus oil, has been demonstrated.[40] Other potential tick repellents such as Alaska yellow cedar oil, lavender oil, and geranium oil have also been identified.[43,44]

Between 24 and 48 hours of attachment to the host are required before infection occurs, and so diseases can be prevented by early removal of ticks.[3,25] Removal of the tick can be done by applying vertical traction to its body as it is grasped gently. The best results may be achieved through forceps that are angled, medium-tipped, and blunt. Instead of tweezers, there are commercially available devices that may also be used. Passing a needle through the tick, using injected or topical lidocaine, covering the tick with petroleum jelly, nail polish, alcohol, or gasoline, and applying a hot match to the tick body are not recommended as tick-removal methods. Granuloma formation and/or infection may result if parts of the proboscis remain in the skin because of improper technique.[45]

Ninety-five percent of host-seeking *I scapularis* nymphs can be killed by a single, well-timed application of deltamethrin at the forest-lawn interface of residential properties.[46] Human babesiosis, human granulocytic anaplasmosis, and Lyme borreliosis could theoretically be prevented by such an approach, but residents in areas highly endemic for these illnesses decline to use acaricides on their properties because of fears regarding environmental damage and toxicity to humans and animals.[3]

Tests had proved the effectiveness in humans of a recombinant vaccine against the Lyme borreliosis spirochete (*B burgdorferi*) outer surface protein A or OspA, a vaccine that was later approved by the United States Food and Drug Administration (FDA). By 2002, this was withdrawn from the market because of low public demand; uncertainty regarding disease risk; class action lawsuits; a difficult vaccination schedule; potential need for boosters; high cost; concerns of antivaccine groups regarding safety; and suggestions that the vaccine antigen, outer surface protein A, was arthritogenic because it served as an autoantigen.[47,48]

For centuries, vegetation management has been a method of controlling ticks. To reduce tick populations, controlled burns, brush removal, and mowing may be used, although effects may be short-lived.[3] Placing a border between naturally tick-infested forested habitats and adjacent lawns on residential properties may be a more long-lasting landscape management strategy.[49,50] Because it has repellent properties, Alaska yellow cedar sawdust may be an appropriate material for such borders.[49] *I scapularis* is found in forest habitats associated with leaf litter and is the principal vector of *B burgdorferi* in the eastern United States. The population of host-seeking ticks is reduced by removal of leaf litter from the forest floor, which exposes these ticks to desiccation.[51]

CONCURRENT INFECTIONS

Although beyond the scope of this article, 1 bite from 1 tick may transmit different infectious pathogens and may result in concurrent infections, resulting in a clinical picture that may be mixed or more complicated.[52] Babesiosis, Lyme disease, and ehrlichiosis can all be transmitted by *I scapularis* concurrently. Lyme disease can occur concurrently with babesiosis in 23% of patients diagnosed with the former.[53] Babesiosis and/or Lyme disease may occur concurrently in 10% to 30% of patients with ehrlichiosis, whereas 10% to 30% of patients with Lyme disease may have ehrlichiosis. More severe symptoms seem to result from such combined infections.[25,52]

REFERENCES

1. Bratton RL, Corey GR. Tick-borne disease. Am Fam Physician 2005;71: 2323–30, 2331–2.
2. Gayle A, Ringdahl E. Tick-borne diseases. Am Fam Physician 2001;64:461–6.
3. Piesman J, Eisen L. Prevention of tick-borne diseases. Annu Rev Entomol 2008; 53:323–43.
4. Raoult D, Fournier PE, Eremeeva M, et al. Naming of rickettsiae and rickettsial diseases. Ann N Y Acad Sci 2005;1063:1–12.
5. Mandl CW. Steps of the tick-borne encephalitis virus replication cycle that affect neuropathogenesis. Virus Res 2005;111:161–74.
6. Ellis J, Oyston PC, Green M, et al. Tularemia. Clin Microbiol Rev 2002;15: 631–46.
7. Goddard J. Tick-borne diseases. In: Georgiev VS, editor. Infectious diseases and arthropods. 2nd edition. Totowa (NJ): Humana Press; 2008. p. 81–129.

8. Centers for Disease Control and Prevention. Tick-borne relapsing fever. Available at: http://www.cdc.gov/relapsing-fever/clinicians/#treatment. Accessed March 16, 2013.

9. Kazzi MG. Colorado tick fever. In: Kulkarni R, editor. Medscape. Available at: http://emedicine.medscape.com/article/786688-medication. Accessed March 16, 2013.

10. Centers for Disease Control and Prevention. Parasites: babesiosis. Available at: http://www.cdc.gov/parasites/babesiosis/health_professionals/index.html#tx. Accessed March 16, 2013.

11. Diaz JH. Ticks, including tick paralysis. In: Mandell GL, Bennett JE, Dolin R, editors. Mandell, Douglas, and Bennett's principles and practice of infectious diseases. 7th edition. Philadelphia: Elsevier Churchill Livingstone; 2010. p. 3649–62.

12. Centers for Disease Control and Prevention. Abstract: Consensus statement: tularemia as a biological weapon: medical and public health management. Available at: http://www.bt.cdc.gov/agent/tularemia/tularemia-biological-weapon-abstract.asp#4. Accessed March 16, 2013.

13. Cunha BA. Ehrlichiosis. In: Bronze M, editor. Medscape. Available at: http://emedicine.medscape.com/article/235839-medication. Accessed March 16, 2013.

14. Wormser GP, Dattwyler RJ, Shapiro ED, et al. The clinical assessment, treatment, and prevention of Lyme disease, human granulocytic anaplasmosis, and babesiosis: clinical practice guidelines by the Infectious Diseases Society of America. Clin Infect Dis 2006;43:1089–134.

15. Centers for Disease Control and Prevention. Rocky Mountain spotted fever (RMSF). Available at: http://www.cdc.gov/rmsf/symptoms/index.html. Accessed March 16, 2013.

16. Steve AC. Lyme borreliosis. In: Kasper DL, Harrison TR, editors. Harrison's manual of medicine. 16th edition. New York: McGraw-Hill; 2005. p. 995–9.

17. Gilbert DN, Moellering RC, Eliopoulos GM, et al. Antimicrobial therapy. The Sanford guide to antimicrobial therapy. 34th edition. Hyde Park (VT): Blackwell Publishing; 2004. p. 39.

18. Byrd RP Jr, Vasquez J, Roy TM. Respiratory manifestations of tick-borne diseases in the southeastern United States. South Med J 1997;90:1–4.

19. Emmons RW. An overview of Colorado tick fever. Prog Clin Biol Res 1985;178: 47–52.

20. Drugs for parasitic infections. Med Lett Drugs Ther, 2010. Available at: http://secure.medicalletter.org/system/files/private/parasitic.pdf. Accessed February 17, 2013.

21. Evans ME, Gregory DW, Schaffner W, et al. Tularemia: a 30-year experience with 88 cases. Medicine 1985;64:251–69.

22. Miller RP, Bates JH. Pleuropulmonary tularemia: a review of 29 patients. Am Rev Respir Dis 1969;99:31–41.

23. Rubin SA. Radiographic spectrum of pleuropulmonary tularemia. Am J Roentgenol 1978;131:277–81.

24. Dennis DT, Inglesby TV, Henderson DA, et al. Tularemia as a biological weapon: medical and public health management. JAMA 2001;285:2763–73.

25. Beers MH, Berkow R. The Merck manual of diagnosis and therapy. 17th edition. Whitehouse Station (NJ): Merck Research Laboratories; 1999.

26. Dumler JS, Walker DH. *Ehrlichia chaffeensis* (human monocytotropic ehrlichiosis), *Anaplasma phagocytophilum* (human granulocytotropic anaplasmosis),

and other Anaplasmataceae. In: Mandell GL, Bennett JE, Dolin R, editors. Mandell, Douglas, and Bennett's principles and practice of infectious diseases. 7th edition. Philadelphia: Elsevier Churchill Livingstone; 2010. p. 2531–8.

27. Belman AL. Tick-borne diseases. Semin Pediatr Neurol 1999;6:249–66.
28. Centers for Disease Control and Prevention. Human ehrlichiosis in the United States. Available at: http://gov/ncidod/dvrd/ehrlichia/index.htm. Accessed February 19, 2013.
29. Shapiro ED. Tick-borne diseases. Adv Pediatr Infect Dis 1997;13:187–218.
30. Piesman J, Mather TN, Sinsky RJ, et al. Duration of tick attachment and *Borrelia burgdorferi* transmission. J Clin Microbiol 1987;25:557–8.
31. Piesman J, Maupin GO, Campos EG, et al. Duration of adult female *Ixodes dammini* attachment and transmission of *Borrelia burgdorferi*, with description of a needle aspiration isolation method. J Infect Dis 1991;163:895–7.
32. Piesman J. Dynamics of *Borrelia burgdorferi* transmission by nymphal *Ixodes dammini* ticks. J Infect Dis 1993;167:1082–5.
33. Falco RC, Fish D, Piesman J. Duration of tick bites in a Lyme disease endemic area. Am J Epidemiol 1996;143:187–92.
34. Centers for Disease Control and Prevention. Lyme disease. Available at: http://www.cdc.gov/lyme/. Accessed February 20, 2013.
35. Bacon RM, Biggerstaff BJ, Schriefer ME, et al. Serodiagnosis of Lyme disease by kinetic enzyme-linked immunosorbent assay using recombinant VlsE1 or peptide antigens of *Borrelia burgdorferi* compared with 2-tiered testing using whole-cell lysates. J Infect Dis 2003;187(8):1187–99.
36. Magid D, Schwartz B, Craft J, et al. Prevention of Lyme disease after tick bites: a cost-effectiveness analysis. N Engl J Med 1992;327:534–41.
37. Treatment of Lyme disease. Med Lett Drugs Ther 2000;42:37–9.
38. Centers for Disease Control and Prevention. Provisional cases of selected notifiable diseases, week ending December 29, 2007. MMWR Morb Mortal Wkly Rep 2008;56:1360–71.
39. Walker DH. Tick-transmitted infectious diseases in the United States. Annu Rev Public Health 1998;19:237–69.
40. Kwitkowski VE, Demko SG. Infectious disease emergencies in primary care. Lippincotts Prim Care Pract 1999;3:108–25.
41. Thorner AR, Walker DH, Petri WA Jr. Rocky Mountain spotted fever. Clin Infect Dis 1998;27:1353–9.
42. Gardulf A, Wohlfart I, Gustafson R. A prospective cross-over field trial shows protection of lemon eucalyptus extract against tick bites. J Med Entomol 2004;41:1064–7.
43. Dietrich G, Dolan MC, Peralta-Cruz J, et al. Repellent activity of fractioned compounds from *Chamaecyparis nootkatensis* essential oil against nymphal *Ixodes scapularis* (Acari: Ixodidae). J Med Entomol 2006;43:957–61.
44. Jaenson TG, Garboui S, Palsson K. Repellency of oils of lemon eucalyptus geranium, and lavender and the mosquito repellent MyggA natural to *Ixodes ricinus* (Acari: Ixodidae) in the laboratory and field. J Med Entomol 2006;43:731–6.
45. Gammons M, Salam G. Tick removal. Am Fam Physician 2002;66:643–5.
46. Schulze TL, Jordan RA, Hung RW, et al. Efficacy of granular deltamethrin against *Ixodes scapularis* and *Amblyomma americanum* (Acari: Ixodidae) nymphs. J Med Entomol 2001;38:344–6.
47. Steere AC, Sikand VK, Meurice F, et al. Vaccination against Lyme disease with recombinant *Borrelia burgdorferi* outer-surface lipoprotein A with adjuvant. N Engl J Med 1998;339:209–15.

48. Poland GA. Vaccines against Lyme disease: what happened and what lessons can we learn? Clin Infect Dis 2011;52(Suppl 3):s253–8.
49. Maupin GO, Fish D, Zultowsky J, et al. Landscape ecology of Lyme disease in a residential area of Westchester County, New York, USA. Am J Epidemiol 1991; 133:1105–13.
50. Piesman J. Response of nymphal *Ixodes scapularis*, the primary tick vector of Lyme disease spirochetes in North America, to barriers derived from wood products or related home and garden items. J Vector Ecol 2006;31:412–7.
51. Schulze TL, Jordan RA, Hung RW. Suppression of subadult *Ixodes scapularis* (Acari: Ixodidae) following removal of leaf litter. J Med Entomol 1995;32:730–3.
52. Walker DH, Barbour AG, Oliver JH, et al. Emerging bacterial zoonotic and vector-borne diseases: ecological and epidemiological factors. JAMA 1996; 275:463–9.
53. Meldrum SC, Birkhead GS, White DJ, et al. Human babesiosis in New York state: an epidemiological description of 136 cases. Clin Infect Dis 1992;15:1019–23.

Methicillin-Resistant Staphylococcus Aureus Infections

Abraham R. Taylor, MD

KEYWORDS

- Methicillin-resistant • *Staphylococcus aureus* • MRSA • Review
- Antibiotic-resistant

KEY POINTS

- Methicillin-resistant *Staphylococcus aureus* (MRSA) is an increasingly common clinical pathogen with a genetic mutation that alters the penicillin binding protein, rendering beta lactam antibiotics ineffective (with the newer ceftaroline and ceftobiprole as notable exceptions).
- Gold standard identification of MRSA strains from clinical specimens is by culture and sensitivity; in general, however, newer proprietary rapid MRSA tests are available for surveillance, blood, and wound specimens and demonstrate high sensitivity and specificity.
- Despite emerging resistance, vancomycin is still the recommended first-line antibiotic for all forms of serious infections if MRSA is suspected or confirmed; uncomplicated skin and soft tissue infections can still be treated with a trial of trimethoprim-sultamethoxazole, doxycycline, and clindamycin, especially if community-associated MRSA is suspected.
- Simple abscesses without surrounding cellulitis can frequently be treated with incision and drainage alone without adjunct antibiotics.

INTRODUCTION

An increasingly common clinical pathogen, methicillin-resistant *Staphylococcus aureus* (MRSA) refers to bacterial strains that confer resistance to a variety of penicillins through the gene *mecA*, which resides on staphylococcal cassette chromosome mec (SCCmec), a mobile bacterial chromosomal element that is transferable between *S aureus* cells. Although the penicillinlike antibiotics confer antimicrobial properties through their ability to selectively and permanently bind the active site of penicillin-binding proteins (PBPs), which are also essential bacterial enzymes used in peptidoglycan linking during cell wall synthesis, the *mecA* gene allows the formation of a mutated PBP, dubbed PBP2a, which has significantly reduced affinity to bind beta-lactam antibiotics. Thus, the resistance patterns in MRSA are caused by antibiotic inability to bind at its active site rather than through breakdown by beta-lactamase,

Department of Family and Community Medicine, Penn State Milton S. Hershey Medical Center, 500 University Drive, Hershey, PA 17033, USA
E-mail address: ataylor3@hmc.psu.edu

Prim Care Clin Office Pract 40 (2013) 637–654
http://dx.doi.org/10.1016/j.pop.2013.06.002
0095-4543/13/$ – see front matter © 2013 Elsevier Inc. All rights reserved.

as in an alternative means of beta-lactam resistance. For this reason, specific beta-lactam antibiotics that are either beta-lactamase stable or contain beta-lactamase inhibitors confer no antimicrobial activity against MRSA strains.

Although it is important to remember that the incidence and prevalence of MRSA vary geographically, much information exists about the emerging and growing clinical problem of MRSA. Prevalence of MRSA United States in 2005 was 31.8 per 100,000 population.[1] Based on data from a cross-sectional study of a single day at 590 institutions in 2010, 6.6% of hospitalized patients will be found to have MRSA isolates, either colonization or infection; compared with a prior study from 2006, the point prevalence of MRSA isolates had increased from 4.6%.[2,3] Although the rates of MRSA isolates in colonization increased, at least in part because of the detection bias related to more wide-spread active surveillance programs, rates of MRSA infection decreased.[3] Patients hospitalized with MRSA infections have a 5-fold increased risk of death during hospitalization than patients without MRSA infection.[4] Furthermore, based on outpatient data from yearly National Ambulatory Medical Care Surveys conducted between 2001 and 2003, 11.6 million visits or 410.7 visits per 10,000 persons occurred per year for skin and soft tissue infections.[5] Emergency department visits for skin and soft tissue infection increased by 31% from 2001 to 2003.[5] Additionally, about 60% of emergency department visits for skin and soft tissue infections (SSTIs) are caused by MRSA, suggesting that, of all staphylococcal infections, an increasing proportion is caused by MRSA.[6]

The broad category of MRSA can be divided into 2 strain types: either community-associated MRSA (CA-MRSA) or hospital-associated MRSA (HA-MRSA). HA-MRSA infections generally have broader resistances given the presence of other regulatory and resistance genes as part of a larger genomic island within the bacterial genetic code. The presence or absence of other genes, like the presence of Panton-Valentine leukocidin or type IV staphylococcal cassette chromosome, may also affect virulence, allowing many strains of CA-MRSA to generally be more virulent than strains of HA-MRSA; this difference in virulence may explain the ease with which CA-MRSA is spread compared with HA-MRSA in the community.[7] Still, according to a Centers for Disease Control and Prevention (CDC) expert panel, this classical association between these microbiological characteristics and differences between MRSA transmission in the community and health care settings may be blurring.[7] More clinically practical than identifying the genomics of the MRSA strains, however, is the use of varying diagnostic criteria that can be used to predict the likelihood that the clinician is dealing with either CA-MRSA or HA-MRSA. The CDC defines CA-MRSA as MRSA infections that comprise a certain set of characteristics as shown in **Box 1**.[8,9]

It is hypothesized that the ubiquitous nature of MRSA ability to cause infection really in any location or indwelling device is related to its ability to form a biofilm. The clinical relevance of CA-MRSA is usually restricted to skin and soft tissue infections; because of the classically increased virulence, outbreaks can occur among close contacts, such as relatives in the same household.[7] Still, CA-MRSA can cause more invasive

---

Box 1
The CDC's clinical criteria for CA-MRSA

Outpatient diagnosis or isolation in inpatients within 48 hours of hospitalization

Absence of hospitalization, long-term care residence, surgery, or dialysis in the last year

No indwelling catheter site

No prior history of MRSA

infections or serious complications such as with postinfluenza pneumonias, necrotizing fasciitis, pyomyositis, and Waterhouse-Friderichsen syndrome.[10–12] HA-MRSA, although also a potential pathogen for skin and soft tissue infections, is a more likely cause of MRSA pneumonia, bacteremia, infective endocarditis, bone and joint infections, and other invasive complications. This invasiveness is likely at least partially caused by the effects of patient characteristics, such as mechanical ventilation, dialysis, recent surgery, indwelling catheters or other devices, immune suppression, and other risks, rather than strictly microbial characteristics.

Prevention

In the transmission of MRSA, the reservoir is asymptomatic patients who are colonized with the nares, the most common site. Approximately one-third of the US population have nasal colonization of S aureus; data from 2001 suggested that 0.8% of the population had MRSA nasal colonization with a more recent study suggesting that the proportion of S aureus isolates confirmed as MRSA may be increasing.[13,14] Dissemination of MRSA from person to person is primarily through contaminated hands. Thus, risk factors for infection or colonization are related to the high probabilities of encountering hosts in people who live or operate in close proximity to others. Such situations can involve athletes; prisoners; group-home, nursing-home, or other facility residents; soldiers; students; day-care attendees; recently hospitalized patients; and other risky subpopulations.[7] **Box 2** contains the CDC-recommended clinician and patient strategies that may limit spread among close contacts and prevent future infections.[7]

Hand hygiene and other standard precautions are critically important measures to combat MRSA.[15] To prevent the spread of MRSA from infected or colonized patients, the CDC also lists contact precautions and isolation as core measures.[15] In single centers or high-risk populations, infection control bundles are supported by limited evidence.[16–18] Still, research of such institutional bundles have major limitations, including their observational design, lack of comparator groups, before-and-after

---

Box 2
Precautionary measures for prevention of SSTIs

1. Wash hands with soap and water or with alcohol-based sanitizer (when unsoiled) with regularity, between patients, notwithstanding the use of gloves, and after touching contaminated surfaces or infected bodily secretions.

2. Wear gloves when dealing with contaminated or infected body sites.

3. Wear eye protection when splatter is likely when dealing with infected body sites.

4. Dress draining wounds with clean, dry bandages when possible; when not possible, avoid skin-to-skin contact until the wound has healed.

5. Ensure greater spatial separation in facilities of patients with documented MRSA; for instance, board them in a private room or cohort with patients of similar infection status.

6. Use gowns, gloves, and dedicated equipment when feasible for patients with documented MRSA for patient care, especially in facilities.

7. Avoid sharing likely contaminated items, such as towels, razors, soaps, clothing, bedding, and athletic equipment.

8. Thoroughly launder contaminated clothing after each use.

9. Clean contaminated surfaces and equipment with labels that specify activity against Staphylococcus aureus.

10. Maintain appropriate general hygiene.

design and resultant threats to internal validity, and assessment of multiple interventions; additionally, concerns about the costs have also been raised.[19–21] For these reasons, the CDC does not recommend universal screening for colonization; instead, the use of active surveillance cultures is based on risk.[15]

With focus on appropriate infection control measures, circumstantial evidence suggests that facilities are able to improve outcomes related to MRSA. For instance, invasive or life-threatening MRSA infections both acquired in health care settings and diagnosed in community settings in patients with recent hospitalization declined 28% from 2005 through 2008.[22] Greater reductions in hospital-acquired or associated infections were found in the subcategory of MRSA bacteremia specifically.[22] These results are in line with a report from the CDC's National Health Safety Network, which demonstrated a 50% decrease in MRSA bacteremia from 1997 to 2007.[23] Although the total disease burden of invasive MRSA seems to be declining in health care facilities, little data exist that supports similar reductions in the community.

Diagnosis and Laboratory Testing

To appropriately identify the pathogen in suspected MRSA infections, clinicians should routinely obtain specimens for culture and antimicrobial sensitivity testing when practical. Appropriate specimens would include respiratory secretions; purulent fluid from weeping cellulitis or from abscess drainage; blood; or other specimens from normally sterile sites, such as synovial fluid or bone biopsies. Traditionally, routine processes for the detection of MRSA used gram stain and culture for S aureus on blood agar, mannitol-salt agar, or Baird-Parker agar with preliminary microbial results reported in 24 to 48 hours. Once S aureus is identified, an additional 24 hours would be needed to confirm antimicrobial resistance, identified using disk susceptibility testing on Mueller-Hinton agar.

The reason for waiting a full 24 hours to determine disk-diffusion susceptibility testing and, indeed, for much of the difficulty in the accurate identification of MRSA is related to concerns of hetero-resistance. Essentially, heteroresistant MRSA strains will grow separate colonies with differing MRSA susceptibilities; this is in contrast to homo-resistance whereby all colonies seem either resistant or susceptible on routine disk susceptibility testing. Hypothetically, hetero-resistance involves varying levels of mecA gene expression across cell lines such that some colonies of MRSA strains with the mecA gene may phenotypically seem susceptible. In practice, most strains of MRSA display high degrees of hetero-resistance making the accurate identification of the antimicrobial sensitivity patterns difficult.

To optimize accurate laboratory identification of methicillin-susceptible and resistant S aureus, the Clinical and Laboratory Standards Institute (CLSI) publishes the guidelines for laboratory identification of all pathogens, including MRSA, and for subsequent susceptibility testing. Included in these recommendations are detailed, complicated laboratory procedures to ensure appropriate handling of specimens and culture samples to ensure acceptable accuracy of test results.

According to the CLSI, the clinical laboratory definition of MRSA during routine susceptibility testing involves testing for oxacillin resistance; strains are considered resistant when the minimum inhibitory concentration (MIC) for the S aureus strain is 4 µg/mL or greater. Methicillin is no longer used in susceptibility testing because it denatures more quickly in storage than oxacillin and because oxacillin is a more accurate predictor of the heteroresistant strains. In addition to oxacillin testing, cefoxitin susceptibility testing is probably now more clinically relevant because it is a more potent inducer of the mecA gene than oxacillin; because disk diffusion tests using cefoxitin are easier to read and have no intermediate susceptibility values because of wider zones of inhibition; and because cefoxitin may, therefore, better help determine heter-oresistant MRSA strains from susceptible *S aureus*.

To combat the delay in the identification of MRSA isolates for diagnosis of MRSA isolates, MRSA rapid testing is available for nasal contaminations, blood samples, and for staphylococcal SSTI drainage samples. Rapid testing for MRSA is based on evidence that such testing can reduce isolation precaution times and reduce the trans-mission of MRSA in hospital settings during active surveillance measures. In addition, earlier identification of MRSA in blood cultures or gram stains suspicious for *S aureus* shows a trend toward reduction in length of hospitalization and may reduce mortality.[24,25]

Two prevalent means of quickly identifying MRSA from clinical samples involve rapid culture on chromogenic agars, which are available in several proprietary varieties, and molecular amplification testing for bacterial genetic targets, such as *mecA* and other SCCmec elements. Rapid culture techniques contain substrate in the media that change color in the presence of *S aureus* and can also identify MRSA specifically when an antibiotic, such as cefoxitin, is present in the agar. The results from chromo-genic agar testing are generally available in 18 to 24 hours for active surveillance spec-imens.[26] They have also been used, although to a limited extent, in identifying MRSA in blood samples.[27] The sensitivity and the specificity of these media vary depending on the specific media used, the gold standard comparison, and the incubation time.

Molecular techniques are also available in several commercially available and in-house varieties and generally involve amplification of samples using some form or polymerase chain reaction followed by screening for SCCmec genetic elements with chromosomally linked genetic elements that are species specific to *S aureus*.[26] Molec-ular testing has been proposed for use in active surveillance specimens, blood sam-ples, and wound specimens.[28,29] In general, these tests also demonstrate reasonably high sensitivity (91%–100%) and specificity (95%–100%).[30] The accuracy of these tests, however, does vary in different studies and especially between different commer-cially available tests, with at least one commercially available test pulled from the US market for marginal sensitivity and specificity.[30] Additionally, care should be taken in using these tests only for the clinical specimen types for which they are approved. Negative results can be confirmed by awaiting the routine culture and sensitivity results.

Another strategy to rapidly identify MRSA from blood samples of gram positive cocci in clusters involves incubating specimens in 2 tubes of broth medium containing a bacteriophage specific to *S aureus* for 5 hours. Only one of these tubes also contains an antibiotic. If specimens contain *S aureus*, the bacteria will multiply in the tube without the antibiotic and cause replication of the bacteriophage specific to *S aureus*. This sample is plated on a lateral flow assay to detect high levels of phage proteins, similar to the assays used in home pregnancy tests. Therefore, positives tests confirm the presence of *S aureus*. Samples positive for *S aureus* warrant further testing to anti-biotic susceptibility by using the antibiotic-containing tube. In this second tube, only *S aureus* sensitive to beta lactams will grow and allow phage replication. Thus, similar plating on the lateral flow assay will only demonstrate the presence of phage proteins if the clinical specimen contains MRSA. This test system, commercially available as MicroPhage KeyPath Assay (MicroPhage, Longmont, CO, USA), demonstrated a sensitivity of 91.8% and a specificity of 98.3% in the detection of *S aureus* and distin-guished Methicillin-sensitive Staphylococcus aureus (MSSA) from MRSA in 99.1% of correctly identified *S aureus* samples.[31]

A final option in the rapid diagnosis of MRSA includes combining peptic nucleic acid probes with fluorescent in situ hybridization to rapidly and accurately diagnosis *S aureus* paired with another in vitro lateral flow immunochromatographic assay for

PBP2a. Sensitivity and specificity of the assay for PBP2a are 100% and 95.24%, respectively.[32] This testing system is marketed as the BinaxNOW PBP2a assay (Alere, Waltham, MA).

Treatment

Antibiotics

Clindamycin Food and Drug Administration (FDA)-approved for treatment of serious *S. aureus* infections, clindamycin is an oral or parenteral antibiotic that commonly retains antimicrobial activity against CA-MRSA but not typically HA-MRSA.[33] This antibiotic is appropriate for a variety of staphylococcal infections, including SSTI, pneumonias, osteomyelitis, and septic arthritis—and is safe in pediatric and obstetric patients. Infectious Diseases Society of America's (IDSA) recommendations are to avoid clindamycin in bacteremia, endocarditis, and other blood stream infections because of its bacteriostatic pharmacodynamics.[34] Pharmacokinetically, clindamycin has poor cerebral spinal fluid (CSF) penetration; therefore, it is not recommended in central nervous system (CNS) MRSA infections. Antibiotic-associated diarrhea is a common adverse drug event. More seriously, *Clostridium difficile* colitis may occur more frequently with clindamycin than with other antibiotics.[35,36]

Similar to macrolide antibiotics, clindamycin, a lincosamide, operates through the inhibition of bacterial protein synthesis by binding and inhibiting the 50S subunit of the bacterial ribosome. To predict the potential of inducible resistance through macrolide-lincosamide-streptogramin B cross-resistance related to this similar mechanism, the double-disk diffusion test or D test is recommended in erythromycin-resistant, clindamycin-sensitive MRSA strains. D testing is performed by placing a disk infused with erythromycin within 20 mm of a disk infused with clindamycin. Positive testing is indicated if the circular zone of inhibition around the clindamycin disk is flattened or warped on the side closest to the erythromycin disk; with the clindamycin disk oriented to the right, the appearance of the zone of inhibition around clindamycin will appear D shaped. Although clinical significance of inducible clindamycin resistance in vivo is less clear, positive D testing would raise doubts about the use of clindamycin in that strain, especially in cases of complicated, severe, or serious infections.

Trimethoprim-sulfamethoxazole Trimethoprim-sulfamethoxazole (TMP-SMX) is a non-FDA-approved option for CA-MRSA but is clinically efficacious in the management of CA-MRSA infections because most strains are susceptible on disk diffusion testing.[37,38] Typically, the use of TMP-SMX is restricted to SSTIs; still, some evidence exists that TMP-SMX may have efficacy, albeit seemingly inferior to vancomycin, in invasive blood stream infections and bone and joint infections.[7,34] TMP-SMX is appropriate for children older than 2 months and in obstetric patients in the first and second trimester. Limited evidence exists that synergistic use of rifampin can improve outcomes in SSTIs caused by CA-MRSA.[7] TMP-SMX is obviously contraindicated in sulfa allergy and should be used cautiously in the setting of chronic kidney disease and concomitant use of renin-angiotensin system inhibitors or potassium-sparing diuretics because of the potential risks of acute kidney injury and hyperkalemia. Another common cause of SSTIs and the most common cause of nonpurulent cellulitis, beta hemolytic streptococci are almost uniformly resistant to TMP-SMX.

Vancomycin Vancomycin prevents the formation of molecular bonds involved in cross-linking the molecular subunits comprising cell walls in gram-positive bacteria. Adverse drug reactions include the red man syndrome, which can be tempered by dosing with an antihistamine and by prolonging the infusion time, and acute kidney injury. Dose adjustments are necessary in situations of poor glomerular filtration due to renal excretion. Pharmacokinetics of vancomycin suggest limited penetration to bone, lung epithelia, and CSF and varied penetration, dependent on degrees of inflammation, into other tissues. Vancomycin is appropriate for pediatric patients and is labeled as pregnancy category C. Because vancomycin displays concentration-dependent killing, therapeutic monitoring involves assessment of trough blood levels only, which are drawn before the fourth or fifth dose when the medication has reached steady state. For serious infections, therapeutic trough concentrations are recommended in the 15- to 20-μg/mL range.[34] Although vancomycin displays bacteriocidal properties, its antimicrobial kill rate of staphylococci is slower than beta lactams making vancomycin a clearly inferior antibiotic to several types of MSSA infections.[34,39]

Even though the use of vancomycin in MRSA infections is off label, this antibiotic is a staple of intravenous MRSA treatment and is the treatment of choice for serious MRSA infections; oral treatments are contraindicated because of the exceedingly poor absorption of the antibiotic from the intestines. Although most strains of CA-MRSA and HA-MRSA are typically susceptible to vancomycin, vancomycin-intermediate Staphylococcus aureus (VISA) and vancomycin-resistant Staphylococcus aureus (VRSA) strains have emerged beginning in the 1990s.[40–42] Intermediate sensitivity to vancomycin is possibly caused by thicker cell walls that impede antibiotic penetration of the cell wall, especially in areas of low antibiotic concentrations.[40] Immediate resistance is mediated through mutation leading to an amino acid substitution in the chemical involved in molecular cross-linking of the cell wall such that vancomycin will no longer bind and impede synthesis.[41] Emerging concerns that vancomycin MIC increases among susceptible strains have lead to recommendations to increase the blood levels that are considered therapeutic.[34] Furthermore, MRSA treatment failures in seemingly susceptible strains have been reported and are thought either to be caused by heteroresistant VISA strains or to be related to the accessory gene regulator (agr) group II polymorphism.[43,44] Because of these difficulties in identifying vancomycin susceptibility, clinical always trumps antimicrobial MIC reporting from the microbiology laboratory.

Tetracyclines Although clindamycin and streptogramin B antibiotics prevent bacterial protein synthesis through binding the 50S ribosomal subunit, the tetracyclines similarly prevent synthesis but bind the 30S subunit. Active in vitro against susceptible MRSA, tetracyclines are bacteriostatic and have limited evidence supporting in vivo effectiveness in clinical MRSA infections.[45] Thus, their use is primarily restricted to SSTIs and to other noninvasive, uncomplicated MRSA infections.[7,34] Common adverse drug reactions within this class include gastrointestinal upset and photosensitivity. These medications are generally not recommended for children younger than 8 years and are pregnancy category D.

Although doxycycline is the only tetracycline with FDA approval for the treatment of staphylococcal infections, it is not specifically approved for MRSA infections; additionally, both minocycline and tetracycline also retain some activity against the S aureus, including MRSA. These antibiotics, however, are generally viable options in vitro for only CA-MRSA. Many microbiology laboratories will test for resistance using only tetracycline. Unfortunately, this practice likely overestimates resistance to minocycline, and perhaps to doxycycline, because some bacteria will carry the tetK gene, which confers tetracycline resistance and the potential for inducible doxycycline resistance; only the tetM gene confers broader resistance to the entire class of antibiotics.[7,34,46,47] CA-MRSA resistance is rare and primarily mediated through tetK; thus, minocycline may still be an option when susceptibility testing suggests only tetracycline resistance. Only limited data, however, support the use of minocycline in such situations.[48]

Linezolid Linezolid is a bacteriostatic antibiotic that inhibits protein synthesis by binding the 50S ribosomal subunit and carries FDA approval for complicated MRSA SSTIs (cSSTIs) and for MRSA pneumonias. Oral bioavailability is high, and parenteral therapy is relegated to patients who have gastrointestinal issues or who are unable to take oral medications. This common oral alternative to intravenous vancomycin and daptomycin effectively treats a variety of HA-MRSA infections, and strains of VISA and VRSA typically retain susceptibility. Although rare, resistance to linezolid has been described and generally occurs with prolonged use.[49] Long-term use can result in toxicities, including reversible thrombocytopenia, anemia, neutropenia; irreversible or partially reversible optic neuropathy and peripheral neuropathy; and lactic acidosis.[7,34] Treatment longer than 2 weeks typically requires monitoring of complete blood counts.[7] Episodes of serotonin syndrome have been reported in this weak inhibitor of monoamine oxidase.[50] The CDC generally advises consultation with an infectious disease specialist for use of this agent in SSTIs.[7] Because of its bacteriostatic pharmacodynamics, linezolid treatment failures have occurred in the treatment of blood stream infections.[51,52] Linezolid is appropriate for children and is pregnancy category C.

Daptomycin The only FDA-approved antibiotic for MRSA blood stream infections, daptomycin, disrupts cellular membrane function in a bacteriocidal fashion and is also approved for complicated SSTIs. The IDSA's guidelines recommend avoiding this agent in MRSA pneumonia because pulmonary surfactant may render it inert.[34] Insusceptible strains of MRSA are rare but do occur and can lead to treatment failures.[53,54] Exposed to vancomycin, some MRSA strains can demonstrate inducible resistance to daptomycin, suggesting that resistance mechanisms may be similar.[53,55,56] Typical dosing is 4 mg/kg per dose daily for cSSTI and 6 mg/kg per dose for blood stream infections.[34] Because of concerns of reduced susceptibility in left-sided endocarditis and during deep-seeded infections, however, some experts have recommended higher doses of 8 to 10 mg/kg per dose.[34] Even higher doses may be required in bacteremic treatment failures.[34] Although outcome data are lacking, this strategy is sound in theory given that daptomycin is a concentration-dependent killing antibiotic that exhibits greater antimicrobial activity at higher peak values. Elevations in creatine phosphokinase (CPK) have occurred, raising concerns of rhabdomyolysis; monitoring CPK is recommended weekly and more frequently with concomitant renal disease or statin therapy.[34] Daptomycin is pregnancy category B; despite ongoing investigations of pediatric pharmacokinetics, dosing regimens are available for children older than 2 years.

Others Several other antibiotics bear mentioning in the clinical management of MRSA. First, ceftaroline and ceftobiprole, 2 novel cephalosporins, have exhibited binding to both traditional PBP and PBP2a and demonstrated activity against MRSA; the former is FDA approved for MRSA cSSTI.[34,57,58] Formerly, tigecycline, a tetracycline derivative, was a possible option for MRSA cSSTI; however, a recent FDA warning suggesting increased risk of mortality with the use of tigecycline has led to the preference of alternate options.[34,57] Telavancin and newer lipoglycopeptides, like dalbavancin and oritavancin, have shown activity against MRSA, VISA, and VRSA.[34,57] To provide synergy, use of rifampin is occasionally used but not as a sole agent because MRSA commonly becomes rapidly resistant.[34] Quinupristin-dalfopristin can be used in invasive MRSA when vancomycin fails, but adverse reactions limit its use as an initial treatment option.[34]

MRSA SSTIS

The most common MRSA infections are SSTIs. The recommended empiric treatments for SSTIs are dependent on classification of the infection into 1 of 3 categories: abscesses, purulent cellulitis, and nonpurulent cellulitis. **Table 1** describes the recommended antibiotics that can be used for SSTI.

To definitively treat simple abscesses, incision and drainage alone seems adequate. Several observational studies and RCTs suggest that cure rates after incision and drainage are similar when comparing adjunct antibiotics active against MRSA with placebo.[59–61] Although antibiotics seem to reduce the development of early recurrence after index SSTI, no difference is found at 90 days.[60] **Box 3** describes several clinical situations whereby adjunct antibiotic treatments would be recommended.[34] When antibiotics are used as adjuncts to incision and drainage, empiric treatment should be directed against CA-MRSA, pending culture results, unless clinical criteria for HA-MRSA are present.

Per the IDSA's recommendations, coverage for MRSA in cellulitis primarily depends on whether or not the cellulitis is purulent or nonpurulent.[34] For cellulitis with purulent drainage or exudates without clearly defined fluctuance or suspected abscess, MRSA coverage is indicated pending culture results; however, for nonpurulent cellulitis, coverage for beta-hemolytic streptococci may be sufficient. Because the main challenge in nonpurulent cellulitis is difficulty in identifying microbial pathogens, treatment failure with agents targeted at beta-hemolytic streptococci or MSSA may warrant empiric treatment to cover for possible CA-MRSA. Oral options for the treatment of CA-MRSA in this situation are described in **Table 1**. The treatment duration should generally be at least 5 to 10 days but may require longer treatments in individual patients, especially the elderly or those with significant comorbidities, such as edema, malnutrition, immunodeficiency, vascular disease, or diabetes.

To adequately treat more complicated SSTIs, the standard oral antibiotics for CA-MRSA may not be sufficient. Obvious complications of SSTIs can include systemic symptoms, rapidly advancing disease, sepsis, deeper or larger SSTIs, wound infections, and infected ulcers or burns. The IDSA's recommended treatment options for cSSTIs appear in **Table 2**; ceftaroline has also recently become FDA approved for such infections.

The IDSA defines recurrent MRSA SSTIs as 2 or more discrete MRSA infections at separate sites within a 6-month time frame.[34] Providers should educate and counsel patients with recurrent MRSA SSTIs regarding preventative strategies of personal and environmental hygiene as described in **Box 2**.[7,34] When preventative measures have been optimized and have failed, the IDSA recommends that decolonization procedures may be considered, but evidence regarding the efficacy is sparse. Although a Cochrane review of 9 trials involving patients with nasal *S aureus* found that mupirocin

Table 1				
Oral antibiotics for MRSA simple SSTIs				
Antibiotic	**Adult Dose**	**Route**	**Frequency**	**Use**
Clindamycin	300–450 mg	PO	TID	D test if erythromycin resistant
TMP-SMX	1–2 DS tabs	PO	BID	Ineffective against GAS
Doxycycline	100 mg	PO	BID	—
Minocycline	100 mg	PO	BID	Load with 200 mg dose × 1
Linezolid	600 mg	PO	BID	Expensive

Abbreviations: DS, double strength; GAS, group A Streptococcus.

> **Box 3**
> **Indications for antibiotics in abscess**
>
> 1. Severe, extensive, widespread, or rapidly progressive disease
> 2. Abscess with associated cellulitis
> 3. Systemic symptoms
> 4. Severe comorbidities or immunosuppression
> 5. Extremes of age
> 6. Abscess in sites that are difficult to drain
> 7. Associated septic phlebitis
> 8. Poor response to incision and drainage alone

performed statistically better than placebo at eradication of colonization and prevention of infection especially in surgical patients and those receiving dialysis, most of the effect was found in MSSA.[62] Another review of studies strictly involving MRSA has found no effect of decolonization with either topical or systemic treatments.[63] In community settings or within families, the evidence supporting decontamination regimens to eliminate colonization or prevent infection is very limited, and the overall application and adherence to all facets of the regimen is usually poor.[7,64,65]

MRSA Bacteremia and Endocarditis

Bacteremia and potentially ensuing endocarditis are serious forms of MRSA infections, and their mortality rate is 30% to 37%.[66,67] Confronted with MRSA bacteremia, a source of infection should be verified with risk factors including intravenous (IV) drug use, indwelling catheters, endocarditis, unidentified abscesses, pneumonia, or infective endocarditis. Additionally, hematogenous spread of the bacteria can occur in patients who are bacteremic. Endocarditis particularly can be associated with embolic and immunologic complications. One study suggests that roughly 12% of all MRSA bacteremia is associated with the complication of endocarditis.[68] If indwelling catheters are present, they should be removed if possible with culture of the catheter tip. Likewise, other inciting sources of the bacteremia should be addressed. If catheters must be retained, trials of antibiotic lock therapy are possible, with the removal of the catheter required if bacteremia persists or if clinical deterioration occurs.[69]

Although less effective for MSSA bacteremia, vancomycin is the treatment of choice for MRSA bloodstream infections. An alternative treatment to vancomycin is

Table 2
Antibiotics for MRSA-complicated SSTIs

Antibiotic	Adult Dose	Route	Frequency	Use
Vancomycin	15–20 mg/kg per dose	IV	Q 8–12 h	First line
Linezolid	600 mg	PO/IV	BID	Oral option; expensive
Daptomycin	4 mg/kg per dose	IV	Daily	
Clindamycin	600 mg	PO/IV	TID	Initiate IV; oral option; inexpensive
Telavancin	10 mg/kg per dose	IV	Daily	
Tigecycline	50 mg	IV	Q 12 h	Increased mortality; load with 100 mg

Abbreviation: IV, intravenous.

daptomycin. Because of emergent MRSA strains with reduced daptomycin suscepti-bility and treatment failures, dosages as high as 8 to 10 mg/kg per dose daily have been considered for left-sided endocarditis and during deep-seeded infections, although further studies need to evaluate safety and efficacy of this practice.[34] Ac-cording to expert recommendations, treatment duration for simple bacteremia without endocarditis can be maintained for 2 weeks.[34] With complications, such as endocar-ditis, metastatic spread, the presence of prostheses, persistent bacteremia despite an initial 2 to 4 days of therapy, and the symptom of fever despite an initial 72 hours of therapy, the treatment duration increases to 4 to 6 weeks.[34]

Occasionally, rifampin or gentamicin will be added for synergistic effect, although data suggesting clinically superior outcomes with adopting this strategy are lacking; in fact, the combination of these synergistic antibiotics may even be more harm-ful.[70–72] Adjunct therapy with these antibiotics in prosthetic valve endocarditis, how-ever, is still recommended but is based on retrospective data of methicillin-resistant coagulase negative staphylococcus infections.[34,73] **Table 3** displays the initial treat-ment options for MRSA bacteremia and endocarditis. Treatment failures with vanco-mycin or daptomycin with or without synergistic adjuncts may require salvage therapy with TMP-SMX, quinupristin-dalfopristin, linezolid, or telavancin.[34] Other agents have also been proposed as treatment options for salvage therapy.[74]

MRSA Pneumonia

Even though MRSA is a rare cause of community-acquired pneumonia, the conse-quences of MRSA pneumonia are severe. Opportunistically, MRSA can cause invasive pneumonia in immune-competent patients with influenza or influenzalike illness. Also, MRSA is significantly more common among ventilator-associated pneumonia. Empiric therapy for MRSA in community-acquired pneumonias is recommended when the illness requires admission to the intensive care unit, when the infection is necrotizing, or it involves cavitary infiltrates or empyema.[34] MRSA empiric therapy can be discon-tinued if sputum and blood cultures do not identify MRSA, especially when another inciting organism is isolated.

Vancomycin and linezolid are the mainstays of the treatment of MRSA pneumonia. Because vancomycin seems to offer poor lung penetration, failure of monotherapy is relatively common. The synergistic use of rifampin with vancomycin has been shown to have some additional utility.[75] Penetrating the lung well and possessing good oral bioavailability, linezolid is an excellent alternative option and has demonstrated cure rates comparable with or better than vancomycin.[76–78] These treatment options for MRSA pneumonia are summarized in **Table 4**. Not recommended by the IDSA, fluo-roquinolones, in the past, have shown activity to CA-MRSA; but resistance is becoming more common and emerges readily with monotherapy.[34] The treatment duration for MRSA pneumonia is typically 7 to 21 days.[34]

Table 3
Antibiotics for MRSA bacteremia and endocarditis

Antibiotic	Adult Dose	Route	Frequency	Use
Vancomycin	15–20 mg/kg per dose	IV	Q 8–12 h	First line
Daptomycin	6 mg/kg per dose	IV	Daily	Alternate (perhaps 8–10 mg/kg)
Gentamicin	1 mg/kg per dose	IV	Q 8 h	Synergy in prosthetic valves
Rifampin	300 mg	PO/IV	Q 8 h	Synergy in prosthetic valves

Table 4
Antibiotics for MRSA pneumonia

Antibiotic	Adult Dose	Route	Frequency	Use
Vancomycin	15–20 mg/kg per dose	IV	Q 8–12 h	Consider rifampin synergy
Linezolid	600 mg	PO/IV	BID	Oral option; expensive
Clindamycin	600 mg	PO/IV	TID	Alternate oral option

MRSA Bone and Joint Infections

Most bone and joint infections with MRSA most commonly occur because of iatrogenic or traumatic inoculations or because of direct extension from more superficial SSTIs. Relatively strong evidence exists that magnetic resonance imaging with contrast is the best initial test in evaluating patients with suspected osteomyelitis; for joint infections, culture of synovial fluid confirms the diagnosis. Purulent collections within joints will need surgical drainage and irrigation, whereas debridement of necrotic bone is standard. High-quality comparative studies are generally lacking; some recommendations, as in SSTIs, are extrapolated from the data of MSSA infections. The optimal route of antibiotic administration and even duration of treatment are largely based on expert opinion rather than evidence.[34] Strategies for route of administration include primary oral treatments, primary intravenous treatment, or initial intravenous treatment with transition to oral therapy; no consistent, high-quality evidence exists to demonstrate superiority among these approaches.

Even though the IDSA's guidelines on MRSA management highlight several concerning issues with vancomycin, this intravenous agent is still generally the standard first-line treatment in bone and joint infections.[34] Some of the issues mentioned include poor efficacy in animal models, poor bone penetration, and reports of high failure rates. Additionally, vancomycin is seemingly inferior to beta lactams in MSSA osteomyelitis and septic arthritis. Synergistic use of rifampin, which has excellent bone and biofilm penetration, may mitigate some of these deficiencies with vancomycin; moreover, this approach is strongly recommended in MRSA-infected joint infections that meet the criteria for device retention.[34] Such criteria include symptoms of less than 3 weeks in either an implant less than 2 months old or a stable implant with documented acute hematogenous spread.[79] Additional treatment options include parenteral daptomycin, oral or parenteral clindamycin, linezolid, and TMP-SMX with rifampin.[34]

Although the antibiotic recommendations, displayed in **Table 5**, are similar for treating MRSA osteomyelitis and septic arthritis, the recommended treatment times differ.[34] Septic arthritis should typically be treated for 3 to 4 weeks. Although typical treatment times of uncomplicated osteomyelitis are at least 8 weeks, some experts

Table 5
Antibiotics for MRSA osteomyelitis and septic arthritis

Antibiotic	Adult Dose	Route	Frequency	Use
Vancomycin	15–20 mg/kg per dose	IV	Q 8–12 h	Typical first line; consider rifampin
Daptomycin	6 mg/kg per dose	IV	Daily	Alternate
Linezolid	600 mg	PO/IV	BID	Oral alternative
Clindamycin	600 mg	PO/IV	TID	Oral alternative
TMP-SMX	4 mg/kg per dose (TMP)	PO/IV	Q 8–12 h	With rifampin 600 mg QD for osteomyelitis

Table 6
Antibiotics for MRSA meningitis, brain abscess, and other CNS infections

Antibiotic	Adult Dose	Route	Frequency	Use
Vancomycin	15–20 mg/kg per dose	IV	Q 8–12 h	Typical first line; consider rifampin
Linezolid	600 mg	PO/IV	BID	Oral alternative
TMP-SMX	5 mg/kg per dose (TMP)	PO/IV	Q 8–12 h	With rifampin 600 mg QD

routinely recommend an additional 1 to 3 months of oral therapy.[34] Prolonged treatment times of 3 to 6 months are recommended for retained joint prostheses in septic arthritis and of an unspecified duration in osteomyelitis that is chronic, did not receive adequate debridement, or persists with elevated inflammatory markers.[34]

MRSA CNS Infections

CNS invasion by MRSA usually results from hematogenous spread or neurosurgical procedures. Neurosurgical treatments, such as incision and drainage, irrigation, shunt removal, and the administration of intrathecal and intraventricular antibiotics are generally required. Outcomes with MRSA CNS infections are typically poor because the antimicrobial options have poor penetration of the blood-brain barrier. The typical treatment of vancomycin has yielded disappointing outcomes likely for this reason. Although the synergistic addition of rifampin is an option, scant evidence exists to demonstrate that superior outcomes. **Table 6** lists the antibiotics with recommendations from the IDSA[31]; given the difficulty with treatment and the poor CSF penetration of many antibiotics, reasonable consideration should be given to intrathecal and intraventricular administration of antibiotics with goals to maintain appropriate bactericidal CSF drug concentrations. Although not commonly used in the United States, chloramphenicol, which has good CNS penetration, is recommended by at least one guideline from outside the United States in the management of MRSA strains sensitive to this antibiotic; evidence to support this practice seems scarce.[80]

REFERENCES

1. Klevens RM, Morrison MA, Nadle J, et al. Invasive methicillin-resistant Staphylococcus aureus infections in the United States. J Am Med Assoc 2007;298: 1763–71.
2. Jarvis WR, Schlosser J, Chinn RY, et al. National prevalence of methicillin-resistant Staphylococcus aureus in inpatients at US healthcare facilities, 2006. Am J Infect Control 2007;35:631–7.
3. Jarvis WR, Jarvis AA, Chinn RY. National prevalence of methicillin-resistant Staphylococcus aureus in inpatients at United States health care facilities, 2010. Am J Infect Control 2012;40:194–200.
4. Noskin GA, Rubin RJ, Schentag JJ, et al. The burden of Staphylococcus aureus infections on hospitals in the United States: an analysis of the 2000 and 2001 nationwide inpatient sample database. Arch Intern Med 2005;165:1756–61.
5. McCraig LF, McDonald LC, Mandal S, et al. Staphylococcus aureus-associated skin and soft tissue infections in ambulatory care. Emerg Infect Dis 2006;12(11): 1715–23.
6. Moran GJ, Krishnadasan A, Gorwitz RJ, et al. Methicillin-resistant S. aureus infections among patients in the emergency department. N Engl J Med 2006;355: 666–74.

7. Gorwitz RJ, Jernigan DB, Powers JH, et al. Participants in the CDC-Convened Experts' Meeting on Management of MRSA in the Community. Strategies for clinical management of MRSA in the community: summary of an experts' meeting convened by the Center for Disease Control and Prevention. 2006. Available at: http://www.cdc.gov/ncidod/dhqp/ar_mrsa_ca.html. Accessed February 17, 2013.

8. Morrison MA, Hageman JC, Klevens RM. Case definition for community-associated methicillin-resistant Staphylococcus aureus. J Hosp Infect 2006; 62:241.

9. CDC. Methicillin-resistant Staphylococcus aureus (MRSA) infections: diagnosis and testing. Centers for Disease Control and Prevention; 2010. Available at: http://www.cdc.gov/mrsa/diagnosis/index.html. Accessed February 17, 2013.

10. Francis JS, Doherty MC, Lopatin U, et al. Severe community-onset pneumonia in healthy adults caused by methicillin-resistant Staphylococcus aureus carrying the Panton-Valentine leukocidin genes. Clin Infect Dis 2005;40:100–7.

11. Kaplan SL. Implications of methicillin-resistant Staphylococcus aureus as a community-acquired pathogen in pediatric patients. Infect Dis Clin North Am 2005;19:747–57.

12. Adem PV, Montgomery CP, Husain AN, et al. Staphylococcus aureus sepsis and the Waterhouse-Friderichsen syndrome in children. N Engl J Med 2005;353: 1245–51.

13. Kuehnert MJ, Kruszon-Moran D, Hill HA, et al. Prevalence of Staphylococcus aureus nasal colonization in the United States, 2001-2002. J Infect Dis 2006; 193:172–9.

14. Creech CB 2nd, Kernodle DS, Alsentzer A, et al. Increasing rates of nasal carriage of methicillin-resistant Staphylococcus aureus in healthy children. Pediatr Infect Dis J 2005;24(7):617–21.

15. Seigel JD, Rhinehart E, Jackson M, et al. Management of multidrug-resistant organisms in healthcare settings, 2006. Am J Infect Control 2007;35:S165–93. Available at: http://www.cdc.gov/hicpac/mdro/mdro_0.html. Accessed February 19, 2013.

16. Ellingson K, Muder RR, Jain R, et al. Sustained reduction in the clinical incidence of methicillin-resistant Staphylococcus aureus colonization or infection associated with a multifaceted infection control intervention. Infect Control Hosp Epidemiol 2011;32(1):1–8.

17. Huang SS, Yokoe DS, Hinrichsen VL, et al. Impact of routine intensive care unit surveillance cultures and resultant barrier precautions on hospital-wide methicillin-resistant Staphylococcus aureus bacteremia. Clin Infect Dis 2006;43: 971–88.

18. Robicsek A, Beaumont JL, Paule SM, et al. Universal surveillance for methicillin-resistant Staphylococcus aureus in 3 affiliated hospitals. Ann Intern Med 2008; 148(6):409–18.

19. Cooper BS, Stone SP, Kibbler CC, et al. Systematic review of isolation policies in the hospital management of methicillin-resistant Staphylococcus aureus: a review of the literature with epidemiological and economic modeling. Health Technol Assess 2003;7(39):1–194.

20. Cooper BS, Stone SP, Kibbler CC, et al. Isolation measures in the hospital management of methicillin resistant Staphylococcus aureus (MRSA): systematic review of the literature. BMJ 2004;329(7465):533.

21. McGinigle KL, Gourlay ML, Buchanan IB. The use of active surveillance cultures in adult ICUs to reduce methicillin-resistant Staphylococcus aureus-related

morbidity, mortality and costs: a systematic review. Clin Infect Dis 2008;46: 1717–25.

22. Kallen AJ, Mu Y, Bulens S, et al. Health care–associated invasive MRSA infections, 2005-2008. J Am Med Assoc 2010;304(6):641–7.

23. Burton DC, Edwards JR, Horan TC, et al. Methicillin-resistant Staphylococcus aureus central line–associated bloodstream infections in US intensive care units, 1997-2007. J Am Med Assoc 2009;301(7):727–36.

24. Bauer KA, West JE, Balada-Llasat JM, et al. An antimicrobial stewardship program's impact with rapid polymerase chain reaction methicillin-resistant Staphylococcus aureus/S. aureus blood culture test in patients with S. aureus bacteremia. Clin Infect Dis 2010;51:1074–80.

25. Brown J, Paladino JA. Impact of rapid methicillin-resistant Staphylococcus aureus polymerase chain reaction testing on mortality and cost effectiveness in hospitalized patients with bacteraemia: a decision model. Pharmacoeconomics 2010;28(7):567–75.

26. Malhotra-Kumar S, Haccuria K, Michiels M, et al. Current trends in rapid diagnostics for methicillin-resistant Staphylococcus aureus and glycopeptide-resistant Enterococcus species. J Clin Microbiol 2008;46:1577.

27. Pape J, Wadlin J, Nachamkin I. Use of BBL CHROMagar MRSA medium for identification of methicillin-resistant Staphylococcus aureus directly from blood cultures. J Clin Microbiol 2006;44:2575.

28. Wolk DM, Picton E, Johnson D, et al. Multicenter evaluation of the cepheid Xpert methicillin-resistant Staphylococcus aureus (MRSA) test as a rapid screening method for detection of MRSA in nares. J Clin Microbiol 2009;47:758–64.

29. Wolk DM, Struelens MJ, Pancholi P, et al. Rapid detection of Staphylococcus aureus and methicillin-resistant S. aureus (MRSA) in wound specimens and blood cultures: multicenter preclinical evaluation of the Cepheid Xpert MRSA/SA skin and soft tissue and blood culture assays. J Clin Microbiol 2009;47:823–6.

30. Geiger K, Brown J. Rapid testing for methicillin-resistant Staphylococcus aureus: implications for antimicrobial stewardship. Am J Health Syst Pharm 2013;70:335–42.

31. Bhowmick T, Mirrett S, Reller LB, et al. Controlled multicenter evaluation of a bacteriophage based method for the rapid detection of Staphylococcus aureus in positive blood cultures. J Clin Microbiol 2013;51:1226–30.

32. Romero-Gómez MP, Quiles-Melero I, Navarro C, et al. Evaluation of the Binax-NOW PBP2a assay for the direct detection of methicillin resistant Staphylococcus aureus from positive blood cultures. Diagn Microbiol Infect Dis 2012; 72:282–4.

33. Tsuji BT, Rybak MJ, Chenug CM, et al. Community- and health care-associated methicillin-resistant Staphylococcus aureus: a comparison of molecular epidemiology and antimicrobial activities of various agents. Diagn Microbiol Infect Dis 2007;58:41–7.

34. Liu C, Bayer A, Cosgrove SE, et al. Clinical practice guidelines by the Infectious Disease Society of America for the treatment of methicillin-resistant Staphylococcus aureus infections in adults and children. Clin Infect Dis 2011;52(3): e18–55.

35. Center for Disease Control and Prevention. Severe clostridium difficile-associated disease in populations previously at low risk-four states, 2005. MMWR Morb Mortal Wkly Rep 2005;54(47):1201–5.

36. Raveh D, Rabinowitz B, Breuer GS, et al. Risk factors for clostridium difficile toxin-positive nosocomial diarrhoea. Int J Antimicrob Agents 2006;28:231–7.

37. Naimi TS, LeDell KH, Como-Sabetti K, et al. Comparison of community- and health care-associated methicillin-resistant Staphylococcus aureus infection. J Am Med Assoc 2003;290:2976–84.

38. Fridkin SK, Hageman JC, Morrison M, et al. Methicillin-resistant Staphylococcus aureus disease in three communities. N Engl J Med 2005;352:1436–44.

39. Strausbaugh LJ, Jacobson C, Sewell DL, et al. Antimicrobial therapy for methicillin-resistant Staphylococcus aureus colonization in residents and staff of a Veterans Affairs nursing home care unit. Infect Control Hosp Epidemiol 1992;13:151–9.

40. Howden BP, Davie JK, Johnson PD, et al. Reduced vancomycin susceptibility in Staphylococcus aureus, including vancomycin-intermediate and heterogenous vancomycin-intermediate strains: resistance mechanisms, laboratory detection, and clinical implications. Clin Microbiol Rev 2010;23:99–139.

41. Chang S, Sievert DM, Hageman JC, et al. Infection with vancomycin-resistant Staphylococcus aureus containing the vanA resistance gene. N Engl J Med 2003;348:1342–7.

42. Appelbaum PC. Reduced glycopeptides susceptibility in methicillin-resistant Staphylococcus aureus (MRSA). Int J Antimicrob Agents 2007;30:398–408.

43. Liu C, Chambers HF. Staphylococcus aureus with heterogeneous resistance to vancomycin: epidemiology, clinical significance, and critical assessment of diagnostic methods. Antimicrobial Agents Chemother 2003;47:1040–5.

44. Moise-Broder PA, Sakoulas G, Eliopoulos GM, et al. Accessory gene regulator group II polymorphism in methicillin-resistant Staphylococcus aureus is predictive of failure of vancomycin therapy. Clin Infect Dis 2004;38:1700–5.

45. Ruhe JJ, Monson T, Bradsher RW, et al. Use of long-acting tetracyclines for methicillin-resistant Staphylococcus aureus infectiosn: case series and review of the literature. Clin Infect Dis 2005;40:1429–34.

46. Bismuth R, Zilhoa R, Sakamoto H, et al. Gene heterogeneity for tetracycline resistance in multidrug-resistant, community-associated methicillin-resistant Staphylococcus spp. Antimicrobial Agents Chemother 1990;34:1611–4.

47. Schwartz BS, Graber CJ, Diep BA. Doxycycline, not minocycline, induces its own resistance in multidrug-resistant, community-associated methicillin-resistant Staphylococcus aureus clone USA300. Clin Infect Dis 2009;48:1483–4.

48. Alausa KO, Cooke AR, Montefiore D, et al. A comparative trial of minocycline and cloxacillin in the treatment of soft tissue infections due to tetracycline resistant Staphylococcus aureus. West Afr J Pharmacol Drug Res 1976;3:103–10.

49. Tsiodras S, Gold HS, Sakoulas G. Linezolid resistance in a clinical isolate of Staphylococcus aureus. Lancet 2001;358:207–8.

50. Wigen CL, Goetz MB. Serotonin syndrome and linezolid. Clin Infect Dis 2002;34:1651–2.

51. Corne P, Marchandin H, Macia JC, et al. Treatment failure of methicillin-resistant Staphylococcus aureus endocarditis with linezolid. Scand J Infect Dis 2005;37:946–9.

52. Ruiz ME, Guerrero IC, Tuazon CU. Endocarditis caused by methicillin-resistant Staphylococcus aureus: treatment failure with linezolid. Clin Infect Dis 2002;35:1018–20.

53. Boucher HW, Sakoulas G. Perspectives on daptomycin resistance, with emphasis on resistance in Staphylococcus aureus. Clin Infect Dis 2007;54:601–8.

54. Marty FM, Yeh WW, Wennersten CB, et al. Emergence of a clinical daptomycin-resistant Staphylococcus aureus isolate during treatment of methicillin-resistant

Staphylococcus aureus bacteremia and osteomyelitis. J Clin Microbiol 2006;44: 595–7.

55. Sakoulas G, Alder J, Thauvin-Eliopoulos C, et al. Induction of daptomycin heterogeneous susceptibility in Staphylococcus aureus by exposure to vancomycin. Antimicrobial Agents Chemother 2006;50:2137–45.
56. Patel JB, Jevitt LA, Hageman J, et al. An association between reduced susceptibility to daptomycin and reduced susceptibility to vancomycin in Staphylococcus aureus. Clin Infect Dis 2006;42:1652–3.
57. Kollef MH. New antimicrobial agents for methicillin-resistant Staphylococcus aureus. Crit Care Resusc 2009;11:282–6.
58. Kanafani ZA, Corey GR. Ceftaroline: a cephalosporin with expanded gram-positive activity. Future Microbiol 2009;4:25–33.
59. Rajendran PM, Young D, Maurer T, et al. Randomized, double-blind, placebo-controlled trial of cephalexin for treatment of uncomplicated skin abscesses in a population at risk for community-acquired methicillin-resistant Staphylococcus aureus infection. Antimicrobial Agents Chemother 2007;51: 4044–8.
60. Duong M, Markwell S, Peter J, et al. Randomized, controlled trial of antibiotics in the management of community-acquired skin abscesses in the pediatric patient. Ann Emerg Med 2010;55:401–7.
61. Schmitz GR, Bruner D, Pitotti R, et al. Randomized controlled trial of trimethoprim-sulfamethoxazole for uncomplicated skin abscesses in patients at risk for community-associated methicillin-resistant Staphylococcus aureus infection. Ann Emerg Med 2010,56:283–7.
62. Van Rijen M, Bonten M, Wenzel R, et al. Mupirocin ointment for preventing Staphylococcus aureus infections in nasal carriers. Cochrane Database Syst Rev 2008;(4):CD006216.
63. Loeb MB, Main C, Eady A, et al. Antimicrobial drugs for treating methicillin-resistant Staphylococcus aureus colonization. Cochrane Database Syst Rev 2003;(4):CD003340.
64. Laupland KB, Conly JM. Treatment of Staphylococcus aureus colonization and prophylaxis for infection with topical intranasal mupirocin: an evidenced-based review. Clin Infect Dis 2003;37(7):933–8.
65. Raz R, Miron D, Colonder R, et al. A 1-year trial of nasal mupirocin in the prevention of recurrent staphylococcal nasal colonization and skin infection. Arch Intern Med 1996;156(10):1109–12.
66. Miro JM, Anguera I, Cabell CH, et al. Staphylococcus aureus native valve infective endocarditis: report of 566 episodes from the International Collaboration on Endocarditis Merged Database. Clin Infect Dis 2005;41:507–14.
67. Fowler VG Jr, Miro JM, Hoen B, et al. Staphylococcus aureus endocarditis: a consequence of medical progress. J Am Med Assoc 2005;293:3012–21.
68. Fowler VG Jr, Olsen MK, Corey GR, et al. Clinical identifiers of complicated Staphylococcus aureus bacteremia. Arch Intern Med 2003;163:2066–72.
69. Mermel LA, Farr BM, Sherertz RJ, et al. Guidelines for the management of intra-vascular catheter–related infections. Clin Infect Dis 2001;32:1249–72.
70. Levine DP, Fromm BS, Reddy BR. Slow response to vancomycin or vancomycin plus rifampin in methicillin-resistant Staphylococcus aureus endocarditis. Ann Intern Med 1991;115:674–80.
71. Riedel DJ, Weekes E, Forrest GN. Addition of rifampin to standard therapy for treatment of native valve infective endocarditis caused by Staphylococcus aureus. Antimicrobial Agents Chemother 2008;52:2463–7.

72. Korzeniowski O, Sande MA. Combination antimicrobial therapy for Staphylococcus aureus endocarditis in patients addicted to parenteral drugs and in nonaddicts: a prospective study. Ann Intern Med 1982;97:496–503.

73. Baddour LM, Wilson WR, Bayer AS, et al. Infective endocarditis: diagnosis, antimicrobial therapy, and management of complications: a statement for healthcare professionals from the Committee on Rheumatic Fever, Endocarditis, and Kawasaki Disease, Council on Cardiovascular Disease in the Young, and the Councils on Clinical Cardiology, Stroke, and Cardiovascular Surgery and Anesthesia, American Heart Association: endorsed by the Infectious Diseases Society of America. Circulation 2005;111:e394–434.

74. Cosgrove SA, Fowler VG Jr. Management of methicillin-resistant Staphylococcus aureus bacteremia. Clin Infect Dis 2008;46(S5):S386–93.

75. Jung YJ, Koh Y, Hong SB, et al. Effect of vancomycin plus rifampin in the treatment of nosocomial methicillin-resistant Staphylococcus aureus pneumonia. Crit Care Med 2010;38:175–80.

76. Wunderink RG, Cammarata SK, Oliphant TH, et al. Continuation of a randomized, double-blind, multicenter study of linezolid versus vancomycin in the treatment of patients with nosocomial pneumonia. Clin Ther 2003;25:980–2.

77. Rubinstein E, Cammarata SK, Oliphant TH, et al. Linezolid (PNU-100766) versus vancomycin in the treatment of hospitalized patients with nosocomial pneumonia: a randomized, double-blind, multicenter study. Clin Infect Dis 2001;32:402–12.

78. Wunderink RG, Rello J, Cammarata SK, et al. Linezolid vs vancomycin: analysis of two double-blind studies of patients with methicillin-resistant Staphylococcus aureus nosocomial pneumonia. Chest 2003;124:1789–97.

79. Zimmerli W, Widmer AF, Blatter M, et al. Role of rifampin for treatment of orthopedic implant-related staphylococcal infections: a randomized controlled trial. Foreign-Body Infection (FBI) Study Group. J Am Med Assoc 1998;279:1537–41.

80. Gemmel CG, Edwards DI, Fraise AP, et al. Guidelines for the prophylaxis and treatment of methicillin-resistant Staphylococcus aureus (MRSA) infections in the UK. J Antimicrob Chemother 2006;57:589–608.

Community-Acquired Pneumonia in Adults and Children

Esther Dan-Phuong Ho, MD

KEYWORDS

- Community-acquired pneumonia • Respiratory infection • Lung imaging
- Antimicrobial treatment

KEY POINTS

- Community-acquired pneumonia in adults and children is common.
- The cause of pneumonia often depends on the patient's age, although the exact microorganism is rarely identified.
- Pneumonia is diagnosed by clinical features, along with lung imaging.
- Lung imaging and other diagnostic testing in the appropriate clinical setting may help with informed decision-making, focused antimicrobial treatment and fewer unnecessary tests.
- Treatment of the pneumonia depends on the likely cause and is based on the patient's age.
- Pneumonia can be prevented with appropriate vaccinations and smoking cessation.

INTRODUCTION: NATURE OF THE PROBLEM

Pneumonia is a common lower respiratory tract infection affecting all ages, with significant morbidity and mortality especially among the extremes of age and those with comorbid conditions.

Definitions of pneumonia can vary depending on the organization, institution, or heath care setting.

Some examples of definitions include

- Community-acquired pneumonia (CAP), the primary focus of this article, is broadly defined as an alveolar infection developing in the outpatient setting or within 48 hours of hospitalization, whereas health care-associated pneumonia is associated with recent or current hospitalization of greater than 48 hours, or exposure to long-term care or skilled nursing facility.
- Pneumonia can also be classified as typical (eg, caused by *Streptococcus pneumonia*), or atypical (eg, caused by *Mycoplasma pneumoniae* or *Chlamydophila*

Disclosures: No funding sources or conflicts of interest to disclose.
Hospitalist Program, Department of Family Medicine, University of California, Irvine, 101 The City Drive South, Orange, CA 92868, USA
E-mail address: danphuoh@uci.edu

Prim Care Clin Office Pract 40 (2013) 655–669
http://dx.doi.org/10.1016/j.pop.2013.05.004
0095-4543/13/$ – see front matter © 2013 Elsevier Inc. All rights reserved.

pneumonia), although it is often difficult to distinguish between typical and atypical pneumonia.

The clinical spectrum of pneumonia varies from a mild outpatient illness that resolves rapidly, to severe sepsis with multiorgan failure and death. The burden of disease is as follows:

- Globally: Pneumonia is the leading cause of death in children, killing over 1.5 million children under the age of 5.[1]
- Nationally:
  - The annual incidence of CAP in the United States (US) is estimated at 5 to 11 per 1000 population, although in children younger than the age of 5, the estimated incidence is 30 to 45 cases per 1000 children, a rate that is unparalleled to any other time of life, except perhaps in those older than 75 years of age.[1]
  - In the US in 2009, 1.1 million people were hospitalized for pneumonia and more than 50,000 people died from the infection.[1]
  - Along with influenza, pneumonia is the eighth leading cause of death in the US; broken down by extremes of age, it is the sixth leading cause of death in the US for children 1 to 4 years of age and the seventh leading cause of death in persons greater than 65 years old.[2]
  - The estimated yearly economic burden of CAP in adults in the US exceeds $17 billion, with the estimated direct cost of a single hospitalization for CAP ranging from $3000 to $13,000.[3]

PATIENT HISTORY
Causes

Although the most common organism causing CAP in all patient populations is *S pneumoniae*, the causes of pneumonia can be hard to determine precisely because the lung is rarely sampled directly and obtaining adequate sputum cultures is often impractical and difficult, especially in infants and children. History taking should be directed to detecting symptoms as well as the following characteristics that may help narrow the list of likely causes:

- The patient's age (**Table 1**)
- The time of year (eg, influenza, respiratory syncytial virus)
- Comorbidities and social habits (eg, *Haemophilus influenzae* for smokers and those with COPD)
- Exposure history (eg, tuberculosis)
- Travel history (eg, *Legionella*)
- Animal exposure (eg, psittacosis)
- Geography (eg, coccidioidomycosis).

Presentation

Patients with pneumonia usually present with acute signs and symptoms of 1 to 2 days duration. For those with an intact immune response, common systemic and respiratory symptoms include[8]

- Cough
- Dyspnea (sensitivity of 70%)
- Fever and/or chills (sensitivity of 50%–85%)
- Pleuritic chest pain
- Purulent sputum (sensitivity of 50%).

Table 1		
Common causes of CAP by age		
Age	Pneumonia Severity	Organism (in order of frequency)

0–2 mo	Moderate to severe	Group B streptococcus
		Gram-negative enteric:
		    E coli, Klebsiella pneumoniae
		    Hib
		    S pyogenes, S aureus
		    Listeria monocytogenes

1–3 mo	Afebrile pneumonitis	*Chlamydia trachomatis, Cytomegalovirus* RSV, other respiratory viruses *Bordetella pertussis*
1–24 mo	Moderate to severe, febrile	RSV, other respiratory viruses *S pneumoniae*, Hib, *S aureus*, NTHi *C trachomatis, M pneumonia* *Mycobacterium tuberculosis*
2–5 y	Mild to moderate	Respiratory viruses *S pneumoniae* Hib, NTHi *M pneumoniae, C pneumoniae* *M tuberculosis*
6–18 y	Mild to moderate	*M pneumoniae* *S pneumoniae* *C pneumoniae* NTHi, influenza A or B, adenoviruses, other respiratory viruses *M tuberculosis*
Adults	Mild to moderate	*S pneumoniae* *M pneumoniae* *H influenzae* *C pneumoniae* Influenza A or B Adenoviruses, RSV, Parainfluenza For hospitalized patients: as above, then *Legionella* Aspiration organisms
All ages	Severe (requiring aggressive support in ICU), with empyema or cavitation	Most common: *S pneumoniae, S aureus* After the most common, in children: *S pyogenes*, Hib, *M pneumoniae* Adenoviruses After the most common, in adults: Legionella species, gram-negative bacilli Hib

Abbreviations: Hib, *H influenza* type b; NTHi, nontypeable *H influenzae*; RSV, respiratory syncytial virus.

Data from Refs.[4–7]

Hemoptysis can suggest a necrotizing infection, but is also a common finding in other respiratory illnesses such as bronchitis. For patients with an impaired immune response, such as the elderly, the clinical presentation often involves nonrespiratory and more subtle findings, including functional decline and confusion.[8]

PHYSICAL EXAMINATION

The diagnosis of pneumonia is based primarily on the clinical assessment. The respiratory rate (RR) can be a sensitive indicator of lower respiratory tract involvement in pediatric and elderly patients, with tachypnea occurring in up to 70% of those older than 65 years.[9,10] Along with the RR, the physical examination of the lungs is a useful supplemental tool to detect pathologic conditions of the lung. Pulse oximetry screening should be performed in all adults with suspected pneumonia and in children with pneumonia with suspected hypoxemia.[4,11]

The following are signs of respiratory distress and are more commonly found in the extremes of age (eg, young children and the elderly) with more severe pneumonia[11]:

- Tachypnea
- Dyspnea
- Retractions (suprasternal, intercostal, or subcostal)
- Grunting
- Nasal flaring
- Apnea
- Altered mental status (AMS)
- Pulse oximetry measuring <90% on room air (**Table 2**).

Table 2
Possible physical examination findings (with comparison to pneumothorax)

	Inspection	Palpation	Percussion	Auscultation
Consolidation	Tachypnea Cyanosis Nasal flaring Respiratory splinting	Increased fremitus (decreased with effusion or empyema)	Dullness	Crackles, Rhonchi Egophony Whispered pectoriloquy
Pleural Effusion	Decreased movement on affected side	Decreased movement Decreased fremitus	Dullness	Decreased breath sounds Whispered pectoriloquy
Pneumothorax	Tachypnea Respiratory distress Cyanosis Tracheal deviation	Decreased fremitus	Hyperresonance	Decreased breath sounds Decreased bronchophony

Data from Bates B. The thorax and lungs. In: Bates B, Bickley LS, Hoekelman RA, et al. A guide to physical examination and history taking. 6th edition. Philadelphia: Lippincott; 1995. p. 256–7.

IMAGING AND ADDITIONAL TESTING

According to the Infectious Diseases Society of America (IDSA)/American Thoracic Society (ATS) guidelines, a demonstrable infiltrate by chest radiograph or other imaging technique is required for the diagnosis of pneumonia in adults, in addition to a constellation of suggestive clinical features.[4] Adults with acute respiratory illnesses who may benefit from a chest radiograph include[12]

- Patients with any of the following vital signs
  - Temperature >100°F (37.8°C)
  - Heart rate >100 beats/min
  - RR >20 breaths/min

- Patients with at least two of the following clinical findings
  - Decreased breath sounds
  - Crackles or rales
  - Absence of asthma.

In contrast, the Pediatric Infectious Diseases Society (PIDS)/IDSA guidelines do not recommend chest radiographs routinely for children treated in the outpatient setting. Chest radiographs are recommended for children in the following situations[11]:

- Suspected or documented hypoxemia or significant respiratory distress
- Failed initial antibiotic treatment
- Hospitalization for the management of pneumonia.

Radiographic findings can establish the diagnosis of pneumonia and distinguish it from other respiratory illnesses, such as bronchitis or viral illness, in the appropriate clinical setting and, therefore, minimize the use of inappropriate antibiotics. Radiographs may also help identify the severity of illness and aid point-of-care decisions, including identifying pleural effusions and cavitations that are likely to be bacterial in origin, requiring antibiotics and possibly further treatment. Limitations of radiographs include false-negative results in patients who are substantially volume-depleted and that a great degree of overlap exists between characteristics traditionally thought to distinguish between viral and bacterial pneumonias, or typical and atypical pneumonias.

The accurate and rapid diagnosis of the microorganism responsible for CAP provides for the best patient care with informed decision-making, focused antimicrobial treatment, and fewer unnecessary tests. Unfortunately, there are no single diagnostic tests in the diagnosis of CAP that can be considered the reference standard. Depending on the clinical situation, some diagnostic tests can help supplement the most accurate diagnosis of CAP (**Table 3**).

Acute-Phase Reactants

In recent years, the biomarker procalcitonin (PCT) has been studied to help guide antibiotic use in infections including pneumonia. PCT is released by multiple tissues within 6 to 12 hours in response to bacterial infections under stimulation from cytokines, is more specific than C reactive protein or the white blood cell count, has higher levels with more severe infections, and has a half-life of 24 hours so that the concentration normalizes fairly quickly with the patient's recovery.[13] Because of this, PCT can be used to help guide antibiotic use in the following scenarios in the emergency department (ED) and hospital settings[14]:

- A PCT level <0.25 mcg/L is thought safe to exclude bacterial infection and withhold antibiotics in patients who do not appear significantly ill
- Patients with PCT levels >0.25 mcg/L should be assumed to have bacterial pneumonia and treated with antibiotics
- For severely ill patients who have improved significantly, a decrease in PCT by 90% of its initial value or to <0.5 mcg/L provides reassurance that antibiotic treatment can be stopped safely.

Limitations of PCT include[14]

- Falsely low levels have been found in patients with empyema and parapneumonic effusions
- Falsely positive levels have been found in some cardiac surgery patients and in patients with nonseptic shock
- PCT is not widely available in US hospitals.

Table 3
Clinical indications in adults and children for further diagnostic tests according to IDSA/ATS and PIDS/IDSA guidelines

	Indications for Testing	
Diagnostic Test	In Adults	In Children
Sputum Gram stain & culture	• Hospitalized patients who can provide a good-quality specimen, especially those a. In ICU (an endotracheal aspirate sample for the intubated) b. With cavitary infiltrates c. With active alcohol abuse d. With severe obstructive or structural lung disease e. With asplenia f. With pleural effusion g. With positive *Legionella* or pneumococcal UAT • Those that fail outpatient antibiotic treatment	• Hospitalized children who can produce an adequate specimen • Those who fail outpatient treatment who can produce an adequate specimen
BC	• Optional for all hospitalized patients • Should be performed in the following patients: a. With severe CAP (eg, in ICU) b. With cavitary infiltrates, leukopenia, positive pneumococcal UAT, or pleural effusion c. With chronic severe liver disease, severe obstructive or structural lung disease, asplenia, or active alcoholism	Outpatient: fails to improve clinically or have progressive symptoms after antibiotics are initiated Inpatient: has moderate-severe CAP
Repeat BC	Not addressed	Positive bacteremia caused by *S aureus*
Pneumococcal UAT	• In ICU • Failed outpatient antibiotic treatment • Has leukopenia • Active alcohol abuse • Chronic severe liver disease • Asplenia • Pleural effusion	Not recommended for the diagnosis of pneumococcal pneumonia in children (false positives common)
Legionella UAT	• In ICU • Fail outpatient antibiotic treatment • Active alcohol abuse • Recent travel within 2 wk • Pleural effusion	Not addressed or not applicable
Testing for viral pathogens	Optional	Sensitive & specific tests for rapid diagnosis of influenza & other respiratory viruses recommended in the evaluation of children with CAP

(continued on next page)

Table 3 (continued)		
	Indications for Testing	
Diagnostic Test	**In Adults**	**In Children**
Testing for atypical organisms	Not recommended	Children with signs & symptoms suspicious for *M pneumoniae* should be tested to guide antibiotic selection Diagnostic testing for *C pneumoniae* is not recommended (reliable testing not available)
Fungal & tuberculosis cultures	Cavitary lesions	Not addressed
Acute-phase reactants	Not addressed	ESR, CRP or procalcitonin can be used in conjunction with clinical findings in severe CAP to assess response to treatment

Abbreviations: BC, blood cultures; UAT, urine antigen test.

Data from Mandell LA, Wunderink RG, Anzueto A, et al. IDSA/ATS consensus guidelines on the management of community-acquired pneumonia in adults. Clin Infect Dis 2007;44(2):S27–72; and Bradley JS, Byington CL, Shah SS, et al. The management of community-acquired pneumonia in infants and children older than 3 months of age: clinical practice guidelines by the Pediatric Infectious Diseases Society and the Infectious Diseases Society of America. Clin Infect Dis 2011;53(7):e25–76.

MANAGEMENT
Site-of-Care

The initial management of pneumonia requires assessing the severity of the illness to determine whether the patient needs to be hospitalized because this can have an impact on mortality. The most widely used validated prediction scoring systems in adults include the PSI (Pneumonia Severity Index) and the CURB (Confusion, Uremia, Respiratory rate, Blood pressure)-65 score. These objective scores can help identify patients who are appropriate for outpatient care, but should not supersede the physician's assessment of additional factors, including the ability to adhere to the treatment plan and the availability of outpatient resources.

The PSI assigns points based on 20 factors in five categories including demographic characteristics, comorbid conditions, physical examination findings, laboratory measurements, and radiographic findings. It then stratifies them into five classes of risk (**Table 4**).[15]

The CURB-65 score gives one point for each of the following factors, with a score of two or greater warranting admission[16]:

- Confusion
- Uremia (serum urea nitrogen [BUN]>20)
- Respiration ≥30
- Blood pressure <90 or ≤60
- >65 years of age (**Table 5**).

There are currently no validated scoring systems to predict which children with pneumonia should be hospitalized. In pediatric patients, the following are indications for hospitalization[11]:

- Infants and children who have moderate to severe CAP
- Infants and children with suspected or documented CAP caused by a pathogen with increased virulence, most notably community-associated methicillin-resistant *Staphylococcus aureus* (CA-MRSA)

Table 4
Mortality risk according to PSI score

Risk Class	Points	Mortality (%)	Recommended Site-of-Care
I	No predictors	0.1	Outpatient
II	≤70	0.6	Outpatient
III	71–90	2.8	Clinical judgment re: inpatient vs outpatient
IV	91–130	8.2	Inpatient
V	>130	29.2	Inpatient

- Infants and children for whom there is concern of inability to comply with treatment at home.

Hospitalization is likely to benefit infants younger than 3 to 6 months of age with suspected bacterial CAP. In the United States, infants younger than 3 months are usually admitted to the hospital for initial management.

Admission to ICU

Pediatric and adult patients with septic shock requiring vasopressors or with acute respiratory failure requiring intubation and mechanical ventilation should be admitted to the ICU.[4,11] Adult patients should also be considered for admission to an ICU bed if they meet three or more of the following criteria[4]:

- RR >30/min
- Pao_2 or Fio_2 ratio <250
- Multilobar infiltrates
- Confusion or AMS
- Uremia (BUN>20)
- Leukopenia (white blood cell <4k)
- Thrombocytopenia (platelets<100k)
- Hypothermia (temperature<36°C)
- Hypotension requiring aggressive intravenous fluids resuscitation.

Children should be admitted to an ICU or a unit with continuous cardiorespiratory monitoring in the following situations[11]:

- Requires use of noninvasive positive pressure ventilation
- Has impending respiratory failure
- Has sustained tachycardia or hypotension
- Has a pulse oximetry measurement <92% with inspired oxygen of ≥0.50
- Has AMS due to hypercarbia or hypoxemia.

Table 5
PSI versus CURB-65: advantages & disadvantages

	PSI	CURB-65
Advantages	Most extensively validated prediction score Identifies patients with a low mortality risk	Simple scoring system
Disadvantages	Complex Underestimates severely ill younger patients without comorbid illnesses	Does not specifically account for comorbid conditions

Pharmacologic Treatment Options

Given that the exact organism causing the infection cannot rapidly be determined and, in fact, is often not identified, treatment of CAP is usually empiric and based on the likely cause as well as the clinical setting (outpatient vs inpatient). For children in the outpatient setting[11]

- Because viral causes are the most likely cause of CAP in preschool aged children, antimicrobial therapy is not routinely required in this age group
- Amoxicillin is the first-line outpatient treatment of immunocompetent infants older than 3 months and preschool children with CAP of suspected bacterial origin because it is safe and effective
- For children older than 5 years with presumed bacterial pneumonia, amoxicillin remains the first-line outpatient treatment, with azithromycin added if atypical CAP is suspected.

In adults, the antibiotics of choice include atypical coverage (**Table 6**).

Duration of Treatment

The standard treatment duration for pneumonia is 7 to 10 days, although with shorter treatment courses have been shown to be effective in both adults and children, especially those with mild pneumonia.[11,18]

In a meta-analysis, the following antibiotics demonstrated equal effectiveness with no difference in outcomes in adults[18]:

- Oral or intravenous azithromycin $\times$ 3–5 days
- Levofloxacin $\times$ 5 days
- Cefuroxime $\times$ 7 days
- Intravenous ceftriaxone $\times$ 5 days.

The IDSA/ATS recommends antibiotic treatment for a minimum of 5 days with patients afebrile for 48 to 72 hours, and one or less sign of clinical instability. The following are criteria for clinical stability[4]:

- Temperature $\leq 37.8°C$
- Heart rate ≤ 100 beats per minute
- RR ≤ 24 breaths/min
- Systolic blood pressure ≥ 90 mm Hg
- O_2 saturation $\geq 90\%$ or Po_2 ≥ 60 mm Hg on room air
- Ability to maintain oral intake
- Normal mental status.

On the other hand, patients who have complications from pneumonia, such as empyema or septicemia with positive blood cultures, will require longer courses of antibiotic therapy ranging from 2 to 4 weeks.

Other Treatment Considerations

Time to first antibiotic dose

Two retrospective studies for Medicare patients with pneumonia demonstrated statistically lower mortality among patients who received early antibiotic treatment.[19,20] Although no prospective trials have produced similar results, a delay in antibiotic treatment can have adverse effects in many infections, especially for sicker patients, thus[4]

- Treatment should be administered as soon as possible after CAP diagnosis is considered likely

Table 6
Empiric therapy for bacterial CAP

	Presumed Bacterial CAP	Presumed Atypical CAP	Presumed Influenza CAP
Outpatient			
3 mo to 5 y old	Amoxicillin 90 mg/kg/d po bid Alternative: amoxicillin or clavulanate 90 mg/kg/d po bid	Azithromycin 10 mg/kg PO on day 1, followed by 5 mg/kg po daily on days 2–5 Alternatives: clarithromycin 15 mg/kg po bid for 7–14 d or erythromycin 40 mg/kg/d po in 4 doses	Oseltamivir
Children >5 y old	As above for children with presumed bacterial CAP who do not have evidence distinguishing bacterial CAP from atypical CAP Maximum dose: amoxicillin 4 g/d	As above, with maximum dose of Azithromycin 500 mg on day 1, and 250 mg on days 2–5 Alternatives: maximum dose clarithromycin 1 g/d or doxycycline for children >7 y old	Oseltamivir or zanamivir (for children >7 y old) Alternative: peramivir
Adults	Previously healthy & no antibiotics >3 mo: macrolide or doxycycline Comorbidities or use of antibiotics within 3 mo: respiratory fluoroquinolone, or β-lactam plus macrolide Consider above in regions with >25% macrolide-resistant *S pneumonia*	Coverage included in presumed bacterial CAP	Oseltamivir Alternative: zanamivir
Inpatient			
0–20 d	Ampicillin and gentamicin or cefotaxime For suspected CA-MRSA: addition of vancomycin	—	
1–3 mo old	Cefotaxime For suspected CA-MRSA: addition of vancomycin	—	

Children >3 mo old fully immunized with conjugate vaccines for Hib and S pneumoniae And Minimal local PCN resistance in invasive strains of pneumococcus	Ampicillin or PCN G Alternatives: ceftriaxone or cefotaxime For suspected CA-MRSA: addition of vancomycin or clindamycin	Azithromycin (in addition to β-lactam if bacterial origin still of concern) Alternatives: clarithromycin or erythromycin; doxycycline for children >7 y old; levofloxacin for children who have reached growth maturity or who cannot tolerate macrolides	Oseltamivir or zanamivir (for children >7 y old) Alternative: peramivir
Children >3 mo old not fully immunized with conjugate vaccines for Hib and S pneumoniae And/or Significant local PCN resistance in invasive strains of pneumococcus	Ceftriaxone or Cefotaxime Alternative: levofloxacin[a] For suspected CA-MRSA: addition of vancomycin or clindamycin	As above	As above
Adults	Non-ICU: respiratory fluoroquinolone, or β-lactam plus either macrolide (or doxycycline) ICU: β-lactam plus either azithromycin or respiratory fluoroquinolone PCN allergic: respiratory fluoroquinolone plus aztreonam For suspected Pseudomonas: antipneumococcal antipseudomonal β-lactam plus ciprofloxacin or levofloxacin (750 mg), or above β-lactam plus aminoglycoside plus azithromycin, or above β-lactam plus aminoglycoside plus antipneumococcal fluoroquinolone PCN allergic: substitute β-lactam with aztreonam For suspected CA-MRSA: add vancomycin or linezolid	Coverage included in presumed bacterial CAP	Oseltamivir Alternative: zanamavir

Abbreviations: Hib, *H influenza* type b; PCN, penicillin.

[a] PIDS/IDSA guidelines do not address in detail the controversy of using quinolones in children; its use in infants and children is considered a risk versus benefit decision.

Data from Refs.[4,5,11,17]

- For patients admitted through ED, the first dose should be administered while still in ED
- For patients sick enough to require hospitalization, give oral or intramuscular antibiotic in the clinic before direct admission.

Switching from intravenous to oral therapy

Factors to consider when switching from intravenous to oral therapy include the following:

- When possible, parenteral therapy should be converted to oral outpatient step-down treatment[4,11]
- In general, stay with same agent or drug class[4,11]
- If parental antibiotic treatment is indicated, it should be offered through a skilled nursing home program or at an appropriate outpatient facility able to provide daily intramuscular injections
- Skilled home health programs providing antibiotics through a peripherally inserted central catheter are more often used and preferable to daily intramuscular shots because of ease of use and comfort for patients.

Indications for discharge

Patients who have been hospitalized for pneumonia can be considered for discharge when the following criteria are met[4,11]:

- Overall clinical improvement (decreased fever for at least 12 to 24 hours, adequate level of activity and appetite)
- Pulse oximetry greater than 90% on room air for at least 12 to 24 hours
- Stable or baseline mental status
- No increased work of breathing or sustained tachypnea or tachycardia
- Can tolerate home antiinfective regimen
- Patients (including parents and infant or child) are able to comply with administering and taking antibiotics
- Chest tube has been removed for 12 to 24 hours without deterioration
- Issues of barriers to care are identified and addressed.

Complications or Treatment Resistance

Pulmonary complications associated with CAP include the following[11]:

- Pleural effusion or empyema
- Pneumothorax
- Lung abscess
- Bronchopleural fistula
- Necrotizing pneumonia
- Acute respiratory failure.

Systemic complications include sepsis with systemic inflammatory response syndrome and, in children, hemolytic uremic syndrome. The respiratory infection can also become metastatic, leading to other infections including meningitis, pericarditis, endocarditis, osteomyelitis, septic arthritis, or a central nervous system abscess.[11]

For patients with severe pneumonia, the IDSA/ATS guidelines recommend the following[4]:

- Screen for adrenal insufficiency in hypotensive fluid-resuscitated severe CAP cases
- Cautiously trial noninvasive ventilation for hypoxemia or respiratory distress (unless immediate intubation is required)
- Use low tidal volume ventilation for diffuse bilateral pneumonia or acute respiratory distress syndrome.

To determine if further support and higher levels of care are indicated, patients who do not respond to treatment after 48 to 72 hours should be reassessed with clinical, laboratory, and imaging evaluations and further investigation to identify if the original pathogen persists or has developed resistance, or if there is new secondary infecting agent. Management of nonresponders includes[4]

- A systemic approach to causes of failure to respond
- Consideration of
  - o Other microbiological procedures
  - o Chest CT
  - o Thoracentesis
  - o Bronchoscopy with bronchoalveolar lavage and transbronchial biopsies
  - o Broadening antibiotic regimen.

Prevention or Long-Term Recommendations

CAP can often be prevented with appropriate vaccinations. Vaccinations are ideally given in the outpatient setting but hospital admission is an important trigger for reassessing and administering vaccinations to those who have not received the appropriate immunizations.

Children and their caregivers should receive the following vaccinations per Advisory Committee on Immunization Practices (ACIP) guidelines[11]:

- Vaccines for *S pneumoniae*, *H influenzae* type b (Hib), and pertussis
- Influenza vaccine annually for children 6 months and older
- Palivizumab (Synagis) for high-risk infants including otherwise healthy premature infants, and in those with comorbid conditions such as chronic lung disease of prematurity, congenital abnormalities of the airway, and neuromuscular disease.

Adults should receive the inactivated influenza vaccine annually and the pneumococcal vaccination as per ACIP guidelines. An alternative to the inactivated influenza vaccine for healthy adults and children (ages 5–49) is the intranasal live attenuated vaccine.[4]

Smoking is associated with a significant risk of invasive pneumococcal disease in immunocompetent nonelderly patients.[21] Smoking cessation should be emphasized and encouraged.

SUMMARY

CAP in adults and children is common. The cause of pneumonia often depends on the patient's age, although the exact microorganism is rarely identified. Pneumonia is diagnosed by clinical features, along with chest imaging. Lung imaging and other diagnostic testing in the appropriate clinical setting may help with informed decision-making, including site-of-care decisions, focused antimicrobial treatment, and fewer unnecessary tests. Treatment of the pneumonia depends on the likely cause and is based on the patient's age. Pneumonia can be prevented with appropriate vaccinations and smoking cessation.

REFERENCES

1. Centers for Disease Control and Prevention. Pneumonia can be prevented—vaccines can help. Available at: http://www.cdc.gov/features/pneumonia. Accessed February 5, 2013.
2. US Department of Health and Human Services. Health, United States 2011, with special feature on socioeconomic status and health. Available at: http://www.cdc.gov/nchs/data/hus/hus11.pdf. Accessed February 5, 2013.
3. File TM Jr, Marrie TJ. Burden of community-acquired pneumonia in North American adults. Postgrad Med 2010;122(2):130–41.
4. Mandell LA, Wunderink RG, Anzueto A, et al. IDSA/ATS consensus guidelines on the management of community-acquired pneumonia in adults. Clin Infect Dis 2007;44(2):S27–72.
5. McIntosh K. Community-acquired pneumonia in children. N Engl J Med 2002; 346:429–37.
6. Juven T, Mertsola J, Waris M, et al. Etiology of community-acquired pneumonia in 254 hospitalized children. Pediatr Infect Dis J 2000;19:293–8.
7. Gaston B. Pneumonia. Pediatr Rev 2002;23:132–40.
8. Nair GB, Niederman MS. Community-acquired pneumonia: an unfinished battle. Med Clin North Am 2011;95:1143–61.
9. Shann F, Hart K, Thomas D. Acute respiratory infections in children: possible criteria for selection of patients for antibiotic therapy and hospital admission. Bull World Health Organ 1984;62:749–53.
10. Metlay JP, Schulz R, Li YH, et al. Influence of age on symptoms at presentation in patients with community-acquired pneumonia. Arch Intern Med 1997;157(13): 1453–9.
11. Bradley JS, Byington CL, Shah SS, et al. The management of community-acquired pneumonia in infants and children older than 3 months of age: clinical practice guidelines by the Pediatric Infectious Diseases Society and the Infectious Diseases Society of America. Clin Infect Dis 2011;53(7):e25–76.
12. Ebell MH. Predicting pneumonia in adults with respiratory illness. Am Fam Physician 2007;76(4):562.
13. Schneider HG, Lam QT. Procalcitonin for the clinical laboratory: a review. Pathology 2007;39:383–90.
14. Schuetz P, Amin DN, Greenwald JL. Role of procalcitonin in managing adult patients with respiratory tract infections. Chest 2012;141:1063–73.
15. Fine MJ, Auble TE, Yealy DM, et al. A prediction rule to identify low-risk patients with community-acquired pneumonia. N Engl J Med 1997;336(4):243–50.
16. Lim WS, van der Eerden MM, Laing R, et al. Defining community acquired pneumonia severity on presentation to hospital: an international derivation and validation study. Thorax 2003;58(5):377–82.
17. Centers for Disease Control and Prevention. Antiviral agents for influenza. Available at: http://www.cdc.gov/flu/professionals/antivirals/antiviral-agents-flu.htm. Accessed February 27, 2013.
18. Li JZ, Winston LG, Moore DH, et al. Efficacy of short-course antibiotic regimens for community-acquired pneumonia: a meta-analysis. Am J Med 2007;120:783–90.

19. Houck PM, Bratzler DW, Nsa W, et al. Timing of antibiotic administration and outcomes for Medicare patients hospitalized with community-acquired pneumonia. Arch Intern Med 2004;164:637–44.

20. Meehan TP, Fine MJ, Krumholz HM, et al. Quality of care, process, and outcomes in elderly patients with pneumonia. JAMA 1997;278:2080–4.

21. Nuorti JP, Butler JC, Farley MM, et al. Cigarette smoking and invasive pneumococcal disease. Active Bacterial Core Surveillance team. N Engl J Med 2000; 342:681–9.

Ear Infections
Otitis Externa and Otitis Media

Hobart Lee, MD*, Jeffrey Kim, MD, Van Nguyen, DO

KEYWORDS

- Otitis externa • Otitis media • Diagnosis • Treatment

KEY POINTS

- Otitis externa is an outer ear infection with high morbidity and potential complications, diagnosed by clinical symptoms including ear pain exacerbated by manipulation of the outer ear and discharge.
- The preferred treatment for otitis externa is topical antibiotics, with or without antiseptics or steroids.
- Otitis media is diagnosed by moderate to severe bulging tympanic membrane or ear pain and mild bulging, or intensely erythematous tympanic membrane.
- The preferred treatment for otitis media is high-dose amoxicillin. Patients younger than 2 years should be treated for 10 days; those 2 to 5 years old for 7 days; and those 6 years and older for 5 to 7 days.

INTRODUCTION

The purpose of this article is to review the current available material pertaining to acute otitis externa (AOE) and acute otitis media (AOM), including the development, presentation, and treatment of both disease processes. The correct differentiation between AOE and AOM is crucial because of the difference in the evaluation and treatment of these disorders. The proper diagnosis of these ear infections can decrease the risk of complications including mastoiditis, hearing loss, chondritis, parotiditis, and necrotizing otitis externa.[1]

OTITIS EXTERNA
Background

AOE is characterized by marked inflammation of the external auditory canal, with or without infection. It is sometimes referred to as external otitis or swimmer's ear, and

Funding Sources: None.
Conflict of Interest: None.
Department of Family Medicine, Loma Linda University, 25455 Barton Road, Suite 209B, Loma Linda, CA 92354, USA
* Corresponding author.
E-mail address: holee@llu.edu

Prim Care Clin Office Pract 40 (2013) 671–686
http://dx.doi.org/10.1016/j.pop.2013.05.005
0095-4543/13/$ – see front matter © 2013 Elsevier Inc. All rights reserved.

is commonly caused by an acute bacterial infection. Patients may report extreme (out of proportion) pain, pruritus, discharge, and decreased hearing acuity.

Although rarely a serious condition, AOE is a disease of high morbidity. Dating back to World War II, its severe otalgia has disabled men, women, and children.[2] The annual incidence is 1.3% for females and 1.2% for males, with a peak period in children 7 to 12 years old and again in adults 65 to 74 years old.[1,3,4] In the pediatric population, AOE is rare in children younger than 2 years.[5] In older children aged 5 to 19 years, however, there is a noted increase in incidence, particularly at the end of the summer.[3] It is thought that the intense heat and/or humidity of the summer months predisposes to AOE.[6]

Pathophysiology

Anatomy

Infection of the external auditory canal (EAC) is complicated by the unique anatomy of the EAC, which is approximately 2.5 cm long and 7 to 9 mm wide.[7] Its narrow and torturous anatomy perpetuates debris accumulation created during an infection. It is hypothesized that it is this limited space for expansion of inflamed tissue that perpetuates the pain and itching associated with AOE.[8]

The membranous lateral one-third of the canal is cartilaginous, containing apocrine and sebaceous glands, and hair follicles. The bony medial two-thirds of the external canal are densely filled with nerves and do not contain subcutaneous tissue; it is only covered with skin. The dermis is in direct contact with the periosteum and tympanic membrane. The narrowest portion of the EAC is the junction between the membranous and bony portions of the canal. This junction creates a potential pathway for spread of infection beyond the ear itself.[9]

Cerumen, made by the apocrine glands and epithelial sloughing, is propelled through the canal via a centrifugal migratory process, in a medial to lateral direction. The hydrophobic nature of the cerumen creates a protective layer on the canal to reduce maceration.[9] Moreover, cerumen's naturally acidic nature (pH 6.0–6.5) inhibits bacterial growth. Most bacteria, specifically those implicated in AOE, are ideally sustained at a pH of 8 to 10.[10] Trauma or swimming can disrupt these protective barriers and allow bacteria to penetrate the canal's epithelium. This process causes a localized inflammatory response and subsequent infection, which increases erythema and edema, further perpetuating the infection.[1]

Causes

Microbiological

AOE is considered a bacterial infection of the EAC. Although approximately 50% of cases are polymicrobial in nature, aerobic bacteria were noted in 91% of cases where cultures could be obtained. *Pseudomonas aeruginosa* and *Staphylococcus aureus* are the 2 most common culprits isolated in cultures.[11] The microbiological etiology of otitis externa is summarized in **Table 1**.

Fungal

The topical antibiotics used to treat bacterial AOE may lead to a secondary fungal infection, commonly mistaken for a bacterial infection owing to its extremely pruritic nature.[2] *Aspergillus* and *Candida* are the main yeast and fungi isolated in episodes of AOE, but occur in less than 2% of cases.[1]

Risk Factors

Major risk factors for AOE include obstruction to the ear canal (stenosis, exostoses, cerumen impaction), hearing aids, ear plugs, self-induced trauma, and

Table 1
Microbiology of otitis externa

Pathogen	%
Pseudomonas aeruginosa	38
Staphylococcus epidermidis	9.1
Staphylococcus aureus	7.8
Mycobacterium otitidis	6.6
Mycobacterium alconae	2.9
Staphylococcus capitis	1.4
Staphylococcus haemolyticus	1.3
Aspergillus, Candida	<2

Data from Clark WB, Brook I, Bianki D, et al. Microbiology of otitis externa. Otolaryngol Head Neck Surg 1997;116:23–5; and Klein JO. Otitis externa, otitis media, and mastoiditis. In: Mandell GL, Bennett JB, Dolin R, editors. Principles and practice of infectious diseases. 7th edition. Philadelphia: Elsevier Churchill Livingstone; 2009.

swimming. Predisposing factors for AOE, most likely multifactorial, are summarized in **Table 2**.

Clinical Symptoms and Signs

AOE most commonly presents with severe pain, exacerbated by traction on the auricle and/or tragus. The pain is caused by pressure on the sensory nerves of the bony portion of the canal.[12] Itching may be a precursor to the pain. Decreased auditory acuity and full sensation is most likely secondary to edema of the skin and tympanic membrane, as well as occlusion of the canal by secretions. Otorrhea is often thick and clumpy with soft, white cerumen.[1] Common symptoms are noted in **Table 3**.

AOE can be divided into 3 stages:

1. Early bacterial otitis externa is characterized by a canal that is erythematous but with scant discharge; this will then develop into an edematous canal with purulent-squamous debris.
2. Moderate bacterial otitis externa has increased pain and edema, with otorrhea becoming more purulent.
3. Severe bacterial otitis externa is intensely painful, and the canal is completely obstructed with otorrhea and debris. This stage may be associated with periauricular edema and adenopathy.[13]

Table 2
Predisposing factors for acute otitis externa

Predisposing Factors	
Genetic	Narrow external auditory canal, amount of ear wax production, hairy ear canal, type A blood
Environmental	Temporal, humidity, heat, prolonged exposure to water, sweating
Trauma	Cotton swabs, hearing aids, ear plugs, instrumentation, foreign body
Dermatologic	Eczema, psoriasis, seborrhea, inflammatory dermatoses
Other	Purulent otorrhea from otitis media, soap, stress

Data from Peterkin GA. Otitis externa. J Laryng & Oto 1974;88(1):15–21; and Schaefer P, Baugh RF. Acute otitis externa: an update. Am Fam Physician 2012;86(11):1055–61.

| Table 3 | |
| Common symptoms of otitis externa | |
Symptoms	Cases (%)
Otalgia	70
Itching	60
Fullness, with or without hearing loss	22

Data from Rosenfeld RM, Brown L, Cannon CR, et al, for the American Academy of Otolaryngology—Head and Neck Surgery Foundation. Clinical practice guideline: acute otitis externa. Otolaryngol Head Neck Surg 2006;134(Suppl 4):S4–23.

Left untreated, AOE can develop into chronic otitis externa (COE), defined as a single episode that lasts longer than 4 weeks or with 4 or more episodes in 1 year.[1]

Diagnosis

Evaluation of the ear should start with a thorough history, including details of onset, severity of pain, water exposure, and signs and symptoms of ear-canal inflammation. Evaluation for AOE should also include visualization and manipulation of the auricle and pinna, otoscopy, and tympanometry. Although the differentiation of AOE from AOM provides few problems to the experienced physician, there are several conditions that need to be considered. Chronic supportive otitis media is characterized by chronic otorrhea and perforated tympanic membrane. Viral infections, particularly Ramsay Hunt syndrome, can present with otalgia and a vesicular rash. Eczema and contact dermatitis can mimic the itching and swelling associated with AOE. Allergic reactions to topical antibiotics (see the section on treatment) and malignant otitis externa (see the section on complications) can appear similar to AOE.[2,6,14]

Treatment

Pain management is an important component of AOE treatment. Mild to moderate pain can be treated with acetaminophen or nonsteroidal anti-inflammatory medications, whereas moderate to severe pain may require opiate medications. Individual pain tolerance, availability, and cost may determine which pain medication should be given.[15] Topical benzocaine otic solution is commonly prescribed for analgesia; however, there are no clinical trials that prove its efficacy for AOE. Topical steroids have shown mixed effectiveness in improving pain in AOE.[16,17]

Topical antibiotic therapy is the first-line treatment for AOE. Systematic treatment is not recommended unless complicating factors such as immunosuppression or extension of infection occur. Topical antibiotic therapy is highly effective, with a number needed to treat (NNT) of 2.[15]

Inappropriate oral antibiotics may lead to persistence or reoccurrence of infection.[3] Several nonantibiotic topical treatments have been shown to be efficacious in the treatment of AOE, including acetic acid, aluminum acetate, boric acid, silver nitrate, antifungal medications, and topical steroids.[15] **Table 4** lists common topical medications for AOE. There are no significant differences in clinical improvement between antiseptic/acidifying agents and antibiotic topical regimens, quinolone and nonquinolone antibiotics, and the use of antibiotics with steroids versus antibiotics alone. Regardless of topical agent, 65% to 90% of patients achieved clinical cure in 7 to 10 days. The current recommendation is that patients be treated for 7 days, with possible extension of therapy as needed.[15] Topical steroids alone were 20% more effective than antibiotics, although heterogeneity of steroid potency and low numbers

Table 4		
Topical products for otitis externa		
Product	**Brand Name (USA)**	**Dosing**
Acetic acid, aluminum acetate	Otic Domeboro	Twice to 4 times daily
Acetic acid	VoSol	Three to 4 times daily
Acetic acid, hydrocortisone	VoSol HC	Three to 4 times daily
Ciprofloxacin, hydrocortisone	Cipro HC	Twice daily
Ciprofloxacin, dexamethasone	Ciprodex	Twice daily
Neomycin, polymyxin B, hydrocortisone	Cortisporin otic solution, suspension	Three to 4 times daily
Ofloxacin	Floxain Otic	Once daily

Data from Osguthorpe JD, Shaughnessy AF. Otitis externa. In: Essential evidence plus [Internet]. Hoboken (NJ): John Wiley & Sons, Inc; 2012. Available at: https://www.essentialevidenceplus. com/content/eee/107. Accessed February 27, 2013.

of patients studied limit generalizability.[18] Acetic acid alone, however, has been noted to be less effective than antibiotics with steroids after 2 or 3 weeks of therapy, and took 2 days longer to improve patient symptoms.[19]

For patients with suspected or known perforation of the tympanic membrane, ototoxic antiseptic and antibiotic regimens should be avoided. Short-term therapy (14 days) with neomycin/polymyxin B/dexamethasone did not appear to affect hearing[20]; however, severe hearing loss has been attributed to excessive, prolonged use of these medications.[21] Visualization of the tympanic membrane or tympanometry should be performed to confirm perforation. Children with tympanostomy tubes within 12 months should be assumed to still have them present. Patients who can taste topical otic medicines after placement in the ear or can expel air from their ear canal should be treated as having a perforation.[15] For these patients, experts have recommended avoiding topical medications that contain alcohol, acidifying agents, or aminoglycosides.[22] The choice of initial topical treatment should be determined by the risk of ototoxicity, the patient's allergies, local antibiotic resistance patterns, availability, cost, and ease of dosing.

Providers should instruct patients on how to use the topical medications. The patient should lie down with the affected ear upward, and drops should be administered until the canal is filled. The pinna and outer ear may need to be manipulated to ensure complete filling. The medication should be left in place for 3 to 5 minutes. Aural toilet (eg, ear lavage) or use of an ear wick may be considered if the ear canal is obstructed by cerumen or very edematous; however, there are no trials confirming the efficacy of ear wick.[15]

Patients should also reduce water exposure into the ear, including avoiding water sports for 7 to 10 days during treatment. Earplugs or cotton with petroleum jelly when bathing, and the use of a hair dryer on the lowest setting after water exposure, can reduce moisture.[15]

Complementary and Alternative Therapies

Home remedies such as a 1:1 combination of isopropyl alcohol and white vinegar have not been formally assessed, but are chemically similar to commercial products with acetic acid. An in vitro study of tea-tree oil was 71% effective against common AOE pathogenic organisms except *P aeruginosa*, which was 75% resistant.[23] Ear candling has not been shown to be effective, and can result in serious injury.[24] Naturopathic herbal extract ear drops appear to be effective in reducing ear pain in children.[25] Although hyperbaric oxygen has been recommended for AOE, a Cochrane review found no randomized controlled trials and a lack of clear evidence in support of hyperbaric oxygen therapy.[26]

Prognosis

Patients should improve within 2 to 3 days of starting treatment. Symptom pain scores on ofloxacin improved as soon as 1 day of treatment,[27] and the majority of patients taking either steroid only or steroid with antibiotics reported no or minimal pain after 4 days of treatment.[28] If patients do not improve, providers can consider ear culture (to differentiate between bacterial or fungal infections), placement of an ear wick, or a change to systematic oral antibiotic that treats *P aeruginosa* and *S aureus*. Patients with continued symptoms should be assessed for other causes (eg, cancer, cellulitis, contact dermatitis, fungal infection, malignant otitis externa) and contact sensitivity from the topical medications. Neomycin is the most common topical agent to cause contact sensitivity, with 20% to 30% prevalence.[29,30] Based on epidemiologic data, only 3% of patients needed secondary evaluation by otolaryngology.[3]

Complications

Malignant otitis externa (MOE) is a rare, severe infection of the auditory canal and surrounding anatomic structures, including bone. It predominantly happens in elderly diabetics or patients infected with human immunodeficiency virus.[31] Pediatric MOE is extremely rare.[32] *P aeruginosa* is the causative agent in more than 90% of MOE.[31] Patients can present with similar symptoms to AOE, making it difficult to distinguish between the two diseases. Patients with MOE, however, will usually report severe disproportionate pain, high fever, possible vertigo and meningeal signs, and classically granulation tissue along the EAC.[13] One retrospective analysis of 23 MOE patients found that 43% had cranial nerve palsies.[33] Imaging is crucial to confirm the diagnosis. Computed tomography (CT) can confirm disease involvement outside the EAC, and characterize bony erosion and soft-tissue involvement.[34] Magnetic resonance imaging (MRI) appears to better identify soft-tissue abnormalities, with 93% of MOE patients having retrocondylar fat infiltration.[35] Ciprofloxacin, 750 mg orally twice daily, is considered first-line therapy, with a duration of at least 4 weeks for osteomyelitis.[36] Most patients will need surgical consultation for possible debridement and initial parenteral antibiotics.

OTITIS MEDIA
Background

AOM is characterized by signs and symptoms of ear pain, inflammation, and middle ear effusion. In 2010, AOM was the 13th most common diagnosis for office visits in the United States, accounting for more than 14 million visits.[37] In 2006, an estimated $2.8 billion was spent on AOM treatment in children,[38] with 76% to 80% of children receiving prescription antibiotics for AOM.[39]

It is important to distinguish AOM from otitis media with effusion (OME). AOM refers to symptomatic inflammation of the middle ear (eg, bulging tympanic membrane), whereas OME is a middle ear effusion without acute signs of inflammation.

Incidence

By age 1 year, 62% to 78% of children had at least one episode of AOM, which increases to 83% to 91% by age 2 or 3.[40,41] The peak incidence appears to be between 6 and 18 months, with a secondary peak at 5 years of age associated with starting school.[42] There are no available data regarding incidence in adults. Risk factors for AOM are listed in **Table 5**. Antibiotics for AOM before the age of 2 appear to increase the risk of recurrent AOM (adjusted odds ratio 2.5).[43]

Certain ethnic groups such as Alaskan Eskimos and Native Americans appear to be at high risk for chronic suppurative otitis media (CSOM).[44] Limited medical services also appear to increase the risk of CSOM.[45]

Pathogenesis

AOM is the result of a confluence of events, including infectious, inflammatory, and immunologic factors. The Eustachian tube sits between the nasal cavities and middle ear, regulating middle ear pressure and clearing secretions. Infants and younger children are at higher risk for AOM because of the shorter length of the Eustachian tube. The shorter tube creates a higher risk for infected secretions to reach the middle ear.

AOM occurs frequently after a viral upper respiratory infection. The congestion and inflammation of the Eustachian tube leads to a buildup of mucosal secretions and blockage of the Eustachian tube. Patients are subsequently infected by bacteria, which often are already colonized in the nasopharynx.[46] The bacteria are transported from the nasopharynx to the middle ear by the negative pressure built up in the Eustachian tube, leading to AOM.[47]

Microbiology

Classically the most common causes of AOM are *Streptococcus pneumoniae*, *Haemophilus influenzae*, and *Moraxella catarrhalis*. Middle ear fluid culture, however, was positive for these 3 bacteria only 61% of the time, and no pathogen was identified in 29% of cultures.[48] In pediatric patients, middle ear fluid cultures were positive for viruses 41% to 75% of the time, with both viral and bacterial coinfection occurring between 45% and 65% of the time.[49,50] Concomitant viral infection with bacterial AOM appears to increase clinical or bacteriologic failure and decrease amoxicillin plasma concentrations in comparison with bacterial infection alone.[51,52]

S pneumoniae used to be the most common pathogen in AOM, accounting for up to 44% of AOM bacterial infections.[53] The 7-valent pneumococcal conjugate vaccine (PCV7) vaccine has reduced the incidence of AOM by 6% to 7%.[54] *S pneumoniae* serotypes included in the PCV7 were 60% to 70% of all *S pneumoniae* AOM in 6- to 59-month-old children.[55] The vaccine does not appear to help older children with recurrent AOM.[56] Subsequent studies have shown that non-PCV7 serotypes have replaced the PCV serotypes as causes of *S pneumoniae* infection.[57] Specifically, serotype 19A has been implicated as multidrug resistant and a cause of

Table 5 Risk factors	
Risk Factor	**Relative Risk**
Family member with acute otitis media	2.63
Day care outside the home	2.45
Parental smoking	1.66
Family day care	1.59
Pacifier use	1.24
Breastfeeding at least 3 mo	0.87

Data from Uhari M, Mäntysaari K, Niemelä M. A meta-analytic review of the risk factors for acute otitis media. Clin Infect Dis 1996;22:1079–83.

treatment failure.[58] The 13-valent pneumococcal conjugate vaccine (PCV13) contains the 19A serotype; however, the impact of the vaccine on the incidence of AOM is unknown.

H influenzae accounts for 56% to 57% of AOM infections. The prevalence has increased from 41% to 43%, presumably from the decrease in *S pneumoniae* infections from the PCV7 vaccine.[59] Bilateral AOM is more likely to be caused by *H influenzae*.[60,61] Most AOM infections caused by *H influenzae* are nontypeable, therefore the *H influenzae* type B vaccine does not decrease the incidence as the PCV7 vaccine has done for *S pneumoniae*.

M catarrhalis is responsible for approximately 14% of AOM.[62] Other causes of AOM include Group A streptococcus, *S aureus*, and viruses.

Clinical Signs and Symptoms

Otalgia is the most common symptom of AOM. Eighty-two percent of children with AOM complained of ear pain, but children younger than 2 years were significantly less likely to report pain.[63] Fever occurs in 23% of children with AOM, with only 0.3% having fever greater than 40.5°C.[64] While earache, night restlessness, and fever have classically been associated with AOM,[65] there is conflicting evidence as to whether any symptom is predictive of AOM. Parental suspicion of AOM, ear pain, ear rubbing, fever, irritability, restless sleep, severe rhinitis, or cough was not significantly different for AOM versus non-AOM patients.[66] However, a validated 7-item symptom scale that included ear pain, ear tugging, irritability, difficulty sleeping, eating less, being less playful, and fever appeared to correlate both with diagnosis and clinical improvement.[67] Although certain symptoms appear to be suggestive of AOM, in itself this is not sufficient for a diagnosis of AOM.

Examination of the tympanic membrane appears to be the most reliable means of predicting AOM. The most commonly reported signs of AOM are bulging tympanic membrane (89%), injected tympanic membrane (57%), and cloudy tympanic membrane (52%).[68] The signs with the highest positive predictive values are bulging tympanic membrane (89%–96%), cloudy tympanic membrane (80%–96%), and distinctly impaired mobility (78%–94%). Red or retracted tympanic membranes did not appear to strongly correlate with AOM.[69]

Despite the specific signs associated with AOM, pediatric otolaryngologists demonstrated only fair agreement ($\kappa = 0.32$) with tympanometry.[70] The *New England Journal of Medicine*'s Videos in Clinical Medicine demonstrate cerumen removal and otoscopy techniques (subscription required).[71] The Johns Hopkins University School of Medicine and the Institute for Johns Hopkins Nursing also have produced clinical videos for review.[72]

Diagnosis

Otitis media is diagnosed by history and physical examination findings. AOM should be diagnosed in children with:

1. Moderate to severe bulging tympanic membrane or new otorrhea not caused by AOE
2. Ear pain and mildly bulging or intensely erythematous tympanic membrane

Children without middle ear effusion should be diagnosed with AOM.[73] There are no differing recommendations for the diagnosis of AOM in adults.

The presence of a middle ear effusion can be determined by several different methods, including visualization of a bulging tympanic membrane on otoscopy, little or no movement of the tympanic membrane on pneumatic otoscopy, tympanometry, clinical otorrhea, or an observed air-fluid level behind the tympanic membrane. Pneumatic otoscopy also allows evaluation of the contour, color, translucency, and mobility of the tympanic membrane.[73] The use of tympanometry, in addition to pneumatic otoscopy, increased the sensitivity of determining a middle ear effusion but did not change clinicians' antibiotic-prescribing habits.[74] Middle ear inflammation can be confirmed on direct otoscopy, including erythema of the tympanic membrane or definitive otalgia. Opacification and cloudiness of the tympanic membrane also supports the diagnosis of AOM.

The differential diagnosis for otitis media includes determining whether the patient has OME. Middle ear pain can also be a consequence of viral upper respiratory syndrome or Eustachian tube dysfunction not related to AOM. OME should be monitored at 3-month intervals and a referral made to otolaryngology if evidence of a mucoid effusion or anatomic damage to the middle ear is suspected. Otherwise, observation is recommended if no developmental or behavioral problems are noted.[75] Antibiotics have not been shown to be effective in quickening resolution of OME.[76] Clinicians should also be aware of eosinophilic otitis media, which is characterized by eosinophils present in fluid aspiration from myringostomy. Eosinophilic otitis media does not respond to classic AOM or OME treatments but does respond to corticosteroid therapy. It is often associated with bronchial asthma.[77] CSOM is defined as a chronic inflammation of the middle ear and mastoid cavity, which presents with recurrent ear discharges or otorrhea through a tympanic perforation.[78] The complications of this disease include perisigmoid intracranial abscess and meningitis.[79]

Treatment

All patients with AOM should be assessed for pain and treated with appropriate oral analgesic medications such as ibuprofen or acetaminophen.[80] Topical ear drops have shown limited effectiveness in older children, and are generally not recommended for AOM.[81]

A 2013 Cochrane review showed a small benefit for antibiotics, with a mild reduction in pain at 2 to 7 days but no change in abnormal tympanometry or AOM reoccurrence rates. Antibiotics did appear to reduce the risk of tympanic membrane perforation and contralateral AOM infection.[82]

The greatest benefit of antibiotics appears to be in children younger than 2 years with bilateral AOM or AOM with otorrhea. In children younger than 2 years, treatment with amoxicillin-clavulanate produced a clinically significant reduction in treatment failure at 10 to 12 days, with an NNT of 2.9.[83]

Current guideline recommendations from the American Academy of Pediatrics (AAP) and American Academy of Family Physicians (AAFP) for the treatment of AOM differ based on age and diagnosis severity.[73] This recommendation is based on trials that showed a 9% difference in 14-day success rates between ampicillin or amoxicillin versus placebo. In children aged 6 to 23 months, antibiotics are recommended for AOM with otorrhea, AOM with severe symptoms, or bilateral AOM. For unilateral AOM without otorrhea, patients can be either started on immediate antibiotics or observed for 2 to 3 days for clinical improvement. In children older than 2, antibiotics are recommended for AOM with otorrhea or AOM with severe symptoms; and for unilateral or bilateral AOM, initial observation for 2 to 3 days can also be done.

Delayed antibiotics (eg, parental discretion and starting antibiotics after waiting 2–3 days) began with the observation that approximately 50% of pediatric AOM patients given placebo rather than antibiotics clinically improved. One prospective clinical study showed that AOM as many as 81% of patients did not require antibiotic initiation.[84] Delayed antibiotics resulted in a 66% reduction in antibiotic use[85] and no change in fever, earache, or unscheduled medical visits.[86] AOM illness durations were shortened by 1.1 days by antibiotics, but did not affect school absence rates.[87] Common side effects of antibiotics such as rash and diarrhea can be avoided with the delayed antibiotic approaches.[59]

Treatment should begin with high-dose amoxicillin, 80 to 90 mg/kg/d divided twice daily. In patients who have taken amoxicillin within the last 30 days or have concurrent conjunctivitis, amoxicillin-clavulanate (90 mg/kg/d of amoxicillin divided twice daily) is recommended.[73] The maximum dose of amoxicillin is 1000 mg per dose. For patients allergic to penicillins, alternative initial therapy includes cefdinir (14 mg/kg/d), cefuroxime (30 mg/kg/d divided twice daily), cefpodoxime (10 mg/kg/d divided twice daily), or ceftriaxone (50 mg/kg/d intramuscular). It is important to bear in mind that no oral cephalosporin is superior to amoxicillin.[59,73] In patients with severe penicillin or cephalosporin allergies, alternative options would then include clindamycin or azithromycin. Clindamycin and azithromycin, however, have limited efficacy against *H influenzae* and penicillin-resistant *S pneumoniae*.[73]

Patients should be reassessed in 2 to 3 days. Patients failing amoxicillin should be switched to amoxicillin-clavulanate. Patients failing amoxicillin-clavulanate or oral cephalosporin should start intramuscular ceftriaxone, 50 mg/kg/d for 3 days. In patients failing therapy, tympanocentesis or nasopharyngeal culture and referral to otolaryngology should be considered.

The duration of therapy depends on the age of the patient. Patients younger than 2 years should be treated for 10 days, patients 2 to 5 years old should be treated for 7 days, and those aged 6 years and older may be treated for 5 to 7 days.[73]

Patients with recurrent AOM or persistent OME may benefit from surgical intervention.[88] A 2006 Cochrane review found that prophylactic antibiotics reduced recurrent AOM by approximately 50% (1.5 episodes per year).[89] This benefit must be balanced against the potential side effects of antibiotics and increasing antibiotic resistance. For this reason, the AAP and AAFP do not recommend prophylactic antibiotics to reduce the incidence of recurrent AOM.[73] Tympanostomy tubes appeared to reduce recurrent AOM episodes by 1.5 episodes per 6 months after placement.[90] The AAP and AAFP currently recommend evaluation for possible tympanostomy tubes for recurrent AOM: 3 episodes within 6 months or 4 episodes in the last year, with 1 episode in the last 6 months.

For OME, national guidelines currently recommend monitoring at 3- to 6-month intervals with hearing tests for effusions lasting longer than 3 months or any signs of developmental delay. Candidates for tube placement include patients with a middle ear effusion lasting longer than 4 months, patients at higher risk, and patients with structural ear damage along with OME.[91] Decongestants and antihistamines have not been shown to be helpful for side effects in the management of OME.[92] Entities such as eosinophilic otitis media and CSOM should be referred to a specialist for evaluation and treatment.

Complications

The long-term sequelae of AOM, OME, and other entities such as CSOM can be divided into extracranial and intracranial complications. Extracranial or intratemporal complications include recurrent episodes of pain, vestibular/balance problems, eardrum perforation with episodes of otorrhea, hearing impairment, tympanosclerosis, cholesteatoma, and mastoiditis. Rarer intracranial complications include epidural or brain abscess, meningitis, subdural empyema, and lateral sinus thrombosis.[93]

Before widespread access to antibiotics, acute mastoiditis was a leading cause of hospitalizations for infants and children.[94] Today, more severe complications are likely to occur in children with limited access to care.[95] Global mortality is highest in young children aged 1 to 4 years, with mortality as high as 101.1 deaths per 10 million in parts of the developing world.[96]

Hearing impairment from AOM complications has been estimated to be as high as 6 per 1000 children in South Asia, versus 0.64 per 10,000 children in North America. Worldwide, about 50% of patients develop mild to moderate conductive hearing loss as a consequence of CSOM.[78] The pathologic progression from AOM to CSOM is unclear, and the evidence to justify treatment of AOM to prevent complications such as mastoiditis is insufficient.[97] One retrospective cohort study did show a 50% decrease in the risk of developing mastoiditis in patients with AOM treated with antibiotics, but the NNT was more than 4800.[98]

Mastoiditis occurs as a consequence of the spread of infection from the middle ear to the mastoid air cells. This process can involve the bone, and thus becomes mastoiditis with either osteitis or periostitis. The diagnosis is made by physical examination and imaging such as CT or MRI, and treatment involves intravenous antibiotics and surgery if necessary.[93]

A cholesteatoma is a cyst of keratinized material that forms as a consequence of chronic otitis media in either the middle ear or mastoid sinus. It can have several consequences, including erosion in the structures of the middle ear causing hearing loss. The expansion of the cholesteatoma can also lead to facial paralysis by compression of the facial nerve, or even brain herniation. These cysts are prone to infection and have a bacterial make-up different to that of AOM, often including pseudomonal species. Cholesteatomas are usually managed surgically.[99]

REFERENCES

1. Beers SL, Abramo TJ. Otitis externa review. Pediatr Emerg Care 2004;20:250–6.
2. McDowall GD. External otitis: otological problems. J Laryngol Otol 1974;88(1): 1–13.
3. Rowlands S, Devalia H, Smith C, et al. Otitis externa in UK general practice: a survey using the UK General Practice Research Database. Br J Gen Pract 2001;51:533–8.
4. Hajioff D, MacKeith S. Otitis externa. Clin Evid (Online) 2010. Available at: http://www.ncbi.nlm.nih.gov/pmc/articles/PMC3217807/.
5. Stone KE. Otitis Externa. Pediatr Rev 2007;28:77–8.
6. Peterkin GA. Otitis externa. J Laryng & Oto 1974;88(1):15–21.
7. Guss J, Ruckenstein MJ. Infections of the external ear. In: Cummings CW, Flint PW, Haughey BH, et al, editors. Otolaryngology: head & neck surgery. 5th edition. Philadelphia: Mosby Elsevier; 2010.
8. Klein JO. Otitis externa, otitis media, and mastoiditis. In: Mandell GL, Bennett JE, Dolin R, editors. Principles and Practice of Infectious Diseases. 7th edition. Philadelphia: Elsevier Churchill Livingstone; 2009.
9. Francis HW. Anatomy of the temporal bone, external ear, and middle ear. In: Cummings CW, Flint PW, Haughey BH, et al, editors. Cummings otolaryngology: head & neck surgery. 5th edition. Philadelphia: Mosby Elsevier; 2010.
10. Aminifarshidmehr N. The management of chronic suppurative otitis media with acid media solution. Am J Otol 1996;17:24–5.
11. Clark WB, Brook I, Bianki D, et al. Microbiology of otitis externa. Otolaryngol Head Neck Surg 1997;116:23–5.

12. Leung AK, Fong JH, Leong AG. Otalgia in children. J Natl Med Assoc 2000;92: 254–60.
13. Osguthorpe JD, Nielsen DR. Otitis externa: review and clinical update. Am Fam Physician 2006;74:1510–6.
14. Schaefer P, Baugh RF. Acute otitis externa: an update. Am Fam Physician 2012; 86(11):1055–61.
15. Rosenfeld RM, Brown L, Cannon CR, et al, for the American Academy of Otolaryngology—Head and Neck Surgery Foundation. Clinical practice guideline: acute otitis externa. Otolaryngol Head Neck Surg 2006;134(Suppl 4):S4–23.
16. Pistorius B, Westberry K, Drehobl M, et al. Prospective, randomized, comparative trial of ciprofloxacin otic drops, with or without hydrocortisone, vs. polymyxin B-neomycin-hydrocortisone otic suspension in the treatment of acute diffuse otitis externa. Infect Dis Clin Pract 1999;8:387–95.
17. Psifidis A, Nikolaidis P, Tsona A, et al. The efficacy and safety of local ciprofloxacin in patients with external otitis: a randomized comparative study. Mediterranean J Otol Audiol 2005;1. Available at: www.mediotol.org/mjo.htm. Accessed February 2, 2013.
18. Rosenfeld RM, Singer M, Wasserman JM, et al. Systematic review of topical antimicrobial therapy for acute otitis externa. Otolaryngol Head Neck Surg 2006; 134:S24.
19. Kaushik V, Malik T, Saeed SR. Interventions for acute otitis externa. Cochrane Database of Systematic Reviews. John Wiley and Sons, Ltd; 2010. http://dx.doi.org/10.1002/14651858.CD004740.pub2. Issue 1.
20. Rakover Y, Keywan K, Rosen G. Safety of topical ear drops containing ototoxic antibiotics. J Otolaryngol 1997;26:194–6.
21. Linder TE, Zwicky S, Brandle P. Ototoxicity of ear drops: a clinical perspective. Am J Otol 1995;16:653–7.
22. Roland PS, Stewart MG, Hannley M, et al. Consensus panel on role of potentially ototoxic antibiotics for topical middle-ear use: introduction, methodology, and recommendations. Otolaryngol Head Neck Surg 2004;130(Suppl 3):S51–6.
23. Farnan TB, McCallum J, Awa A, et al. Tea tree oil: in vitro efficacy in otitis externa. J Laryngol Otol 2005;119:198–201.
24. Seely DR, Quigley SM, Langman AW. Ear candles: efficacy and safety. Laryngoscope 1996;106:1226–9.
25. Sarrell EM, Cohen HA, Kahan E. Naturopathic treatment of ear pain in children. Pediatrics 2003;111:e574–9.
26. Phillips JS, Jones SE. Hyperbaric oxygen as an adjuvant treatment for malignant otitis externa. Cochrane Database of Systematic Reviews. John Wiley and Sons, Ltd; 2005. http://dx.doi.org/10.1002/14651858.CD004617.pub2. Issue 2.
27. Torum B, Block SL, Avila H, et al. Efficacy of ofloxacin otic solution once daily for 7 days in the treatment of otitis externa: a multicenter, open-label, phase III trial. Clin Ther 2004;26:1046–54.
28. Emgard P, Hellstrom S. A group III steroid solution without antibiotic components: an effective cure for external otitis. J Laryngol Otol 2005;119:342–7.
29. Devos SA, Mulder JJ, van der Valk PG. The relevance of positive patch test reactions in chronic otitis externa. Contact Derm 2000;42:354–5.
30. Rutka J. Acute otitis externa: treatment perspectives. Ear Nose Throat J 2004; 83(Suppl 4):20–2.
31. Grandis JR, Branstetter BF, Yu VL. The changing face of malignant (necrotising) external otitis: clinical, radiological, and anatomic correlations. Lancet Infect Dis 2004;4:34–9.

32. Nir D, Nir T, Danino J, et al. Malignant external otitis in an infant. J Laryngol Otol 1990;104(6):488–90.
33. Mani N, Sudhoff H, Rajagopal S, et al. Cranial nerve involvement in malignant external otitis: implications for clinical outcome. Laryngoscope 2007;117: 907–10.
34. Sudhoff H, Rajagopal S, Mani N, et al. Usefulness of CT scans in malignant external otitis: effective tool for the diagnosis, but of limited value in predicting outcome. Eur Arch Otorhinolaryngol 2008;265(1):53–6.
35. Kwon BJ, Han MH, Oh SH, et al. MRI findings and spreading patterns of necrotizing external otitis: is a poor outcome predictable? Clin Radiol 2006;61(6): 495–504.
36. Handzel O, Halperin D. Necrotizing (malignant) otitis externa. Am Fam Physician 2003;68:309–12.
37. National ambulatory medical care survey: 2010 summary tables. In: Centers for Disease Control and Prevention. Available at: http://www.cdc.gov/nchs/data/ahcd/namcs_summary/2010_namcs_web_tables.pdf. Accessed February 7, 2013.
38. Soni A. Ear infections (otitis media) in children (0-17): use and expenditures, 2006. Statistical Brief No. 228. Agency for Healthcare Research and Quality Website. Available at: http://www.meps.ahrq.gov/mepsweb/data_files/publications/st228/stat228.pdf. Accessed February 7, 2013.
39. Grijalva CG, Nuorti JP, Griffin MR. Antibiotic prescription rates for acute respiratory tract infections in US ambulatory settings. JAMA 2009;302(7):758–66.
40. Teele DW, Klein JO, Rosner B. Epidemiology of otitis media during the first seven years of life in children in greater Boston: a prospective, cohort study. J Infect Dis 1989;160:83–94.
41. Paradise JL, Rockette HE, Colborn DK, et al. Otitis media in 2253 Pittsburgh-area infants: prevalence and risk factors during the first two years of life. Pediatrics 1997;99:318–33.
42. Daly KA, Giebink GS. Clinical epidemiology of otitis media. Pediatr Infect Dis J 2000;19:S31–6.
43. Bezakova N, Damoiseaux RA, Hoes AW, et al. Recurrence up to 3.5 years after antibiotic treatment of acute otitis media in very young Dutch children: survey of trial participants. BMJ 2009;338:b2525.
44. Bluestone CD. Epidemiology and pathogenesis of chronic suppurative otitis media: implications for prevention and treatment. Int J Pediatr Otorhinolaryngol 1998;42:207–23.
45. Minja BM, Machemba A. Prevalence of otitis media, hearing impairment and cerumen impaction among school children in rural and urban Dar es Salaam, Tanzania. Int J Pediatr Otorhinolaryngol 1996;37:29–34.
46. Revai K, Mamidi D, Chonmaitree T. Association of nasopharyngeal bacterial colonization during upper respiratory tract infection and the development of acute otitis media. Clin Infect Dis 2008;46:e34–7.
47. Bluestone CD, Klein JO. Physiology, pathophysiology, and pathogenesis. In: Otitis media in infants and children. 3rd edition. Philadelphia: W.B. Saunders Company; 2001. p. 34–57.
48. Kaur R, Adlowitz DG, Casey JR, et al. Simultaneous assay for four bacterial species including Alloiococcus otitidis using multiplex-PCR in children with culture negative acute otitis media. Pediatr Infect Dis J 2010;29:741–5.
49. Ruohola A, Meurman O, Nikkari S, et al. Microbiology of acute otitis media in children with tympanostomy tubes: prevalences of bacteria and viruses. Clin Infect Dis 2006;43:1417–22.

50. Pitkäranta A, Virolainen A, Jero J, et al. Detection of rhinovirus, respiratory syncytial virus, and coronavirus infections in acute otitis media by reverse transcriptase polymerase chain reaction. Pediatrics 1998;102(2 Pt 1):291–5.
51. Chonmaitree T, Owen MJ, Patel JA, et al. Effect of viral respiratory tract infection on outcome of acute otitis media. J Pediatr 1992;120:856–62.
52. Canafax DM, Yuan Z, Chonmaitree T, et al. Amoxicillin middle ear fluid penetration and pharmacokinetics in children with acute otitis media. Pediatr Infect Dis J 1998;17:149–56.
53. Casey JR, Pichichero ME. Changes in frequency and pathogens causing acute otitis media in 1995-2003. Pediatr Infect Dis J 2004;23(9):824–8.
54. Eskola J, Kilpi T, Palmu A, et al. Efficacy of a pneumococcal conjugate vaccine against acute otitis media. N Engl J Med 2001;344:403–9.
55. Hausdorff WP, Yothers G, Dagan R, et al. Multinational study of pneumococcal serotypes causing acute otitis media in children. Pediatr Infect Dis J 2002;21: 1008–16.
56. Jansen AG, Hak E, Veehoven RH, et al. Pneumococcal conjugate vaccines for preventing otitis media. Cochrane Database Syst Rev 2009;(2):CD001480. http://dx.doi.org/10.1002/14651858.CD001480.pub3.
57. Casey JR, Adlowitz DG, Pichichero ME. New patterns in the otopathogens causing acute otitis media six to eight years after introduction of pneumococcal conjugate vaccine. Pediatr Infect Dis J 2010;29:304–9.
58. Couloigner V, Levy C, François M, et al. Pathogens implicated in acute otitis media failures after 7-valent pneumococcal conjugate vaccine implementation in France: distribution, serotypes, and resistance levels. Pediatr Infect Dis J 2012;31:154–8.
59. Coker TR, Chan LS, Newberry SJ, et al. Diagnosis, microbial epidemiology, and antibiotic treatment of acute otitis media in children: a systematic review. JAMA 2010;304:2161–9.
60. McCormick DP, Chandler SM, Chonmaitree T. Laterality of acute otitis media: different clinical and microbiologic characteristics. Pediatr Infect Dis J 2007;26: 583–8.
61. Leibovitz E, Asher E, Piglansky L, et al. Is bilateral acute otitis media clinically different than unilateral acute otitis media? Pediatr Infect Dis J 2007;26: 589–92.
62. Bluestone CD, Stephenson JS, Martin LM. Ten-year review of otitis media pathogens. Pediatr Infect Dis J 1992;11:S7–11.
63. Hayden GF, Schwartz RH. Characteristics of earache among children with acute otitis media. Am J Dis Child 1985;139:721–3.
64. Schwartz RH, Rodriguez WJ, Brook I, et al. The febrile response in acute otitis media. JAMA 1981;245:2057–8.
65. Kontiokari T, Koivunen P, Niemelä M, et al. Symptoms of acute otitis media. Pediatr Infect Dis J 1998;17:676–9.
66. Laine MK, Tähtinen PA, Ruuskanen O, et al. Symptoms or symptom-based scores cannot predict acute otitis media at otitis-prone age. Pediatrics 2010; 125:e1154–61.
67. Shaikh N, Hoberman A, Paradise JL, et al. Development and preliminary evaluation of a parent-reported outcome instrument for clinical trials in acute otitis media. Pediatr Infect Dis J 2009;28(1):5–8.
68. Arola M, Ruuskanen O, Ziegler T, et al. Clinical role of respiratory virus infection in acute otitis media. Pediatrics 1990;86(6):848–55.

69. Karma PH, Penttilä MA, Sipilä MM, et al. Otoscopic diagnosis of middle ear effusion in acute and non-acute otitis media. I. The value of different otoscopic findings. Int J Pediatr Otorhinolaryngol 1989;17(1):37–49.
70. Steinbach WJ, Sectish TC, Benjamin DK Jr, et al. Pediatric residents' clinical diagnostic accuracy of otitis media. Pediatrics 2002;109(6):993–8.
71. Shaikh N, Hoberman A, Kaleida PH, et al. Diagnosing otitis media—otoscopy and cerumen removal. N Engl J Med 2010;362:e62. http://dx.doi.org/10.1056/NEJMvcm0904397 [video]. Available at: http://www.nejm.org/doi/full/10.1056/NEJMvcm0904397. Accessed February 27, 2013.
72. American Academy of Pediatrics. Section on Infectious Diseases. A view through the otoscope: distinguishing acute otitis media from otitis media with effusion [video]. Available at: http://www2.aap.org/sections/infectdis/video.cfm. Accessed February 27, 2013.
73. Lieberthal AS, Carroll AE, Chonmaitree T, et al. The diagnosis and management of acute otitis media. Pediatrics 2013;131(3):e964–99.
74. Spiro DM, King WD, Arnold DH, et al. A randomised clinical trial to assess the effects of tympanometry on the diagnosis and treatment of acute otitis media. Pediatrics 2004;114(1):177–81.
75. Linsk RL, Blackwood RA, Cooke JM, et al. UMHS Otitis Media Guideline. July 2007. Available at: http://www.med.umich.edu/1info/fhp/practiceguides/om/OM.pdf. Accessed March 14, 2013.
76. Van Zon A, Van der Heijden GJ, Van Dongen TM, et al. Antibiotics for otitis media with effusion in children. Cochrane Database Syst Rev 2012;(9):CD009163.
77. Lino Y, Tomikoa-Matsutani S, Matsubara A, et al. Diagnostic criteria of eosinophilic otitis media, a newly recognized middle ear disease. Auris Nasus Larynx 2011;38(4):456–61.
78. Acuin J. Chronic suppurative otitis media: burden of illness and management options. WHO; 2004. Available at: http://www.who.int/pbd/deafness/activities/hearing_care/otitis_media.pdf. Accessed March 14, 2013.
79. Yorgancilar E, Yildirim M, Gun R, et al. Complications of chronic suppurative otitis media: a retrospective review. Eur Arch Otorhinolaryngol 2013;270:69–76.
80. American Academy of Pediatrics, Committee on Psychosocial Aspects of Child and Family Health, Task Force on Pain in Infants, Children, and Adolescents. The assessment and management of acute pain in infants, children, and adolescents. Pediatrics 2001;108(3):793–7.
81. Foxlee R, Johansson A, Wejfalk J, et al. Topical analgesia for acute otitis media. Cochrane Database Syst Rev 2006;(3):CD005657.
82. Venekamp RP, Sanders S, Glasziou PP, et al. Antibiotics for acute otitis media in children. Cochrane Database Syst Rev 2013;(1):CD000219.
83. Hoberman A, Paradise JL, Rockette HE, et al. Treatment of acute otitis media in children under 2 years of age. N Engl J Med 2011;364(2):105–15.
84. Stevanovic T, Komazec Z, LemajicKomazec S, et al. Acute otitis media: to follow-up or treat? Int J Pediatr Otorhinolaryngol 2010;74(8):930–3.
85. McCormick DP, Chonmaitree T, Pittman C, et al. Nonsevere acute otitis media: a clinical trial comparing outcomes of watchful waiting versus immediate antibiotic treatment. Pediatrics 2005;115(6):1455–65.
86. Spiro DM, Tay KY, Arnold DH, et al. Wait-and-see prescription for the treatment of acute otitis media: a randomized controlled trial. JAMA 2006;296(10):1235–41.

87. Little P, Gould C, Williamson I, et al. Pragmatic randomised controlled trial of two prescribing strategies for childhood acute otitis media. BMJ 2001;322(7282): 336–42.
88. Grevers G. Challenges in reducing the burden of otitis media disease. An ENT perspective on improving management and prospects for prevention. Int J Pediatr Otorhinolaryngol 2010;74(6):572–7.
89. Leach AJ, Morris PS. Antibiotics for the prevention of acute and chronic suppurative otitis media in children. Cochrane Database Syst Rev 2006;(4):CD004401.
90. McDonald S, Langton Hewer CD, Nunez DA. Grommets (ventilation tubes) for recurrent acute otitis media in children. Cochrane Database Syst Rev 2008;(4):CD004741.
91. American Academy of Family Physicians, American Academy of Otolaryngology-Head and Neck Surgery, American Academy of Pediatrics Subcommittee on Otitis Media with Effusion. Otitis media with effusion. Pediatrics 2004;113:1412–29.
92. Griffin G, Flynn CA. Antihistamines and/or decongestants for otitis media with effusion (OME) in children. Cochrane Database Syst Rev 2011;(9):CD003423.
93. Casselbrant ML, Mandel EM. Acute otitis media and otitis media with effusion. In: Cummings CW, Flint PW, Haughey BH, et al, editors. Otolaryngology: head & neck surgery. 5th edition. Philadelphia: Mosby Elsevier; 2010. p. 2761–77.
94. Thorne MC, Chewaproug L, Elden LM. Suppurative complications of acute otitis media: changes in frequency over time. Arch Otolaryngol Head Neck Surg 2009;135(7):638–41.
95. Klein JO. Is acute otitis media a treatable disease. N Engl J Med 2011;364:168.
96. Monasta L, Ronfani L, Marchetti F, et al. Burden of disease caused by otitis media: systematic review and global estimates. PLoS One 2012;7(4):e36226.
97. Vergison A, Dagan R, Arguedas A, et al. Otitis media and its consequences: beyond the earache. Lancet Infect Dis 2010;10:195–203.
98. Thompson PL, Gilbert RE, Long PF, et al. Effect of antibiotics for otitis media on mastoiditis in children: a retrospective cohort study using the United kingdom general practice research database. Pediatrics 2009;123(2):424–30.
99. Chole RA, Sudhoff HH. Chronic otitis media, mastoiditis, and petrositis. In: Cummings CW, Flint PW, Haughey BH, et al, editors. Otolaryngology: head & neck surgery. 5th edition. Philadelphia: Mosby Elsevier; 2010. p. 1963–78.

Urinary Tract Infections

Alina Wang, MD, Parminder Nizran, MD, Michael A. Malone, MD*,
Timothy Riley, MD

KEYWORDS

- Urinary tract infection • UTI • Pyelonephritis • Complicated UTI

KEY POINTS

- Urinary tract infections (UTI)s are often differentiated into upper and lower: lower UTIs (acute cystitis) refer to infection of the bladder, whereas upper UTIs (pyelonephritis) refers to infection of the kidney. Clinical presentation helps differentiate between upper and lower UTIs. Risk factors for UTIs include female gender, recent sexual intercourse, recent spermicide use, and a history of previous UTI.
- UTIs are classified as either complicated or uncomplicated. Most UTIs are uncomplicated. A complicated UTI is associated with an underlying condition that increases the risk of failing therapy such as urinary obstruction, instrumentation, anatomic abnormality, catheterization, pathogen multiresistance, or underlying conditions that affect the immune system.
- Primary laboratory tests for UTIs consist of urinalysis and urine culture. Imaging studies are not routinely required. The most common pathogen for uncomplicated cystitis and pyelonephritis is *Escherichia coli* (75%–95%).
- Nitrofurantoin, fosfomycin, and trimethoprim-sulfamethoxazole (TMP-SMX) are first-line therapies for acute uncomplicated cystitis. However, because of the increase in TMP-SMX resistance to levels greater than 20% in many regions, local resistance levels should be considered before using TMP-SMX.
- Uncomplicated pyelonephritis can be treated as an outpatient, if it is mild or moderate. Complicated or severe pyelonephritis should be treated as an inpatient with parenteral antibiotics. Decisions regarding antibiotic agents should be individualized based on patients' allergies, tolerability, community resistance rates, cost, and availability.

INTRODUCTION

Urinary tract infection (UTI) is a common condition seen in primary care. It is the 15th most common condition seen by family physicians and is the diagnosis code for 2% of family medicine visits.[1] UTIs are more common in women, because of a shorter urethra and the presence of antibacterial substances in male prostatic fluid, with an annual prevalence in women of 11% and a greater than 50% lifetime prevalence.[2]

Penn State Department of Family and Community Medicine, Hershey, PA, USA
* Corresponding author.
E-mail address: mmalone@hmc.psu.edu

Prim Care Clin Office Pract 40 (2013) 687–706
http://dx.doi.org/10.1016/j.pop.2013.06.005
0095-4543/13/$ – see front matter © 2013 Elsevier Inc. All rights reserved.

The incidence of asymptomatic and symptomatic UTI in young healthy adult men is lower, with an annual incidence of less than 1%.[3,4] Lower UTIs (cystitis) make up most UTIs. Upper UTIs are significantly less common, with an annual incidence of 12 to 13 cases per 10,000 women, according to a review study.[5]

UTIs are most common in young women but also occur in postmenopausal women, at a lower incidence rate. In a prospective cohort study of 1017 postmenopausal women followed for 2 years,[6] the estimated incidence of culture-confirmed acute cystitis was 0.07 episodes per person per year.

UTIs are often divided into upper and lower UTIs.[7] Upper and lower UTIs are often differentiated based on clinical presentation (see section on clinical presentation).

Lower UTI

Acute cystitis is an infection of the bladder. It can occur alone or in conjunction with an upper UTI.

Upper UTI

Pyelonephritis is an infection of the kidney.

UTIs are classified as complicated versus uncomplicated. Most episodes of cystitis and pyelonephritis are considered to be uncomplicated in otherwise healthy nonpregnant adult women. Although UTIs in men have traditionally been considered complicated, acute uncomplicated UTIs occasionally occur in healthy men. A complicated UTI, whether localized to the lower or upper tract, is associated with an underlying condition that increases the risk of recurrent infection or treatment failure.

Complicated UTI is associated with an underlying condition that increases the risk of failing therapy (**Box 1**).

Box 1
Factors associated with complicated UTI

Conditions Associated with Complicated UTI

Diabetes

Pregnancy

History of acute pyelonephritis in the past year

Symptoms for 7 or more days before seeking care

Multidrug-resistant pathogen

Hospital-acquired infection

Renal failure

Urinary tract obstruction (benign prostatic hypertrophy, stenosis, stone)

Presence of an indwelling urethral catheter, stent, nephrostomy tube, or urinary diversion

Recent urinary tract instrumentation

Functional or anatomic abnormality of the urinary tract

History of UTI in childhood

Renal transplantation

Immunosuppression

RISK FACTORS FOR UTI

Indwelling catheter and hospitalization: the most important risk factor for bacteriuria is the presence of a catheter[8]; catheter-associated UTI is the most common nosocomial infection; hospitalized patients have a risk of 5% per day while an indwelling catheter is in place[8,9]

Recent or frequent sexual intercourse[10,11]

Recent spermicide use, particularly associated with increased risk of *Staphylococcus saprophyticus* UTI[10,12]

History of previous UTI[10]

Insertive anal intercourse[13]

Lack of circumcision in men[13]

Pelvic examinations and Pap smear[14]

Urinary tract stent

Intermittent bladder catheterization[8]

Obstructive uropathy, including neurogenic bladder and nephrolithiasis

Vesicoureteric reflux or other functional abnormalities

Chemical or radiation injury of uroepithelium

Recent urinary tract instrumentation[15]

Polycystic renal disease[16]

Renal transplantation

Immunodeficiency or immunosuppression[15]

MICROBIOLOGY

Most UTIs are monomicrobial; the most common pathogen is *Escherichia coli*, accounting for 70% to 95% cases of acute uncomplicated cystitis.[5,17]

The second most common pathogen is *Staphylococcus saprophyticus*, accounting for 5% to 15% of UTIs, and occurs mainly in young women. Other less common pathogens include species of Enterobacteriaceae, such as *Klebsiella pneumoniae* and *Proteus mirabilis*.[2,18] The microbial spectrum of complicated UTIs is broader and also includes *Pseudomonas, Enterococcus, Staphylococcus, Serratia, Providencia,* and fungi.[19,20]

Among otherwise healthy nonpregnant women, the isolation of organisms such as lactobacilli, enterococci, group B streptococci, and coagulase-negative staphylococci (other than *Staphylococcus saprophyticus*) most commonly represents contamination of the urine specimen.[21,22]

ANTIMICROBIAL RESISTANCE

There is significant variability in different areas among *E coli* for in vitro susceptibility. In general, resistance rates greater than 20% were reported in all regions for ampicillin, and in many regions for trimethoprim-sulfamethoxazole (TMP-SMX).[23–26] Fluoroquinolone resistance rates show a consistent trend for increasing resistance over time. In a US study of outpatient *E coli* urinary isolates, resistance rates to ciprofloxacin increased from 3% to 17% between 2000 and 2010.[27]

Resistance rates for first-generation and second-generation oral cephalosporins and amoxicillin-clavulanic acid are regionally variable but generally less than 10%.[23–25] However, community-onset UTIs caused by *E coli* strains that produce CTX-M extended-spectrum β-lactamases are increasing.[28]

Nitrofurantoin and fosfomycin have good in vitro activity in all countries investigated. These patterns suggest these 2 agents are appropriate antimicrobials for empirical therapy for cystitis in most regions.[23–25] Nitrofurantoin is more commonly used antibacterial in primary care clinics in United States.

Local resistance rates reported in hospital antibiograms are often distorted by cultures of samples obtained from hospitalized patients or those with complicated UTI. These antibiograms may not predict susceptibilities in women with uncomplicated community-acquired infection, in whom resistance rates tend to be lower.[29–31]

CLINICAL PRESENTATION

In young children, the only symptom of a UTI may be fever (**Table 1**).[15] Infants may feed poorly, vomit, sleep more, or show signs of jaundice. In older children, new-onset urinary incontinence may occur.[32]

DIAGNOSIS
History and Physical Examination

The diagnosis of uncomplicated cystitis or pyelonephritis begins with assessment of the clinical history. History is an important component in the evaluation of UTIs. In 1 study,[15] women who presented with 1 or more symptoms of UTI had approximately 50% probability of infection. Specific combinations of symptoms, such as dysuria and frequency, increased the probability of UTI to more than 90%, effectively ruling in the diagnosis of UTI based on history alone. However, history taking, physical examination, and dipstick urinalysis were not able to reliably rule out UTI when a patient presented with 1 or more symptoms.

Obtaining a history of previous sexually transmitted disease and risky sexual behavior is useful in the assessment of dysuria and urinary symptoms. Vaginal discharge reported on history suggests that vaginitis, cervicitis, or pelvic inflammatory disease may be the cause of the dysuria, and a pelvic examination should be performed in these patients.

Physical examination in all patients should include:

Vital signs to check for fever
Evaluation for flank pain and costovertebral angle tenderness
Abdominal examination to assess suprapubic tenderness and pelvic discomfort

Table 1	
Presentation of upper and lower UTIs	
Part of Urinary Tract Affected	**Presentation**
Upper urinary tract (pyelonephritis)	Flank pain Costovertebral angle tenderness Fever >38°C Sweats Chills Nausea Vomiting Hematuria Rarely: shock, renal failure
Lower urinary tract	Pelvic pressure Suprapubic abdominal pain Urinary frequency Hematuria Burning with urination

Laboratory Testing

Laboratory diagnostic tools consist of urinalysis, with microscopy or dipstick, and urine culture with susceptibility data. A urine Gram stain may be helpful in guiding the choice of empirical therapy, especially in hospitalized patients. A urine culture should be performed in all patients with risk factors for complicated UTIs. Pregnancy testing is also appropriate in women of childbearing age. All patients with suspected pyelonephritis or renal abscess should have blood cultures obtained. A complete blood count may be useful in determining the severity of infection, but is rarely helpful in determining the diagnosis or the need for admission.

Urinalysis

Urinalysis by dipstick or microscopy in the absence of urine culture is often sufficient for diagnosis of uncomplicated cystitis, if symptoms are consistent with a UTI. Urine specimens may be obtained by midstream clean catch, suprapubic aspiration, or catheterization. Urinalysis for evaluation of pyuria and bacteruria are the 2 most important initial laboratory indicators of UTI. However, pyuria and bacteriuria may be absent if the infection does not communicate with the collecting system or if the collecting system is obstructed. Pyuria is typically present in most women with upper and lower UTIs, and its absence suggests consideration of another diagnosis or an obstructing lesion.[33,34]

Dipstick testing
Dipstick testing with suspected UTI usually includes glucose, protein, blood, nitrite, and leukocyte esterase. However, only nitrite, leukocyte esterase (+1 or greater) and blood seem to independently predict UTI.[35] Pyuria, indicated by a positive result of the leukocyte esterase dipstick test, is found in most patients with UTIs. Leukocyte esterase can rapidly screen for pyuria; in 1 study it had a sensitivity of 75% to 96% and specificity of 94% to 98%.[36]

In 1 study,[37] dipstick diagnosis based on findings of nitrite or both leukocyte esterase and blood was 77% sensitive and 79% specific, with a positive predictive value of 81% and a negative predictive value of 65%. However, results of the dipstick test provide little useful information when the history is strongly suggestive of UTI, because even negative results for both tests do not reliably rule out the infection in such cases.[15]

Microscopy
Pyuria In quantifying pyuria by microscopy, the finding of greater than or equal to 10 leukocytes/mL of urine by direct microscopy correlates highly with symptomatic, culture-proven UTIs.

Bacteriuria The determination of bacteriuria by direct microscopy is inaccurate, particularly at lower levels of bacteriuria. Significant bacteriuria, previously defined as greater than or equal to 10^5 CFU/mL of urine, has been redefined with the observation that as few as 10^2 CFU/mL can be associated with significant pyuria and symptoms suggestive of cystitis.[36]

Other urinalysis findings
White blood cell casts The presence of white blood cell casts in the urine is diagnostic of upper tract infection and likely pyelonephritis.

Hematuria The presence of hematuria is helpful because it is common in the setting of UTI but not in urethritis or vaginitis. Hematuria is not a predictor for complicated infection and does not warrant extended therapy. In developing countries, hematuria is suggestive of schistosomiasis.

Proteinuria Proteinuria is commonly observed in infections of the urinary tract, and is typically low grade. More than 2 g of protein per 24 hours suggests glomerular disease.

Nitrite Nitrite reflects the presence of Enterobacteriaceae (gram-negative bacteria), which convert urinary nitrate to nitrite. The nitrite test is sensitive and specific for detecting 10^5 or more CFU of Enterobacteriaceae per milliliter of urine, although it lacks adequate sensitivity for detection of other organisms, so negative results should be interpreted with caution. This test has a sensitivity and specificity of 22% and 94% to 100%, respectively. False-positive nitrite tests can occur with substances that turn the urine red, such as phenazopyridine or ingestion of beets.[34,36]

Urine culture

Urine culture remains the standard for the diagnosis of UTI. A few decades ago, most experts believed that urine cultures were unnecessary in young women with probable cystitis because almost all were caused by pansusceptible isolates of *E coli*. The causative pathogens and their susceptibility profiles are frequently predictable in women with uncomplicated UTI. However, antibiotic resistance in uropathogenic *E coli* has become a significant concern. Therefore, the need for routine and posttreatment urine cultures in nonpregnant women with acute dysuria is controversial, although there is little evidence for routine urine cultures on all patients with dysuria.[7,36,38,39]

The 2010 Infectious Disease Society of America consensus limits for cystitis and pyelonephritis in women: more than 1000 CFU/mL and more than 10,000 CFU/mL, respectively, for clean catch midstream urine specimens. Historically, the definition of UTI was based on the finding at culture of 100,000 CFU/mL of a single organism.[7] However, this definition missed up to 50% of symptomatic infections, and therefore, the lower colony rate of greater than 1000 CFU/mL is now accepted.[40] The definition of asymptomatic bacteriuria still uses the historical threshold and is defined as a urine culture (clean catch or catheterized specimen) growing greater than 100,000 CFU/mL in an asymptomatic individual.[7]

Any amount of pathogen on a culture from a suprapubic aspirate should be considered evidence of a UTI.

Indications for a urine culture[2,36,39,41]:
    Symptoms are atypical
    Risk factor(s) for a complicated UTI are present
    Pregnancy
    Patient treated for a UTI within 3 months with recurrence or persistence of
        symptoms
    Suspected or diagnosed pyelonephritis

Imaging Studies

Imaging studies are not routinely required for the diagnosis of acute uncomplicated pyelonephritis, but may be helpful in patients with known urinary tract structural abnormality or renal insufficiency. Computed tomography (CT) and ultrasonography are useful modalities to evaluate for the presence of an underlying anatomic abnormality or abscess, but CT is generally the study of choice to detect complicated UTIs.[42–45] CT is more sensitive than excretory urography or renal ultrasonography for detecting renal abnormalities caused by infection and in delineating the extent of disease.[42–44]

Renal ultrasonography is appropriate in patients for whom exposure to contrast or radiation is undesirable. Magnetic resonance imaging is not advantageous over CT except when avoidance of contrast dye or ionizing radiation is necessary.[46]

Imaging should be obtained or considered if the patient has pyelonephritis and[47,48]:
    Persistent clinical symptoms after 48 to 72 hours of appropriate antibiotic therapy
    Symptoms consistent with renal stones
    Diabetes
    Highly virulent pathogen
    History of urologic surgery
    Immunosuppression
    Recurrent pyelonephritis

LOWER UTI TREATMENT
Asymptomatic Bacteriuria

Prospective, randomized trials consistently conclude that antimicrobial therapy for asymptomatic bacteriuria is not beneficial in most populations.[49-55] The main exception is in pregnant women, who benefit from treatment of asymptomatic bacteriuria.

Nonantibiotic Treatments

Phenazopyridine
For some patients with cystitis, a urinary analgesic such as over-the-counter oral phenazopyridine 3 times daily as needed may be useful to relieve discomfort caused by severe dysuria. A 2-day course is usually sufficient to allow time for symptomatic response to antimicrobial therapy and minimize inflammation. Dysuria is usually diminished within a few hours after the start of antimicrobial therapy.[56] Phenazopyridine should not be used chronically because it may mask clinical symptoms requiring clinical evaluation.

Antibiotics for Cystitis

Without treatment, 25% to 42% of uncomplicated acute cystitis cases in women resolve spontaneously.[57] Even without effective treatment, the likelihood that uncomplicated acute cystitis progresses to pyelonephritis is only around 2%.[58] However, the standard therapy for all UTIs is antibiotic treatment.

Considerations in selecting an antibiotic agent for treatment of acute cystitis includes efficacy, risk of adverse effects, resistance rates, propensity to cause ecological adverse effects of antimicrobial therapy, cost, and drug availability. None of the antimicrobials available clearly outweighs the others in terms of optimizing each of these factors for treatment of acute cystitis. The optimal antibiotic may also differ based on geographic region.

Appropriate antimicrobials for treatment of acute uncomplicated cystitis in women
First-choice agents for treatment of uncomplicated acute cystitis in the United States include:

- Nitrofurantoin monohydrate/macrocrystals
- TMP-SMX
- Fosfomycin

Nitrofurantoin (100 mg orally twice daily for 5–7 days): nitrofurantoin is a reasonable first-line therapy for uncomplicated acute cystitis based on clinical efficacy and cost.[59] It is bactericidal in urine at therapeutic doses. Clinical efficacy rate with a 5-day to

7-day regimen is 90% to 95% based on randomized trials with minimal resistance and ecological adverse effects.[60–62] Nitrofurantoin should be avoided if there is suspicion for early pyelonephritis and is contraindicated when creatinine clearance is less than 60 mL/min.

TMP-SMX (1 double-strength tablet [160/800 mg] twice daily for 3 days): TMP-SMX has shown early clinical efficacy rate with a 3-day to 7-day regimen of 86% to 100% based on randomized trials, although more recent studies show higher resistance.[60–64] However, the conclusion from a more recent study notes that TMP-SMX may no longer be acceptable for the treatment of acute uncomplicated cystitis in the United States because of high resistance rates greater than 20% in many regions.[65] Although there is some debate on the use of empirical TMP-SMX for acute cystitis, it should be avoided as empirical treatment if the prevalence of resistance is known to be high in the area or if the patient has taken TMP-SMX for cystitis in the preceding 3 months. However, use of TMP-SMX is acceptable if the infecting strain is known to be susceptible.[66]

In some instances, trimethoprim, at a dose of 100 mg twice daily × 3 days, is used in place of TMP-SMX and is considered equivalent. This dose could be considered as a regimen in patients who are sulfa-allergic and have sensitivity on culture to TMP-SMX.[38]

Resistance to TMP-SMX has been associated with concomitant resistance to other antibiotics. Because of the importance of maintaining the effectiveness of TMP-SMX for treatment of serious infections, German national guidelines no longer recommend this agent as first-line empirical treatment of uncomplicated cystitis.[67]

Fosfomycin trometamol in a 3-g single dose: fosfomycin is a bactericidal agent with a clinical efficacy rate that seems to be similar to that of nitrofurantoin.[62,68] Fosfomycin has minimal resistance and ecological adverse effects. Fosfomycin should be avoided if there is suspicion for early pyelonephritis.

Pivmecillinam at 400 mg orally twice daily for 3 to 7 days: pivmecillinam is an extended gram-negative spectrum penicillin used only for treatment of UTI. It is not available in the United States, but is a therapy for choice in many Nordic countries because of low resistance rates and low propagation of resistance.[69] Pivmecillinam should be avoided if there is suspicion for early pyelonephritis.

Fluoroquinolones: 3-day regimens are reasonable alternative second-line agents. Multiple randomized trials have shown that fluoroquinolones are effective for treatment of acute cystitis, although increased resistance is mitigating the usefulness of the fluoroquinolone class.[61,70–72] When possible, fluoroquinolones should be reserved for important uses other than acute cystitis and are therefore not first-line agents for uncomplicated acute cystitis.[73]

Oral β-lactams: β-lactam antibiotics may be used when usual first-line agents are not appropriate.[7,67] However, oral β-lactams seem to be less effective than fluoroquinolones and TMP-SMX (**Table 2**).[74,75]

Treatment of complicated lower UTIs (cystitis)

Patients with complicated cystitis who can tolerate oral therapy may be treated with an oral fluoroquinolone such as ciprofloxacin for 5 to 14 days. Nitrofurantoin, TMP-SMX, fosfomycin, and oral β-lactams are poor choices for empirical oral therapy in complicated cystitis because of high prevalence of resistance among causative pathogens. However, use of these antibiotics is acceptable if the isolate is known to be susceptible. Presence of gram-positive cocci is suggestive of enterococci, which is typically treated empirically with penicillins such as amoxicillin, ampicillin, or amoxicillin-clavulanate.

The optimal duration of antimicrobial therapy for the treatment of acute symptomatic complicated UTIs has not been systematically studied. A uniform

Table 2
Treatment of uncomplicated cystitis in nonpregnant women

First-Line Therapy	Second-Line/Alternative Therapy

Fosfomycin[a]
    3 g orally as a single dose
	Quinolones (ciprofloxacin, levofloxacin)
	    Ciprofloxacin or levofloxacin 250 mg orally BID for 3 d

Nitrofurantoin[a]
    100 mg orally BID for 5–7 d
	Cephalosporin
	    Cefdinir 300 mg orally BID for 7 d, cefaclor 500 mg
	    orally TID for 7 d, cefuroxime 250 mg orally BID for
	    7–10 d

TMP-SMX[b]
    160 mg/800 mg orally BID for 3 d
	Amoxicillin-clavulanate
	    500 mg/125 mg orally BID for 3–7 d

[a] In the setting of diagnostic uncertainty regarding cystitis versus early pyelonephritis, nitrofuran-toin and fosfomycin should be avoided because of poor tissue penetration for pyelonephritis.
[b] Use when resistance levels are <20%.
Data from Gupta K, Hooton TM, Naber KG, et al. International clinical practice guidelines for the treatment of acute uncomplicated cystitis and pyelonephritis in women: a 2010 update by the Infectious Diseases Society of America and the European Society for Microbiology and Infectious Diseases. Clin Infect Dis 2011;52(5):e103.

recommendation for treatment duration is likely not appropriate because of variation of the types and severity of complicated UTIs. Most clinical trials have evaluated 7 to 14 days of therapy, but as short as 5 days has been shown to be efficacious.[76–86] However, using a 3-day regimen is not recommended or proved to be effective. For example, a prospective randomized clinical trial of 3 versus 14 days of ciprofloxacin therapy in patients with spinal cord injury reported fewer symptomatic relapses after therapy than with the 14-day treatment.[87]

A 7-day regimen is suggested for patients presenting with symptoms consistent with lower tract infection, and a longer 10-day to 14-day course is recommended for patients with more severe presentations manifested by fever, bacteremia, or hypo-tension (**Box 2**).[88]

Intravenous treatment of complicated cystitis

Parenteral regimens that may be administered once daily include levofloxacin, cipro-floxacin, ceftriaxone, carbapenem, or an aminoglycoside. Dose and duration often vary based on the severity of the infection.[89]

PYELONEPHRITIS

Pyelonephritis is an ascending UTI that has reached the pelvis of the kidney. It is diag-nosed clinically based on history and physical and laboratory findings (see **Table 1** for clinical presentation).

Box 2
First-line oral treatment of complicated lower UTI

First-Line Oral Treatment

Ciprofloxacin

    500 mg orally twice a day x (5) 7–14 days

Levofloxacin

    750 mg orally daily x (5) 7–14 days

Evaluation of Pyelonephritis

Urinalysis/other laboratory tests: see section on urinalysis and evaluation for cystitis.
    Urine culture: should be obtained in all patients with suspected pyelonephritis.
    Blood culture: should be obtained in all patients hospitalized with pyelonephritis.

Treatment of Acute Pyelonephritis

Empirical antibiotic therapy should be started immediately in all patients with suspected pyelonephritis, with a regimen tailored appropriately by susceptibility testing.[7] Hospital antibiotic treatment should use an intravenous (IV) antimicrobial regimen such as fluoroquinolone; aminoglycoside, with or without ampicillin; extended-spectrum cephalosporin or extended-spectrum penicillin, with or without an aminoglycoside; or a carbapenem.

Oral ciprofloxacin at a dose of 500 mg twice daily for 7 days is an appropriate choice for outpatient therapy, when resistance of community uropathogens to fluoroquinolones does not exceed 10%. If the prevalence of fluoroquinolone resistance is believed to be high (>10%), an initial 1-time IV dose of a long-acting parenteral antimicrobial, such as 1 g of ceftriaxone or a consolidated 24-hour dose of an aminoglycoside is recommended. Oral β-lactam agents are less effective than most other agents available for the treatment of pyelonephritis. If an oral β-lactam agent is used, an initial IV dose of a long-acting parenteral antibiotic, such as ceftriaxone or aminoglycoside, is also recommended. The use of nitrofurantoin, fosfomycin, and pivmecillinam should be avoided in the setting of pyelonephritis, because they do not achieve suitable renal tissue levels.[7]

Urine culture and susceptibility testing should be performed in patients with known or suspected pyelonephritis. Initial empirical therapy should be tailored appropriately by the infecting pathogen. The approach to empirical therapy depends on the severity of illness, the prevalence of resistant pathogens in the community, and specific host factors such as allergy or intolerance history.[7]

Complicated Pyelonephritis

All patients with complicated pyelonephritis should initially be managed in the hospital setting. Underlying urinary tract anatomic or functional abnormalities (such as obstruction or neurogenic bladder) should be addressed in consultation with a urologist (**Table 3**).[90]

Table 3 Treatment of complicated pyelonephritis[a]	
Antibiotic	Dosing
Mild to Moderate Complicated Pyelonephritis	
Cefepime or ceftriaxone	1 g daily
Ciprofloxacin	400 mg q 12 h
Levofloxacin	750 mg daily
Aztreonam	1 g q 8 h
Complicated Severe Pyelonephritis	
Meropenem	500 mg q 8 h
Imipenem	500 mg q 6 h

[a] Note that duration of therapy varies, and combinations can be used in severe cases.
    Data from Refs.[76–86]

Pyelonephritis Inpatient Management

Indications for inpatient management:

Complicated pyelonephritis
Severe illness with high fever, pain, and marked debility
Inability to maintain oral hydration or take oral medications
Pregnancy
Concerns about patient compliance

Inpatient antibiotic regimen

Women with pyelonephritis requiring hospitalization should be treated initially with an IV antimicrobial regimen such as a fluoroquinolone, aminoglycoside, extended-spectrum cephalosporin, extended-spectrum penicillin, or a carbapenem.[21] Carbapenems are widely regarded as the drug of choice for pyelonephritis caused by extended-spectrum β-lactamase–producing strains.[91]

Patients initially treated with parenteral therapy, who are able to tolerate fluids and medication orally, can be transitioned to oral antibiotic therapy. Serum fluoroquinolone levels achieved with oral and IV dosing are equivalent, and the modes of delivery are equally effective clinically.[92] The duration of antibiotic therapy does not need to be extended with bacteremia in the absence of other complicating factors, because there is no evidence that bacteremia portends a worse prognosis.[92]

Outpatient Management

Outpatient management is acceptable if none of the indications (listed earlier) for inpatient admission is present. Outpatient management is acceptable for patients with mild to moderate illness, who can be stabilized with rehydration and antibiotics in an outpatient facility and discharged on oral antibiotics under close supervision. In an emergency department study, a 12-hour observation period with IV antibiotics followed by completion of outpatient oral antibiotics was effective for 97% of patients.[93]

Outpatient antibiotic treatment

Fluoroquinolones are the only oral antimicrobials recommended for outpatient empirical treatment of acute uncomplicated pyelonephritis.[7] Fluoroquinolones remain highly effective for treatment of pyelonephritis when the infecting pathogen is susceptible, but there is increasing resistance to this drug class. From 2000 to 2010, the antimicrobial resistance of urinary E coli isolates to ciprofloxacin and TMP-SMX among outpatients increased substantially.[24] In the setting of fluoroquinolone hypersensitivity or known resistance, TMP-SMX or an oral β-lactam could be used, but only in combination with an initial intramuscular/IV dose of a long-acting parenteral cephalosporin or aminoglycoside.[94] Use of nitrofurantoin, fosfomycin, and pivmecillinam should be avoided in the setting of pyelonephritis, because they do not achieve adequate renal tissue levels.[7]

For antibiotic treatment regimens used in complicated pyelonephritis see **Table 3**.

RECURRENT UTIS

Definition: recurrent UTI refers to 2 or more infections in 6 months or 3 or more infections in 1 year.[95]

Recurrent UTI Epidemiology

Recurrent uncomplicated UTIs are common among young, healthy women, even although they generally have anatomically and physiologically normal urinary tracts.[96]

For uncomplicated UTIs, there is no evidence that recurrent UTI leads to chronic health problems such as hypertension or renal disease. When the initial infection is caused by *E coli*, women seem to be more likely to develop a second UTI within 6 months than those with a first UTI caused by another organism.[97] In a Finnish study of women ages 17 to 82 years who had *E coli* cystitis,[98] 44% had a recurrence within 1 year. Recurrent pyelonephritis in healthy women is uncommon.

Evidence-Based Recommendations for Recurrent UTIs

Urinalysis and midstream urine culture and sensitivity should be performed with the first presentation of symptoms to establish the correct diagnosis of recurrent UTI.[95] Patients with persistent hematuria or persistent growth of bacteria aside from *E coli* should undergo cystoscopy and imaging of the upper urinary tract.

Sexually active women suffering from recurrent UTIs and using spermicide should be encouraged to consider an alternative form of contraception. Women with recurrent UTI associated with sexual intercourse should be offered postcoital prophylaxis as an alternative to continuous therapy to minimize cost and side effects.

Pregnant women at risk of recurrent UTI should be offered continuous or postcoital prophylaxis with nitrofurantoin or cephalexin.

Vaginal estrogen should be offered to postmenopausal women who experience recurrent UTIs.

Prophylaxis for recurrent UTI should not be undertaken until a negative culture 1 to 2 weeks after treatment has confirmed eradication of the UTI. Continuous daily antibiotic prophylaxis using cotrimoxazole, nitrofurantoin, cephalexin, trimethoprim, TMP-SMX, or a quinolone during a 6-month to 12-month period should be offered to women with 2 UTIs or more in 6 months or 3 UTIs or more in 12 months. Acute self-treatment should be restricted to compliant and motivated patients in whom recurrent UTIs have been clearly documented.

Patients should be informed that cranberry products are effective in reducing recurrent UTIs. Acupuncture may be considered as an alternative in the prevention of recurrent UTIs in women who are unresponsive to or intolerant of antibiotic prophylaxis. Probiotics and vaccines are not proven therapy for recurrent UTI.

Complications[99]:
   Renal or perinephric abscess
   Bacteremia/sepsis
   Acute kidney injury
   Papillary necrosis
   Emphysematous pyelonephritis

FOLLOW-UP

Follow-up urine cultures are not needed in patients with acute cystitis or pyelonephritis whose symptoms resolve on antibiotics.

Patients with acute cystitis or pyelonephritis who have persistent symptoms after 48 to 72 hours of appropriate antimicrobial therapy or recurrent symptoms within a few weeks of treatment should be changed to a different antibiotic, with imaging if warranted (see section on diagnosis), and a repeat urine culture should be obtained.

FUTURE RESEARCH

Antibiotics represent the standard treatment of UTI; however, even after treatment, patients frequently suffer from recurrent infection with the same or different strains.

In addition, successful long-term treatment has been complicated by an increase in both the number of antibiotic-resistant strains and the prevalence of antibiotic resistance mechanisms. As a result, preventative approaches to UTI, such as vaccination, are being sought and developed, but there are no safe and effective vaccines.[100]

Special Populations

UTI in children

Eight percent of girls and 2% of boys have a UTI by age 2 years. Pathogens are similar in children, with *E coli* predominating. Childhood UTIs can be associated with long-term negative outcomes, including hypertension, toxemia in pregnancy, and chronic renal failure.[101]

Diagnosis and first UTI workup UTI should be suspected in febrile infants without an obvious source. Urine specimens collected with a bag are considered insufficient to make a diagnosis. Transurethral and suprapubic catheterization are accepted methods of urine collection in children. Sensitivity and specificity of urinalysis components are similar in children compared with adults. All children younger than 3 years diagnosed with a first UTI should have a renal ultrasound scan and a voiding cysturethrogram (VCUG). Boys older than 3 years can either have ultrasonography with VCUG or a renal cortical scan with follow-up VCUG as indicated based on the results. Girls between the ages of 3 and 7 years should have either ultrasonography with VCUG or a renal scan if febrile, or observation without imaging if afebrile. Girls older than 7 years can be observed without imaging.[101]

Antibiotic treatment First-line antimicrobial agents include the β-lactams amoxicillin-clavulanate (25–45 mg/kg/d divided every 12 hours), cephalexin (25–50 mg/kg/d, divided every 6–12 hours), and cefpodoxime (10 mg/kg/d divided every 12 hours), as well as TMP-SMX (8–10 mg/kg/d divided every 12 hours). Two-day to 4-day courses have been shown to be as effective as 7 to 14 days.

Acute pyelonephritis can be treated with 10 to 14 days of oral therapy or 2 to 4 days of IV therapy followed by oral antibiotics to complete 10 to 14 days. Hospitalization is indicated for toxic-appearing children or those unable to succeed on oral therapy. An aminoglycoside is recommended if IV therapy is initiated. Fluoroquinolones have traditionally been avoided in children. However, Cipro is now approved by the US Food and Drug Administration for treatment of *E coli*–complicated UTI or pyelonephritis between the ages of 1 and 17 years. Nonetheless, the American Academy of Pediatrics has recommended reserving use of fluoroquinolones for use with multidrug-resistant or *Pseudomonas* infections. Aminoglycosides should be used in their place for hospitalized patients with acute pyelonephritis.[101]

Prevention Prophylactic antibiotics are useful only in cases of severe vesicoureteral reflux. Circumcision decreases the risk of UTI, but benefits do not outweigh risks of surgical complications. Cranberry juice has not been shown to be effective in children.[101]

UTI in pregnancy

Bacteriuria occurs in prevalence and organisms similar to that seen in nonpregnant women.[102] Unlike in nonpregnant patients, in whom asymptomatic bacteriuria is not treated, all bacteriuria in pregnant women should be treated whether it is symptomatic or not. Treatment of bacteriuria in pregnant women reduces the risk of the associated complications in the following list[103–114]:

Preterm birth
Preterm premature rupture of membranes

Low birth weight
Perinatal mortality
Pyelonephritis (75% right-sided in pregnant women)

REFERENCES

1. Pace WD, Dickinson LM, Staton EW. Seasonal variation in diagnoses and visits to family physicians. Ann Fam Med 2004;2(5):411–7.
2. Fihn SD. Clinical practice. Acute uncomplicated urinary tract infection in women. N Engl J Med 2003;349(3):259–66.
3. Krieger JN, Ross SO, Simonsen JM. Urinary tract infections in healthy university men. J Urol 1993;149(5):1046.
4. Vorland LH, Carlson K, Aalen O. An epidemiological survey of urinary tract infections among outpatients in Northern Norway. Scand J Infect Dis 1985;17(3):277.
5. Czaja CA, Scholes D, Hooton TM, et al. Population-based epidemiologic analysis of acute pyelonephritis. Clin Infect Dis 2007;45(3):273.
6. Jackson SL, Boyko EJ, Scholes D, et al. Predictors of urinary tract infection after menopause: a prospective study. Am J Med 2004;117(12):903.
7. Gupta K, Hooton TM, Naber KG, et al. International clinical practice guidelines for the treatment of acute uncomplicated cystitis and pyelonephritis in women: a 2010 update by the Infectious Diseases Society of America and the European Society for Microbiology and Infectious Diseases. Clin Infect Dis 2011;52(5):e103.
8. Hameed A, Chinegwundoh F, Thwaini A. Prevention of catheter-related urinary tract infections. Br J Hosp Med (Lond) 2010;71(3):148–50, 151–2.
9. Klevens RM, Edwards JR, Richards CL Jr, et al. Estimating health care-associated infections and deaths in U.S. hospitals, 2002. Public Health Rep 2007;122(2):160–6.
10. Scholes D, Hooton TM, Roberts PL, et al. Risk factors associated with acute pyelonephritis in healthy women. Ann Intern Med 2005;142(1):20.
11. Hooton TM, Scholes D, Hughes JP, et al. A prospective study of risk factors for symptomatic urinary tract infection in young women. N Engl J Med 1996;335(7): 468–74.
12. Fihn SD, Boyko EJ, Chen CL, et al. Use of spermicide-coated condoms and other risk factors for urinary tract infection caused by Staphylococcus saprophyticus. Arch Intern Med 1998;158(3):281–7.
13. Hooton TM, Stamm WE. Diagnosis and treatment of uncomplicated urinary tract infection. Infect Dis Clin North Am 1997;11(3):551.
14. Tiemstra JD, Chico PD, Pela E. Genitourinary infections after a routine pelvic exam. J Am Board Fam Med 2011;24(3):296–303.
15. Bent S, Nallamothu BK, Simel DL, et al. Does this woman have an acute uncomplicated urinary tract infection? JAMA 2002;287(20):2701–10.
16. Hwang JH, Park HC, Jeong JC, et al. Chronic asymptomatic pyuria precedes overt urinary tract infection and deterioration of renal function in autosomal dominant polycystic kidney disease. BMC Nephrol 2013;14:1.
17. Echols RM, Tosiello RL, Haverstock DC, et al. Demographic, clinical, and treatment parameters influencing the outcome of acute cystitis. Clin Infect Dis 1999; 29(1):113.
18. Grabe M, Bjerklund-Johansen TE, Botto H, et al, European Association of Urology (EAU). Guidelines on urological infections. EAU 2013.
19. Nicolle LE. Complicated urinary tract infection in adults. Can J Infect Dis Med Microbiol 2005;16(6):349–60.

20. Warren JW. Catheter-associated urinary tract infections. Infect Dis Clin North Am 1987;1(4):823–54.
21. Hooton TM. Clinical practice. Uncomplicated urinary tract infection. N Engl J Med 2012;366(11):1028–37.
22. Gupta K, Trautner B. In the clinic. Urinary tract infection. Ann Intern Med 2012; 156(5):ITC3-1–15.
23. Kahlmeter G. An international survey of the antimicrobial susceptibility of pathogens from uncomplicated urinary tract infections: the ECO.SENS Project. J Antimicrob Chemother 2003;51(1):69.
24. Naber KG, Schito G, Botto H, et al. Surveillance study in Europe and Brazil on clinical aspects and Antimicrobial Resistance Epidemiology in Females with Cystitis (ARESC): implications for empiric therapy. Eur Urol 2008;54(5): 1164.
25. Zhanel GG, Hisanaga TL, Laing NM, et al. Antibiotic resistance in *Escherichia coli* outpatient urinary isolates: final results from the North American Urinary Tract Infection Collaborative Alliance (NAUTICA). Int J Antimicrob Agents 2006;27(6):468.
26. Sanchez GV, Master RN, Karlowsky JA, et al. In vitro antimicrobial resistance of urinary *Escherichia coli* isolates among U.S. outpatients from 2000 to 2010. Antimicrobial Agents Chemother 2012;56(4):2181–3.
27. Swami SK, Liesinger JT, Shah N, et al. Incidence of antibiotic-resistant *Escherichia coli* bacteriuria according to age and location of onset: a population-based study from Olmsted County, Minnesota. Mayo Clin Proc 2012;87(8): 753 9.
28. Prakash V, Lewis JS 2nd, Herrera ML, et al. Oral and parenteral therapeutic options for outpatient urinary infections caused by Enterobacteriaceae producing CTX-M extended-spectrum beta-lactamases. Antimicrobial Agents Chemother 2009;53(3):1278–80.
29. Miller LG, Tang AW. Treatment of uncomplicated urinary tract infections in an era of increasing antimicrobial resistance. Mayo Clin Proc 2004;79(8):1048.
30. Schito GC, Naber KG, Botto H, et al. The ARESC study: an international survey on the antimicrobial resistance of pathogens involved in uncomplicated urinary tract infections. Int J Antimicrob Agents 2009;34(5):407.
31. Ho PL, Yip KS, Chow KH, et al. Antimicrobial resistance among uropathogens that cause acute uncomplicated cystitis in women in Hong Kong: a prospective multicenter study in 2006 to 2008. Diagn Microbiol Infect Dis 2010;66(1):87.
32. Bhat RG, Katy TA, Place FC. Pediatric urinary tract infections. Emerg Med Clin North Am 2011;29(3):637–53.
33. Stamm WE. Measurement of pyuria and its relation to bacteriuria. Am J Med 1983;75(1B):53.
34. Wilson ML, Gaido L. Laboratory diagnosis of urinary tract infections in adult patients. Clin Infect Dis 2004;38(8):1150.
35. Little P, Turner S, Rumsby K, et al. Developing clinical rules to predict urinary tract infection in primary care settings: sensitivity and specificity of near patient tests (dipsticks) and clinical scores. Br J Gen Pract 2006;56(529):606–12.
36. Pappas PG. Laboratory in the diagnosis and management of urinary tract infections. Med Clin North Am 1991;75(2):313.
37. Little P, Turner S, Rumsby K, et al. Dipsticks and diagnostic algorithms in urinary tract infection: development and validation, randomised trial, economic analysis, observational cohort and qualitative study. Health Technol Assess 2009; 13(19):iii–iv, ix–xi, 1–73.

38. Warren JW, Abrutyn E, Hebel JR, et al. Guidelines for antimicrobial treatment of uncomplicated acute bacterial cystitis and acute pyelonephritis in women. Infectious Diseases Society of America (IDSA). Clin Infect Dis 1999;29(4):745.

39. McIsaac WJ, Low DE, Biringer A, et al. The impact of empirical management of acute cystitis on unnecessary antibiotic use. Arch Intern Med 2002;162(5): 600.

40. Mehnert-Kay SA. Diagnosis and management of uncomplicated urinary tract infections. Am Fam Physician 2005;72(3):451–6.

41. Gupta K, Hooton TM, Stamm WE. Increasing antimicrobial resistance and the management of uncomplicated community-acquired urinary tract infections. Ann Intern Med 2001;135(1):41.

42. Meyrier A, Condamin MC, Fernet M, et al. Frequency of development of early cortical scarring in acute primary pyelonephritis. Kidney Int 1989;35(2):696.

43. Tsugaya M, Hirao N, Sakagami H, et al. Computerized tomography in acute pyelonephritis: the clinical correlations. J Urol 1990;144(3):611.

44. Kawashima A, LeRoy AJ. Radiologic evaluation of patients with renal infections. Infect Dis Clin North Am 2003;17(2):433.

45. Johnson JR, Vincent LM, Wang K, et al. Renal ultrasonographic correlates of acute pyelonephritis. Clin Infect Dis 1992;14(1):15.

46. Demertzis J, Menias CO. State of the art: imaging of renal infections. Emerg Radiol 2007;14(1):13.

47. Sandberg T, Stokland E, Brolin I, et al. Selective use of excretory urography in women with acute pyelonephritis. J Urol 1989;141(6):1290.

48. Kanel KT, Kroboth FJ, Schwentker FN, et al. The intravenous pyelogram in acute pyelonephritis. Arch Intern Med 1988;148(10):2144.

49. Nicolle LE, Mayhew WJ, Bryan L. Prospective randomized comparison of therapy and no therapy for asymptomatic bacteriuria in institutionalized elderly women. Am J Med 1987;83(1):27–33.

50. Ouslander JG, Shapira M, Schnelle JF, et al. Does eradicating bacteriuria affect the severity of chronic urinary incontinence in nursing home residents? Ann Intern Med 1995;122:749–54.

51. Boscia JA, Kobasa WD, Knight RA, et al. Therapy vs no therapy for bacteriuria in elderly ambulatory nonhospitalized women. JAMA 1987;257:1062–71.

52. Mohler JL, Cowen DL, Flanigan RC. Suppression and treatment of urinary tract infection in patients with an intermittently catheterized neurogenic bladder. J Urol 1987;138:336–40.

53. Warren JW, Anthony WC, Hoopes JM, et al. Cephalexin for susceptible bacteriuria in afebrile, long-term catheterized patients. JAMA 1982;248:454–8.

54. Harding GK, Nicolle LE, Ronald AR, et al. How long should catheter-acquired urinary tract infection in women be treated? A randomized controlled study. Ann Intern Med 1991;114:713–9.

55. Harding GK, Zhanel GG, Nicolle LE, et al, Manitoba Diabetic Urinary Infection Study Group. Antimicrobial treatment in diabetic women with asymptomatic bacteriuria. N Engl J Med 2002;347:1576–83.

56. Klimberg I, Shockey G, Ellison H, et al. Time to symptom relief for uncomplicated urinary tract infection treated with extended-release ciprofloxacin: a prospective, open-label, uncontrolled primary care study. Curr Med Res Opin 2005; 21(8):1241–50.

57. Falagas ME, Kotsantis IK, Vouloumanou EK, et al. Antibiotics versus placebo in the treatment of women with uncomplicated cystitis: a meta-analysis of randomized controlled trials. J Infect 2009;58(2):91–102.

58. Christiaens TC, De Meyere M, Verschraegen G, et al. Randomised controlled trial of nitrofurantoin versus placebo in the treatment of uncomplicated urinary tract infection in adult women. Br J Gen Pract 2002;52(482):729–34.
59. McKinnell JA, Stollenwerk NS, Jung CW, et al. Nitrofurantoin compares favorably to recommended agents as empirical treatment of uncomplicated urinary tract infections in a decision and cost analysis. Mayo Clin Proc 2011;86(6): 480.
60. Gupta K, Hooton TM, Roberts PL, et al. Short-course nitrofurantoin for the treatment of acute uncomplicated cystitis in women. Arch Intern Med 2007;167(20): 2207.
61. Iravani A, Klimberg I, Briefer C, et al. A trial comparing low-dose, short-course ciprofloxacin and standard 7 day therapy with co-trimoxazole or nitrofurantoin in the treatment of uncomplicated urinary tract infection. J Antimicrob Chemother 1999;43(Suppl A):67.
62. Stein GE. Comparison of single-dose fosfomycin and a 7-day course of nitrofurantoin in female patients with uncomplicated urinary tract infection. Clin Ther 1999;21(11):1864.
63. Kavatha D, Giamarellou H, Alexiou Z, et al. Cefpodoxime-proxetil versus trimethoprim-sulfamethoxazole for short-term therapy of uncomplicated acute cystitis in women. Antimicrobial Agents Chemother 2003;47(3):897.
64. Arredondo-García JL, Figueroa-Damián R, Rosas A, et al. Comparison of short-term treatment regimen of ciprofloxacin versus long-term treatment regimens of trimethoprim/sulfamethoxazole or norfloxacin for uncomplicated lower urinary tract infections: a randomized, multicentre, open-label, prospective study. J Antimicrob Chemother 2004;54(4):840.
65. Sanchez GV, Master RN, Bordon J. Trimethoprim-sulfamethoxazole may no longer be acceptable for the treatment of acute uncomplicated cystitis in the United States. Clin Infect Dis 2011;53(3):316–7.
66. Metlay JP, Strom BL, Asch DA. Prior antimicrobial drug exposure: a risk factor for trimethoprim-sulfamethoxazole-resistant urinary tract infections. J Antimicrob Chemother 2003;51(4):963.
67. Wagenlehner FM, Schmiemann G, Hoyme U, et al. National S3 guideline on uncomplicated urinary tract infection: recommendations for treatment and management of uncomplicated community-acquired bacterial urinary tract infections in adult patients. Urologe A 2011;50(2):153–69 [in German].
68. Van Pienbroek E, Hermans J, Kaptein AA, et al. Fosfomycin trometamol in a single dose versus seven days nitrofurantoin in the treatment of acute uncomplicated urinary tract infections in women. Pharm World Sci 1993;15(6):257–62.
69. Graninger W. Pivmecillinam–therapy of choice for lower urinary tract infection. Int J Antimicrob Agents 2003;22(Suppl 2):73.
70. Nicolle LE, Madsen KS, Debeeck GO, et al. Three days of pivmecillinam or norfloxacin for treatment of acute uncomplicated urinary infection in women. Scand J Infect Dis 2002;34(7):487.
71. Richard GA, Mathew CP, Kirstein JM, et al. Single-dose fluoroquinolone therapy of acute uncomplicated urinary tract infection in women: results from a randomized, double-blind, multicenter trial comparing single-dose to 3-day fluoroquinolone regimens. Urology 2002;59(3):334.
72. Fourcroy JL, Berner B, Chiang YK, et al. Efficacy and safety of a novel once-daily extended-release ciprofloxacin tablet formulation for treatment of uncomplicated urinary tract infection in women. Antimicrobial Agents Chemother 2005;49(10):4137.

73. Hooton TM, Besser R, Foxman B, et al. Acute uncomplicated cystitis in an era of increasing antibiotic resistance: a proposed approach to empirical therapy. Clin Infect Dis 2004;39(1):75.

74. Hooton TM, Scholes D, Gupta K, et al. Amoxicillin-clavulanate vs ciprofloxacin for the treatment of uncomplicated cystitis in women: a randomized trial. JAMA 2005;293(8):949.

75. Rodríguez-Baño J, Alcalá JC, Cisneros JM, et al. Community infections caused by extended-spectrum beta-lactamase-producing *Escherichia coli*. Arch Intern Med 2008;168(17):1897.

76. Ulleryd P, Sandberg T. Ciprofloxacin for 2 or 4 weeks in the treatment of febrile urinary tract infection in men: a randomized trial with a 1 year follow-up. Scand J Infect Dis 2003;35:34–9.

77. Jimenez-Cruz F, Josovich A, Cajigas J, et al. A prospective, multicenter, randomized, double-blind study comparing ertapenem and ceftriaxone followed by appropriate oral therapy for complicated urinary tract infections in adults. Urology 2002;60:16–22.

78. Cox CE, Marbury TC, Pittman WG, et al. A randomized, double-blind multicenter comparison of gatifloxacin vs ciprofloxacin in the treatment of complicated urinary tract infection and pyelonephritis. Clin Ther 2002;24:223–36.

79. Tomera KM, Burdmann EA, Pamo Reyna OG, et al. Ertapenem versus ceftriaxone followed by appropriate oral therapy for treatment of complicated urinary tract infections in adults: results of a prospective, randomized double-blind multicenter study. Antimicrobial Agents Chemother 2002;46:2895–900.

80. Naber KG, Savov O, Salmen HC. Piperacillin 2 g/tazobactam 0.5 g is as effective as imipenem 0.5 g/cilastatin 0.5 g for the treatment of acute uncomplicated pyelonephritis and complicated urinary tract infections. Int J Antimicrob Agents 2002;19:95–103.

81. Raz R, Naber NG, Raizenberg C, et al. Ciprofloxacin 250 mg twice daily versus ofloxacin 200 mg twice daily in the treatment of complicated urinary tract infections in women. Eur J Clin Microbiol Infect Dis 2000;19:327–31.

82. Krcmery S, Naber NG. Ciprofloxacin once versus twice daily in the treatment of complicated urinary tract infections. German Ciprofloxacin UTI Study Group. Int J Antimicrob Agents 1999;11:133–8.

83. Klimberg IW, Cox CE II, Fowler CL, et al. A controlled trial of levofloxacin and lomefloxacin in the treatment of complicated urinary tract infection. Urology 1998;51:610–5.

84. Frankenschmidt A, Naber KG, Bischoff W, et al. Once-daily fleroxacin versus twice-daily ciprofloxacin in the treatment of complicated urinary tract infections. J Urol 1997;158:1494–9.

85. Pisani E, Bartoletti R, Trinchieri A, et al. Lomefloxacin versus ciprofloxacin in the treatment of complicated urinary tract infections: a multicenter study. J Chemother 1996;8:210–3.

86. Naber KG, di Silverio F, Geddes A, et al. Comparative efficacy of sparfloxacin versus ciprofloxacin in the treatment of complicated urinary tract infection. J Antimicrob Chemother 1996;37(Suppl A):135–44.

87. Dow G, Rao P, Harding G, et al. A prospective, randomized trial of 3 or 14 days of ciprofloxacin treatment for acute urinary tract infection in patients with spinal cord injury. Clin Infect Dis 2004;39(5):658–64.

88. Nicolle LE. Catheter-related urinary tract infection. Drugs Aging 2005;22(8):627.

89. Stamm WE, Hooton TM. Management of urinary tract infections in adults. N Engl J Med 1993;329(18):1328.

90. Nicolle LE. A practical guide to the management of complicated urinary tract infection. Drugs 1997;53(4):583.
91. Pitout JD. Infections with extended-spectrum beta-lactamase-producing Enterobacteriaceae: changing epidemiology and drug treatment choices. Drugs 2010;70(3):313.
92. Mombelli G, Pezzoli R, Pinoja-Lutz G, et al. Oral vs intravenous ciprofloxacin in the initial empirical management of severe pyelonephritis or complicated urinary tract infections: a prospective randomized clinical trial. Arch Intern Med 1999; 159(1):53.
93. Ward G, Jorden RC, Severance HW. Treatment of pyelonephritis in an observation unit. Ann Emerg Med 1991;20(3):258.
94. Sanchez M, Collvinent B, Miró O, et al. Short-term effectiveness of ceftriaxone single dose in the initial treatment of acute uncomplicated pyelonephritis in women. A randomised controlled trial. Emerg Med J 2002;19(1):19.
95. Epp A, Larochelle A, Lovatsis D, et al. Recurrent urinary tract infection. J Obstet Gynaecol Can 2010;32(11):1082–90.
96. Foxman B. Recurring urinary tract infection: incidence and risk factors. Am J Public Health 1990;80(3):331.
97. Foxman B, Gillespie B, Koopman J, et al. Risk factors for second urinary tract infection among college women. Am J Epidemiol 2000;151(12):1194.
98. Ikäheimo R, Siitonen A, Heiskanen T, et al. Recurrence of urinary tract infection in a primary care setting: analysis of a 1-year follow-up of 179 women. Clin Infect Dis 1996;22(1):91.
99. Shields J, Maxwell AP. Acute pyelonephritis can have serious complications. Practitioner 2010;254(1728):19, 21, 23–4, 2.
100. Brumbaugh AR, Mobley HL. Preventing urinary tract infection: progress toward an effective *Escherichia coli* vaccine. Expert Rev Vaccines 2012;11(6): 663–76.
101. White B. Diagnosis and treatment of urinary tract infection in children. Am Fam Physician 2011;83(4):409–15.
102. Stenqvist K, Sandberg T, Lidin-Janson G, et al. Virulence factors of *Escherichia coli* in urinary isolates from pregnant women. J Infect Dis 1987;156(6):870–7.
103. Naeye RL. Causes of the excessive rates of perinatal mortality and prematurity in pregnancies complicated by maternal urinary-tract infections. N Engl J Med 1979;300:819.
104. Millar LK, Cox SM. Urinary tract infections complicating pregnancy. Infect Dis Clin North Am 1997;11:13.
105. Patterson TF, Andriole VT. Detection, significance, and therapy of bacteriuria in pregnancy. Update in the managed health care era. Infect Dis Clin North Am 1997;11:593.
106. Delzell JE Jr, Lefevre ML. Urinary tract infections during pregnancy. Am Fam Physician 2000;61:713.
107. Kass EH. Bacteriuria and pyelonephritis of pregnancy. Arch Intern Med 1960; 105:194.
108. Smaill F, Vazquez JC. Antibiotics for asymptomatic bacteriuria in pregnancy. Cochrane Database Syst Rev 2007;(2):CD000490.
109. Lang JM, Lieberman E, Cohen A. A comparison of risk factors for preterm labor and term small-for-gestational-age birth. Epidemiology 1996;7:369.
110. Millar LK, DeBuque L, Wing DA. Uterine contraction frequency during treatment of pyelonephritis in pregnancy and subsequent risk of preterm birth. J Perinat Med 2003;31:41.

111. Whalley PJ, Martin FG, Peters PC. Significance of asymptomatic bacteriuria detected during pregnancy. JAMA 1965;193:879.
112. Rouse DJ, Andrews WW, Goldenberg RL, et al. Screening and treatment of asymptomatic bacteriuria of pregnancy to prevent pyelonephritis: a cost-effectiveness and cost-benefit analysis. Obstet Gynecol 1995;86:119.
113. Mittendorf R, Williams MA, Kass EH. Prevention of preterm delivery and low birth weight associated with asymptomatic bacteriuria. Clin Infect Dis 1992;14:927.
114. Zinner SH, Kass EH. Long-term (10 to 14 years) follow-up of bacteriuria of pregnancy. N Engl J Med 1971;285:820.

Meningitis

Katherine Putz, MD[a],*, Karen Hayani, MD[b], Fred Arthur Zar, MD[c]

KEYWORDS

- Aseptic • Meningismus • Blood-brain barrier • Cerebrospinal fluid • Vaccination
- Prophylaxis • Acute meningitis

KEY POINTS

- Meningitis is an important infectious disease that affects different age groups.
- Bacterial meningitis must be distinguished from aseptic meningitis and specific antimicrobial therapy must be provided emergently.
- The incidence of bacterial meningitis has declined significantly since the advent of routine childhood immunizations.
- Although aseptic meningitis usually follows a benign clinical course, occasionally hospitalization and specific therapy is required.

ASEPTIC MENINGITIS

Aseptic Meningitis: Five Key Points for Primary Care
1. Aseptic meningitis caused by enteroviruses is most common in the summer months, is more common than bacterial meningitis, and generally has a benign clinical course.
2. Aseptic meningitis or meningoencephalitis resulting from herpes simplex virus (HSV) can have serious neurologic sequelae, and empiric therapy with acyclovir is warranted if the clinical course and workup are suggestive of HSV.
3. Neonates and children with meningismus require lumbar puncture and empiric antimicrobial therapy until cerebrospinal fluid (CSF) laboratory results become available.
4. Kernig and Brudzinski signs are insensitive yet highly specific, and thus useful in deciding which patients need a lumbar puncture.
5. Computed tomography (CT) is warranted before lumbar puncture in patients greater than 60 years of age, patients with an abnormal level of consciousness, gaze palsy, facial palsy, arm or leg drift, abnormal visual fields, abnormal language,

[a] Department of Family Medicine, University of Illinois at Chicago, 1919 West Taylor Street MC 663, Chicago, IL 60612, USA; [b] Division of Pediatric Infectious Diseases, Children's Hospital of University of Illinois, University of Illinois at Chicago, 840 South Wood Street, M/C 856, Chicago, IL 60612, USA; [c] M2 Clinical Pathophysiology Course, Department of Medicine (MC 718), College of Medicine, University of Illinois Hospital and Health Sciences System, 840 South Wood Street, Room 440 CSN, Chicago, IL 60612, USA
* Corresponding author.
E-mail address: kasiaputz@gmail.com

Prim Care Clin Office Pract 40 (2013) 707–726
http://dx.doi.org/10.1016/j.pop.2013.06.001
0095-4543/13/$ – see front matter © 2013 Elsevier Inc. All rights reserved.

inability to answer 2 consecutive questions or follow 2 consecutive commands correctly, or history of seizure or immunocompromised state.

Introduction

The etiology may be noninfectious and associated with a systemic disease, medication, or other pathologic factor; however, most cases of aseptic meningitis are caused by viruses (**Table 1**).

Epidemiology

Aseptic meningitis is not a reportable disease in the United States and consequently the prevalence, 10 cases per 100,000 persons per year, is likely underestimated (**Boxes 1–4**).[1]

More than 30 different viruses and subtypes have been shown to cause acute meningitis; however, enteroviruses and their subtypes are the leading etiologic agents and cause 85% to 95% of cases.[12,13] Identification of a specific etiologic agent became possible initially with tissue culture in 1949[3] and subsequently with the polymerase chain reaction (PCR) in 1968. The PCR has become the test of choice and is widely available for HSV, enteroviruses, and other viruses (see **Table 3**). Except in cases of HSV, there are no therapeutic modalities specific for different causes of aseptic meningitis. However, identification may be useful for confirmation of viral infection to allow the discontinuation of antibacterial antibiotics, to allow the continuation or discontinuation of acyclovir, and for epidemiologic purposes.

Pathogenesis and Pathophysiology

Viral transmission to the human host occurs by various routes, and several defense mechanisms exist to prevent further viral spread (see **Table 1**). Local viral replication often occurs in lymphoid tissue close to the site of infection, which may act as a reservoir and cause a secondary viremia.[3] The secondary viremia is more commonly responsible for viral spread to the central nervous system (CNS).[11] Viral CNS invasion occurs by crossing the blood-brain barrier (BBB) via cerebral capillary endothelial cells, protected within leukocytes, by direct spread along olfactory nerves, through the choroid plexus epithelium, or by traveling along peripheral nerves.[14,15] This process stimulates a proliferation of mononuclear cells, in some cases initially polymorphonuclear followed by mononuclear cells. Presentation of viral antigens by mononuclear cells further propagates influx of immune cells causing cytokine release, altered permeability of the BBB, and influx of serum immune globulins. Both humoral and cell-mediated immunity play a role in host protection and elimination of the virus from the CNS.[14] This inflammatory process is responsible for the clinical signs that indicate nerve-root irritation often seen in meningitis, including neck stiffness and physical examination findings.[16] Progression of the inflammatory response can lead to vasculitis, cell necrosis, and cerebral edema.

Clinical Manifestations of Aseptic Meningitis

Symptoms, signs, and sequelae of aseptic meningitis vary depending on the virus, the age, and the immune status of the host (**Table 2**). With the exception of HSV meningitis/meningoencephalitis, most cases of aseptic meningitis are characterized by a benign clinical course. Specific populations in which this disease has the potential for significant morbidity and mortality are those that have deficient humoral immunity: neonates and patients with agammaglobulinemia.[22]

Table 1
Epidemiology and transmission of aseptic meningitis[a]

	Enteroviruses	Mumps	Herpesviruses	Flaviviruses	LCMV
Subtypes	Echoviruses 30, 11, 9, 6, 7, 18, 16, 71, 25 Coxsackie B2, A9, B1, B3, B4		HSV-1, HSV-2 CMV-1, EBV-1, VZV, HHV-61	St Louis encephalitis, West Nile virus, La Crosse virus, Jamestown Canyon virus, snowshoe hare virus	
Incidence (% total cases)	85%–95%		0.5%–3%		Rare
Transmission	Fecal-oral → stomach → viremia	Respiratory droplet → upper respiratory lymphatic system	Close contact with mucosal surface of infected person, viral shedding; sexual	Cutaneous inoculation by vector, local tissue replication → lymphatic system	Ingestion of food contaminated with animal urine, exposure of open wounds to dirt
Primary host defense mechanisms	Gastric acidity Bile, digestive enzymes Secretory IgA	Mucociliary clearance Alveolar macrophages			Gastric acidity, bile, digestive enzymes, secretory IgA, neutrophils, macrophages

Abbreviations: CMV, cytomegalovirus; EBV, Epstein-Barr virus; HHV, human herpesvirus; HSV, herpes simplex virus; IgA, immunoglobulin A; LCMV, lymphocytic choriomeningitis virus; VZV, varicella zoster virus.
[a] Other viruses include adenovirus, parainfluenza virus type 3, influenza virus, measles virus, human immunodeficiency virus.

Box 1
Epidemiology of enteroviruses

- Incidence of aseptic meningitis in any given geographic area often mirrors the prevalence of the enteroviruses
- Of more than 70 subtypes, the 2 most common implicated in meningitis are echovirus 30 and coxsackie A1[2]
- Worldwide distribution: in temperate climates, the infections primarily during May to October; in tropical areas, incidence is high throughout all seasons
- Enteroviruses are the most common cause of aseptic meningitis in adults
- Most cases involve children younger than 5 years, which is due to the lack of prior immunity[3,4]

Box 2
Epidemiology of mumps virus

- Routine vaccination
  - 1998: 82 of 215 countries
  - 2002: 121 of 215 countries[5,6]
- Most cases occur in children 5 to 9 years of age

Box 3
Epidemiology of herpesviruses

- Herpes simplex virus (HSV)-1 and HSV-2 are responsible for 0.5% to 3% of all cases of aseptic meningitis
- HSV-1 and HSV-2 are the most common cause of encephalitis in children and adults[7]
- There is concomitant aseptic meningitis in 36% of women and 13% of men suffering from primary genital infection with HSV-2[8]
- HSV-2: most likely to cause neurologic complications, they are most often transient[9,10]

Box 4
Epidemiology of arboviruses

- General term for arthropod-borne viruses; includes flaviviruses
- St Louis encephalitis virus: endemic to Americas; most commonly in southern and eastern states; most common cause of arthropod-transmitted aseptic meningitis in the United States until 2002
- West Nile virus: important agent from 1999 to 2002; in 2012 incidence increased to 5387 cases, 51% involving neuroinvasive disease[11]; more often associated with encephalitis

Table 2
Clinical manifestations of aseptic meningitis in different populations

	Newborns and Infants <3 mo of Age	Children	Adults	Agammaglobulinemia
History	Maternal perinatal fever, prenatal infections, drug use, sexual history[17] Infant with poor feeding, lethargy, irritability, altered sleep pattern, seizures, rash, vomiting, diarrhea, respiratory difficulty[18]	Sudden onset	Symptoms persistent for over a week Fever, headache, photophobia	
Physical	Bulging anterior fontanelle (late) irritability[18]	Nuchal rigidity, fever, vomiting, salivary gland enlargement (50%), abdominal pain	Fever, nuchal rigidity	Dermatomyositis (50%)
Possible associated findings		Exanthemata, myopericarditis, conjunctivitis, pleurodynia, herpangina, hand-foot-and-mouth disease[19]; Parotitis	Acute extremity weakness (WNV), recurrent disease (Mollaret meningitis), pharyngitis, lymphadenopathy, splenomegaly (EBV)	CEMA: headache, seizures
Complications	Meningoencephalitis with multiorgan involvement (hepatic necrosis, myocarditis, necrotizing enterocolitis)[20]	None[21]		Hearing loss, coma, weakness, ataxia, paresthesias, loss of cognitive skills

Abbreviations: CEMA, chronic meningoencephalitis in agammaglobulinemia; EBV, Epstein-Barr virus; WNV, West Nile virus.

History

In patients of all ages, the current season of the year should be taken into account. History of exposure to sick contacts, travel, sexual history, and substance-abuse history should always be elicited and may point to a specific diagnosis. Patients may provide a history of recent or concomitant respiratory or gastrointestinal infection. The clinical history, however, has low sensitivity and specificity for the diagnosis of meningitis.[23]

Risk factors for severe disease in neonates should be considered to identify patients who would benefit from early and aggressive workup and management[24–26]:

- Onset before 1 week of age
- Prematurity
- Low hemoglobin (<10.7 mg/dL)
- High serum white blood cell count
- Premature birth
- Maternal illness

Physical Examination

Vital signs, assessment of mental status, and physical examination should be performed on all patients presenting with history and symptoms outlined in **Table 2**. Fever is almost always present in all age groups and has a sensitivity of 85%.[27] Of note, nuchal rigidity, bulging anterior fontanelle, and/or headache are absent in more than 90% of children younger than 2 years.[18] Even in older patients, the classic sign of nuchal rigidity and symptoms of photophobia may also be absent in 33%.[4] Because over 99% of adult patients present with fever, nuchal rigidity, headache, or altered mental status, absence of all of these symptoms makes meningitis unlikely.[28,29] Nuchal rigidity alone has a sensitivity of 70%.[23] The sensitivity of Kernig and Brudzinski signs ranges from 5% to 14%; however, the specificity for both signs is greater than 90%.[21,23,27,30,31] A headache that becomes worse with active rapid horizontal head turning is termed jolt accentuation of headache. Although one study suggests a high sensitivity,[27] another failed to confirm this.[21] Altered mental status and focal neurologic signs and seizures are uncommon; if present, they should prompt consideration of viral encephalitis or bacterial meningitis (**Box 5**).[31–33]

Diagnosis

Lumbar puncture should be performed when clinical suspicion for meningitis exists after history and physical examination have been performed. However, elevated intracranial pressure from a space-occupying lesion or inflammation can risk cerebral herniation if lumbar puncture is performed. Thus, CT of the head should be done before the lumbar puncture if suspicion exists for a space-occupying lesion.[34,35] Neonates and infants with open fontanelles do not require a CT scan before lumbar puncture.

Box 5
Meningeal signs

Definition: Kernig sign

Inability or reluctance to allow full extension of the knee when the hip is flexed 90°[23]

Definition: Brudzinski neck sign

Spontaneous flexion of the hips during attempted passive flexion of the neck

In adults, clinical features that indicate an increased likelihood of brain herniation after lumbar puncture have been identified. Absence of all of the following features has a negative predictive value of 97% and can be used to determine the situations whereby it is appropriate to perform lumbar puncture without prior imaging[35]:

• Age ≥60 years	• Immunocompromised state
• Seizure within 1 week of presentation	• History of CNS disease
• Abnormal level of consciousness	• Gaze palsy
• Facial palsy	• Abnormal visual fields
• Arm or leg drift	• Abnormal language
• Inability to answer 2 consecutive questions correctly	
• Inability to follow 2 consecutive commands correctly	

CSF should be assayed for cell count, protein, glucose, culture, Gram stain, and selected viral PCR studies, depending on the clinical presentation (**Table 3**). Pleocytosis is almost always present. The promptness of the PCR method for nucleic acid amplification has lessened the utility of tissue culture for etiologic diagnosis; the latter requires a mean of 3 to 8 days of incubation whereas PCR requires less than 1 day.[36,37] If suggested by the history, a PPD skin test, syphilis serology, serum human immunodeficiency virus (HIV) antibody, and serum HIV RNA PCR should be performed. Results of complete blood count and C-reactive protein are similar to those seen in other viral infections; this may aid in differentiation from bacterial meningitis. The bacterial meningitis score, a clinical prediction rule that identifies pediatric patients at very low risk for bacterial meningitis, can be useful to identify patients 1 month to 19 years old who do not require antimicrobial therapy (**Box 6**).[38,39] This rule cannot be used in patients with any of the following present in their clinical history: immunosuppression, history of neurosurgical procedure, purpura on physical examination, antibiotic use in the preceding 48 hours, or a CSF red blood cell count of 0.01×10^6 or more per microliter.

Table 3
Laboratory findings in aseptic meningitis

Parameter	Findings in Aseptic Meningitis	Notes
CSF opening pressure	Normal (<180 mm H_2O) or slightly elevated	Must be measured in lateral recumbent position
CSF cell count	10–1000 cells/μL	Neutrophils may predominate initially (≥50%), gradual shift toward lymphocytes occurs (≥80%)[17]
CSF Protein	Usually normal to mildly elevated (<200 mg/dL)	
CSF Glucose	Usually normal to mildly decreased	Often decreased in LCMV Meningitis
CSF PCR		Commercially available for enterovirus, HSV-1, HSV-2, arboviruses, CMV, EBV, HHV-6, VZV

Abbreviations: CSF, cerebrospinal fluid; PCR, polymerase chain reaction.
Data from Bamberger D. Diagnosis, initial management and prevention of meningitis. Am Fam Physician 2010;82(12):1491–8.

> **Box 6**
> **Bacterial meningitis score**
>
> Likelihood of bacterial meningitis <0.1% in patients who lack all of the following:
>
> - Positive CSF Gram stain
> - CSF absolute neutrophil count ≥1000/μL
> - CSF protein ≥80 mg/dL
> - Peripheral blood ANC ≥10,000/μL
> - History of seizure

Management of Aseptic Meningitis

Antimicrobial therapy should be initiated immediately after lumbar puncture, if bacterial meningitis is a possibility, until initial CSF results and/or PCR results become available. However, empiric antibiotics should not be delayed if the patient is critically ill or requires a CT scan and lumbar puncture cannot be performed in a timely fashion. Consideration of antimicrobial agents and whether to give dexamethasone is discussed further in the next section. If bacterial meningitis and HSV infection have been ruled out, supportive care with pain and fever control is usually the treatment of choice for aseptic meningitis. Acyclovir is the drug of choice if HSV is diagnosed (**Table 4**). Pleconaril, an antipicornaviral agent, was studied in patients with primary immunodeficiency and initially appeared to be effective against enteroviruses; however, drug interactions, side effects, and poor efficacy were a concern, and this drug is not recommended and not available in the United States.[40] Patients with aseptic meningitis do not necessarily require inpatient admission; however, children with CSF pleocytosis, and elderly or immunocompromised patients should be hospitalized.[41] Respiratory droplet isolation precautions should be instituted for hospitalized patients until antimicrobial therapy has been given for 24 hours (as per hospital infection control rules) and/or an etiologic agent is identified. The fecal-oral route is the primary method of transmission in the majority of cases of aseptic meningitis; consequently, hand hygiene is of great importance and sharing of eating or drinking utensils is discouraged. Fecal viral shedding of patients infected with enterovirus can occur for 5 to 6 weeks from exposure.

Complications, Admission, and Referral Criteria

Complications can be severe in neonates, and are reviewed in **Table 2**. Patients who have altered mental status, those requiring antimicrobial therapy, and neonates

Table 4
Treatment of aseptic meningitis

	Rationale	Treatment Agent
All patients	Pain control, fever control Empiric antibiotic therapy while awaiting bacterial culture results	Acetaminophen, ibuprofen, ketorolac See **Tables 11 & 12**
Suspicion for HSV	Possibility of encephalitis	Acyclovir
Suspicion for VZV	Expert opinion[42]	Acyclovir
CEMA		Intravenous immunoglobulin

warrant hospital admission. Intensive care therapy may be required based on clinical status, but is uncommon.

Cost Considerations

Although non-HSV aseptic meningitis is a benign disease in the majority of cases, the morbidity is significant when hospitalization and time off work are considered.[43] An estimated 25,000 to 50,000 patients with aseptic meningitis are hospitalized annually, at an estimated cost of between $234 and $310 million every year.[1,44] Use of clinical history and presentation, lumbar puncture with gram stain and PCR, as well as the bacterial meningitis rule for children can aid clinicians in determining which patients warrant hospital admission and empiric antimicrobial therapy while awaiting CSF culture results. Many stable patients who have history, clinical, and laboratory findings suggestive of aseptic meningitis can be discharged home with instructions for symptom control and follow-up. Adult outpatients presenting with fever and headache without the clinical finding of jolt accentuation of headache or meningismus, no risk factors, and otherwise normal physical examination can likely be managed with close follow-up.

BACTERIAL MENINGITIS

Bacterial Meningitis: Five Key Points for Primary Care
1. The incidence of bacterial meningitis has declined significantly over the past 30 years thanks to routine vaccination of children and selected adults. Primary care clinicians have an important role in patient education regarding the importance of vaccination.
2. Bacterial meningitis should be treated with broad-spectrum antibiotics immediately to prevent rapid clinical deterioration and a poor outcome, with subsequent antibiotic adjustments based on CSF culture results.
3. Chemoprophylaxis for close contacts of patients with Haemophilus influenzae and meningococcal meningitis is an important strategy for prevention of bacterial meningitis.
4. Dexamethasone therapy before or with the initial dose of antibiotics is recommended in children and adults.
5. Patients with bacterial meningitis should be admitted to the intensive care unit for close monitoring.

Introduction

The incidence of bacterial meningitis has been declining in the United States, largely as a result of the increased use of vaccines against H influenzae type B, Streptococcus pneumoniae, and Neisseria meningitidis. Bacterial meningitis, when it occurs, often results in significant morbidity and mortality.

Epidemiology

The incidence of bacterial meningitis was 1.38 per 100,000 persons in the United States in 2007, a significant change from approximately 3.0 per 100,000 persons annually between 1978 and 1981.[45–47] Several preventive measures that targeted 4 of the 5 most common pathogens implicated are largely responsible for this decline. Cumulatively, these advances have caused a shift in the median age of patients with bacterial meningitis from 15 months in 1981 to 39 years in 2003.[48] By contrast, the rates of group B streptococcal (GBS) meningitis in neonates remain stable. Since 2002, the recommended universal screening of pregnant women for GBS vaginal and rectal colonization has been able to identify the 15% to 25% of women who are carriers; however, intrapartum antibiotic prophylaxis has only been shown to decrease rates of neonatal early-onset (<7 days) GBS sepsis.[49] Neonatal GBS meningitis is more commonly a manifestation of late-onset (7–89 days) GBS infection, and these rates have not been affected by the advent of routine maternal GBS screening and prophylaxis. Meningitis caused by *Mycobacterium tuberculosis*, *Treponema pallidum*, and *Borrelia burgdorferi* are very rare in the United States (**Boxes 7–9**).

Despite the overall decline in incidence, the mortality of bacterial meningitis has not changed significantly over the past 20 years and is generally in the range of 15% to 25%.[17] Detailed epidemiologic data can be found in **Tables 5–7**.

Pathogenesis and Pathophysiology of Bacterial Meningitis

In the process of bacterial infection and invasion that eventually results in meningitis, there are several bacterial virulence factors and corresponding host defenses (**Table 8**). A key step in the pathophysiology of meningitis is the crossing of the BBB, which may be more likely in the setting of high-grade bacteremia. Specific pathogens have been shown to possess surface factors that mediate transcellular or intercellular invasion such as OmpA and a protein encoded by *ibe10* in *Escherichia coli*, lipotechoic acid in *Streptococcus agalactiae*, and platelet-activating receptor in *S pneumoniae*.[54] Other pathogens enter monocytes or follow them across the endothelium. A third method of invasion is exemplified by *Listeria monocytogenes*, which is taken up by endothelial cells in phagosomes with the help of In1B surface protein.

The deleterious effects of CNS inflammation resulting from bacterial meningitis are many. Increased intracranial pressure occurs as a result of increased BBB permeability. Leukocyte and bacterial toxins induce cellular swelling as well as obstruction of CSF flow, which can lead to hydrocephalus. Cerebral blood flow may be decreased because of vasculitis and may lead to thrombosis and ischemia. Free radicals produced by granulocytes, endothelial cells, and bacteria contribute to direct neuronal injury.

Clinical Features of Bacterial Meningitis

The clinical presentation of bacterial meningitis is classically more severe and acute compared with that of aseptic meningitis (**Table 9**). The acute onset of fever, headache, and neck stiffness over hours to days is typical, but the presence of all 3 of these symptoms simultaneously is present in less than 50% of cases. Almost all patients have at least 2 of the following 4 symptoms: fever, neck stiffness, headache, or altered mental status (Glasgow Coma Scale score <14).[55] Headache is the most common symptom, seen in more than 85% of patients at presentation, followed by fever in 80%. Nausea and vomiting may also be present. As previously discussed, Kernig and Brudzinski signs are insensitive but highly specific. Cranial nerve (CN) palsies may occur as a result of increased intracranial pressure, and most commonly involve CN III, IV, VI, and VII.[17] Seizures and focal neurologic signs, present in 20% to 30%, can be a result of brain ischemia.[17] Cushing's triad of hypertension, bradycardia,

---

Box 7
Epidemiology of H influenzae

- Previously most common cause of meningitis in children[45]

- Routine immunization since 1990

- Decreased incidence by 55% from 40 to 69 cases per 100,000 to 1 case per 100,000[50,51]

Box 8
Epidemiology of S pneumoniae

- Polysaccharide vaccine introduced 1990
- Meningitis in children declined by 26% overall and by 62% in children 2 to 23 months old

---

and irregular respirations is a manifestation of increased intracranial pressure, which may progress to subsequent herniation, coma, and death.

Diagnosis of Bacterial Meningitis

Indications for lumbar puncture and prior CNS imaging have been previously discussed. CSF analysis should be performed, and provides useful diagnostic information as outlined in **Table 10**. A cloudy appearance of CSF suggests bacterial meningitis. CSF to serum glucose ratio is less than 0.40 in more than 70% of cases. The likelihood of positive Gram stain varies with bacterial concentration, and is positive in at least 60% of cases. Bacterial concentrations of 10^5 correlate with a positive Gram stain in 97% of cases, whereas concentrations of 10^3 decrease the likelihood to 25%. Patients who require imaging before lumbar puncture should receive empiric antimicrobial therapy without delay, even if this affects the utility of CSF Gram stain and culture.

It is unclear as to how quickly appropriate antimicrobial therapy leads to CSF sterilization. Gram stain is more likely to be positive in cases of S pneumoniae, H influenzae, and N meningitidis, and is positive in less than 50% of cases of meningitis attributable to gram-negative bacilli and L monocytogenes. CSF culture is available within 24 to 48 hours and remains the gold standard for the definitive diagnosis of bacterial meningitis, providing specific identification of the organism and antimicrobial sensitivity testing to guide management.

Specific diagnostic tests

Rapid latex agglutination tests are available for H influenzae, S pneumoniae, N meningitidis (except Type B), E coli, and GBS; however, these have not been helpful in antimicrobial management, owing to limitations in sensitivity and specificity. PCR has a high sensitivity and negative predictive value of nearly 100%, and can rapidly detect S pneumoniae, N meningitidis, H influenzae, GBS, L monocytogenes, and M tuberculosis.[58] PCR may be especially useful when CSF Gram stain and culture are negative, but does not provide any information regarding antimicrobial susceptibility, which is determined by CSF culture. In neonates born to mothers with inadequately treated syphilis, lumbar puncture with a CSF-VDRL test is performed, which is helpful in guiding long-term management. In adults, CSF-VDRL is insensitive but highly specific. If CSF-VDRL is positive, therapy for neurosyphilis should be given. With respect to tuberculous meningitis, growth of organisms in CSF mycobacterial culture may take several weeks. CSF acid-fast smear has low sensitivity; however, the yield may be increased with multiple large-volume samples of CSF. PCR has a sensitivity of 85% to 95% and may be used to diagnose, but not exclude, tuberculous meningitis.

Box 9
Epidemiology of N meningitidis

- Conjugate polysaccharide vaccines licensed in 2005
- Meningococcal meningitis declined by 58% from 1998 to 2007

Table 5
Epidemiology of bacterial meningitis in the United States according to organism

	S agalactiae (GBS)	L monocytogenes	S pneumoniae	N meningitidis	H influenzae	Other Gram-Negative Bacilli
Incidence (cases/100,000)	0.25	0.05	0.81	0.19	0.08	
Percentage of all cases of meningitis (%)	5	8	61		7	
Mortality (%)	15–29		19–26	3–13	3–6	7–27

Data from Tunkel AR, van de Beek D, Scheld MW. Acute meningitis. In: Mandell GL, Bennett JE, Dolin R, editors. Mandell, Douglas, and Bennett's principles and practice of infectious diseases. 7th edition. Philadelphia: Churchill Livingstone Elsevier; 2009. p. 1189–229; and Thigpen MC, Whitney CG, Messonier NE, et al. Bacterial meningitis in the United States, 1998-2007. N Engl J Med 2011;364:2016-25.

Table 6							
Epidemiology and empiric therapy by age group							
	S agalactiae (GBS)	E coli	L monocytogenes	S pneumoniae	N meningitidis	H influenzae	Other Gram-Negative Bacilli
Neonates (<3 mo)	+++	++	+				
Children & Adults				+++	++	Rare	
Age >50 y			+	+++	++		+

Table 7
Specific epidemiologic patterns

S agalactiae (GBS)	Decline in early-onset GBS but not late-onset GBS with maternal GBS screening and prophylaxis
N meningitidis	Perpetuated by nasopharyngeal carriage Increased incidence in patients with terminal complement deficiency[52]
S pneumoniae	Highest morbidity and mortality in adults with underlying diabetes, chronic renal disease, chronic hepatic disease, alcoholism Increased incidence in patients with surgical or functional asplenia Increased incidence in patients with cochlear implants with positioners
L monocytogenes	Uncommon; seen in infants <1 y old and adults >50 y and those with cell-mediated immune defects
Staphylococcus aureus	Rare without history of central nervous system (CNS) trauma or surgery Most common cause of meningitis post neurosurgery[53]
Staphylococcus epidermidis	Rare without history of CNS trauma or surgery Most common cause of meningitis post-CSF shunt placement[53]
T pallidum	CNS invasion most common but asymptomatic during primary syphilis, symptomatic during secondary and tertiary syphilis Incidence 0.3%–2.4% in untreated syphilis
B burgdorferi	Overall incidence of Lyme disease 9.7/100,000 persons CNS involvement in 10%–15% of cases, usually within first 6 mo of infection
M tuberculosis	Low incidence in USA due to public health interventions including diagnosis and treatment of latent tuberculosis

Imaging

Head CT or magnetic resonance imaging (MRI) are not routinely recommended, but may be considered in patients who do not respond to therapy and in patients who suffer seizures or focal neurologic deficits, or display other evidence of increased intracranial pressure (see earlier discussion). MRI in tuberculous meningitis can reveal classic features of basal meningeal enhancement and hydrocephalus.

Management

When a patient's presentation is suggestive of bacterial meningitis, empiric antimicrobial therapy should be initiated immediately (**Table 11**). If lumbar puncture can be performed without delay and there are no clinical signs to warrant CNS imaging, blood cultures should be obtained, lumbar puncture performed, and CSF sent for studies including Gram stain, culture, cell count with differential, protein, and glucose. In adults with possible bacterial meningitis, therapy with dexamethasone should be initiated before the first antibiotic dose. This treatment attenuates the inflammatory response in the subarachnoid space and therefore limits cellular damage.[59] However, in adults there is no evidence that dexamethasone therapy before antibiotics is of benefit with pathogens other than S pneumoniae, therefore if S pneumoniae is ruled out as an etiologic agent, dexamethasone therapy may be discontinued. In children, dexamethasone given just before antibiotics decreases the incidence of neurologic deficits and hearing loss caused by H influenzae type B meningitis, and in children

Table 8
Pathogenic factors of bacterial meningitis

Stage of Infection	Host Factors	Bacterial Factors
Mucosal colonization	Secretory IgA inhibition of bacterial adherence Anticapsular antibodies	Fimbriae Polysaccharide capsule IgA protease
Bloodstream invasion	Tight junctions between epithelial cells	Breakdown of tight junctions Pathogen-initiated endocytosis
Bacteremia	Neutrophil phagocytosis Pathogen-specific antibodies Complement pathway	Polysaccharide capsule
Meningeal invasion	BBB	Fimbriae ibe10, OmpA, PAF receptor, In1B
Survival in subarachnoid space	Meningeal inflammation → complement activation (weak), CSF leukocytosis	Polysaccharide capsule
Subarachnoid space inflammation	Inflammatory cytokines and chemokines (IL-1, TNF, PAF) → cerebral edema Increased BBB permeability	Peptidoglycan (gram-positive) Lipo-oligosaccharide (gram-negative)
Increased BBB permeability	Inflammatory cytokines	Lipo-oligosaccharide

Abbreviations: BBB, blood-brain barrier; IL, interleukin; PAF, platelet-activating factor; TNF, tumor necrosis factor.

Data from Tunkel AR, van de Beek D, Scheld MW. Acute meningitis. In: Mandell GL, Bennett JE, Dolin R, editors. Mandell, Douglas, and Bennett's principles and practice of infectious diseases. 7th edition. Philadelphia: Churchill Livingstone Elsevier; 2009. p. 1189–229.

Table 9
Clinical features of bacterial meningitis due to specific pathogens

N meningitidis	Petechiae and purpura of the extremities
T pallidum	Syphilitic meningitis: similar to aseptic meningitis Meningovascular syphilis; vertigo, personality changes, behavioral changes, seizures, focal deficits occurring over weeks to months
B burgdorferi	Headache, photophobia, nausea, vomiting, malaise, fatigue, myalgias, arthralgias, weight loss, neck stiffness (in decreasing order of frequency) Somnolence, emotional instability, behavioral changes, depression, impaired memory & concentration seen in 50% Cranial nerve (CN) palsies in 50%, most commonly CN VII may be bilateral, usually asynchronously
M tuberculosis[56]	Prodromal low-grade fever, malaise, headache, vomiting, personality changes lasting weeks with progression to more severe headache, altered mental status, stroke, hydrocephalus, CN palsies

Data from Tunkel AR, van de Beek D, Scheld MW. Acute meningitis. In: Mandell GL, Bennett JE, Dolin R, editors. Mandell, Douglas, and Bennett's principles and practice of infectious diseases. 7th edition. Philadelphia: Churchill Livingstone Elsevier; 2009. p. 1189–229.

Table 10
Laboratory findings in bacterial meningitis

Organism	S pneumoniae, N meningitidis, S agalactiae, H influenzae	T pallidum	B burgdorferi	M tuberculosis[56]
CSF opening pressure	200–500 mm H_2O	Normal to slightly elevated	Normal to slightly elevated	Normal to slightly elevated
CSF cell count	100–5000 cells/μL, neutrophil pleocytosis	>10 cells/μL, mononuclear pleocytosis	Elevated but usually <500 cells/μL, lymphocytic pleocytosis	100–500 cells/μL, lymphocytic pleocytosis
CSF protein	100–500 mg/dL	>50 mg/dL	<200 mg/dL[57]	100–500 mg/dL
CSF glucose	<40 mg/dL	Slightly decreased	Normal	<45 mg/dL

Table 11
Empiric therapy in suspected bacterial meningitis

Age Group	Antimicrobial Therapy
<1 mo	Ampicillin + gentamicin + cefotaxime
Infants, children, and adults	Vancomycin + ceftriaxone
Age >50 y	Vancomycin + ampicillin + ceftriaxone

Data from Tunkel AR, Hartman BJ, Kaplan SL, et al. Practice guidelines for the management of bacterial meningitis. Clin Infect Dis 2004;39:1267–84.

Table 12
Antimicrobial therapy for specific pathogens

Pathogen	Antimicrobial Agent
S agalactiae	Penicillin G ± gentamicin
S pneumoniae: penicillin susceptible	Penicillin G or ampicillin
S pneumoniae: penicillin intermediate or resistant	Ceftriaxone or cefotaxime plus vancomycin
N meningitidis	Penicillin G or ampicillin
H influenzae	Ceftriaxone or cefotaxime
L monocytogenes	Ampicillin ± gentamicin
T pallidum	Penicillin G
B burgdorferi	Ceftriaxone
M tuberculosis	Isoniazid + rifampin + pyrazinamide + ethambutol

Data from Tunkel AR, Hartman BJ, Kaplan SL, et al. Practice guidelines for the management of bacterial meningitis. Clin Infect Dis 2004;39:1267–84.

with *S pneumoniae* meningitis it may also improve outcome, although this has been less well documented.

Patients with presumed bacterial meningitis should be admitted to an intensive care unit for close monitoring of clinical status. Droplet isolation precautions should be initiated immediately and continued until after 24 hours of antibiotic therapy. When results of CSF cultures and susceptibility testing become available, broad-spectrum antimicrobials can be switched to specific therapy. Chemoprophylaxis for household contacts is recommended for *H influenzae* and *N meningitidis* meningitis.

Supportive care and adjunctive therapies

Patients with bacterial meningitis must be monitored closely for clinical deterioration. Airway support or intubation should be considered in patients with an increased respiratory rate, oxygen saturation less than 90%, or partial pressure of oxygen less than 60 mm Hg.[60] Septic shock is a possibility, and hemodynamic monitoring in this setting is warranted to assess response to fluid resuscitation and/or inotropic agents. Patients may require intensive fluid resuscitation and should be monitored for development of syndrome of inappropriate antidiuretic hormone (SIADH). Proton-pump inhibitors should be given to decrease the incidence of gastric ulceration. Increased intracranial pressure should be suspected based on clinical findings. Elevated CSF pressure can be treated with dexamethasone, elevation of the head of the bed to 30°, use of osmotic diuretics such as mannitol (25%) or hypertonic saline (3%), and hyperventilation.[60] If seizures occur during the clinical course, anticonvulsants should be given, and electroencephalographic monitoring may be performed.

Prophylaxis of close contacts

In cases of bacterial meningitis whereby *H influenzae* or *N meningitidis* are the suspected or proven etiologic agents, close contacts of patients should receive prophylactic antibiotics within 24 hours of diagnosis of the patient.[61] The definition of close contacts differs between the 2 organisms.[62]

Complications and Referral Criteria

The majority of patients with bacterial meningitis who receive appropriate antimicrobial therapy recover without complications. When complications do occur, they can include cardiorespiratory failure, stroke, hyponatremia, SIADH, hearing loss, CN palsies, meningoencephalitis, seizures, and cognitive impairment. The incidence of these decreases with the use of dexamethasone, prompt initiation of antibiotics, and close monitoring in the intensive care unit. Less common complications include hydrocephalus, subdural empyema, and brain abscess, which may require neurosurgical consultation.

Cost-Effective Strategies for Diagnosis and Treatment

Bacterial meningitis is a life-threatening disease whose treatment requires hospitalization, usually in the intensive care unit, and intravenous antimicrobial therapy. Potential strategies for cost-saving involve judicious use of imaging modalities, discharge of patients with a low clinical suspicion for bacterial meningitis, and narrowing of antimicrobial spectrum when susceptibilities become available. Chemoprophylaxis of household contacts of infected individuals is effective in decreasing the incidence of new cases of meningitis. Perhaps the most cost-effective strategy has been the routine and widespread use of *H influenzae* B, meningococcal, and pneumococcal vaccines, which has significantly decreased the incidence of bacterial meningitis.

REFERENCES

1. Khetsuriani N, Quiroz ES, Holman RC, et al. Viral meningitis associated hospitalizations in the United States 1988-1999. Neuroepidemiology 2003;22:345–52.
2. Zaotis T, Klein JD. Enterovirus infections. Pediatr Rev 1998;19:183–91.
3. Rotbart HA. Viral meningitis and the aseptic meningitis syndrome. In: Scheld M, Whitley R, Durack D, editors. Infections of the central nervous system. 2nd edition. New York: Raven; 1997. p. 23–46.
4. Wilfert CM, Lehrman SN, Katz SL. Enteroviruses and meningitis. Pediatr Infect Dis 1983;2:333–41.
5. Galazka AM, Robertson SE, Kraigher A. Mumps and mumps vaccine: a global review. Bull World Health Organ 1999;77(1):3–14.
6. WHO recommended standards for surveillance of selected vaccine preventable diseases. (2003, February). World Health Organization Home Page. Available at: http://www.who.int/vaccines-documents/. Accessed January 8, 2013.
7. Corey L, Spear PG. Infections with herpes simplex viruses (2). N Engl J Med 1986;314:749–57.
8. Corey L, Adams HG, Brown ZA, et al. Genital herpes simplex virus infection: clinical manifestations, course and complications. Ann Intern Med 1983;98: 958–72.
9. Bergstrom T, Vahlne A, Alestig K, et al. Primary and recurrent herpes simplex virus type 2-induced meningitis. J Infect Dis 1990;162:322–30.
10. Mommeja-Marin H, Lafaurie M, Scieux C, et al. Herpes simplex virus type 2 as a cause of severe meningitis in immunocompromised adults. Clin Infect Dis 2003; 37:1527–33.
11. Whitley RJ. Viral infections of the central nervous system. In: Cohen J, Powderly WG, editors. Infectious diseases. 2nd edition. London: Mosby; 2004. p. 267–9.
12. CDC. Enterovirus surveillance—United States, 1997-1999. MMWR Morb Mortal Wkly Rep 2000;49:913–6.
13. Rotbart HA. Enteroviral infections of the central nervous system. Clin Infect Dis 1995;20:971–81.
14. Johnson RT. Pathogenesis of CNS infections. In: Johnson RT, editor. Viral infections of the central nervous system. New York: Raven; 1982. p. 37–60.
15. Cassady KA, Whitely RJ. Pathogenesis and pathophysiology of viral infections of the central nervous system. In: Scheld WM, Whitley RJ, Marra CM, editors. Infections of the central nervous system. 3rd edition. Philadelphia: Lippincott Williams & Wilkins; 2004. p. 57–74.
16. Brody IA, Wilkins RH. The signs of Kernig and Brudzinski. Arch Neurol 1969;21: 215–8.
17. Tunkel AR, van de Beek D, Scheld MW. Acute meningitis. In: Mandell GL, Bennett JE, Dolin R, editors. Mandell, Douglas, and Bennett's principles and practice of infectious diseases. 7th edition. Philadelphia: Churchill Livingstone Elsevier; 2009. p. 1189–229.
18. Norris CM, Danis PG, Garder TD. Aseptic meningitis in the newborn and young infant. Am Fam Physician 1999;59(10):2761–70.
19. Connolly KJ, Hammer SM. The acute aseptic meningitis syndrome. Infect Dis Clin North Am 1990;4:599–622.
20. Rorabaugh ML, Berlin LE, Heldrich F, et al. Aseptic meningitis in infants younger than 2 years of age: acute illness and neurologic complications. Pediatrics 1993;92:206–11.

21. Wagdhare S, Kalantri A, Joshi R, et al. Accuracy of physical signs for detecting meningitis: a hospital-based diagnostic accuracy study. Clin Neurol Neurosurg 2010;112:752–7.
22. McKinney RE, Katz SL, Wilfert CM. Chronic enteroviral meningoencephalitis in agammaglobulinemic patients. Rev Infect Dis 1987;9:334–56.
23. Thomas KE, Hasbun R, Jekel J, et al. The diagnostic accuracy of Kernig's sign, Brudzinski's sign, and nuchal rigidity in adults with suspected meningitis. Clin Infect Dis 2002;35:46–52.
24. Lin TY, Kao HT, Hsieh SH, et al. Neonatal enterovirus infections: emphasis on risk factors for severe and fatal infections. Pediatr Infect Dis J 2003;22:889–94.
25. Modlin JF. Perinatal echovirus infection: insights from a literature review of 61 cases of serious infection and 16 outbreaks in nurseries. Rev Infect Dis 1986; 8:918–26.
26. Azbug MJ. Prognosis for neonates with enterovirus hepatitis and coagulopathy. Pediatr Infect Dis J 2001;20:758–63.
27. Uchihara T, Tsukagoshi H. Jolt accentuation of headache: the most sensitive sign for CSF pleocytosis. Headache 1991;31:167–71.
28. Durand ML, Calderwood SB, Weber DJ, et al. Acute bacterial meningitis in adults: a review of 493 episodes. N Engl J Med 1993;328:21–8.
29. Sigurdardottir B, Bjornsson OM, Jonsdottir KE, et al. Acute bacterial meningitis in adults: a 20-year overview. Arch Intern Med 1997;157:425–30.
30. Attia L, Hatala R, Cook D, et al. The rational clinical examination. Does this adult patient have acute meningitis? JAMA 1999;282:175–81.
31. Rorabaugh ML, Berlin LE, Rosenberg L, et al. Absence of neurodevelopmental sequelae from aseptic meningitis. Pediatr Res 1992;30:177A.
32. Magnussen CR. Meningitis in adults: ten-year retrospective analysis at a community hospital. N Y State J Med 1980;80:901–6.
33. Behrman RE, Meyers BR, Mendelson MR, et al. Central nervous system infections in the elderly. Arch Intern Med 1989;149:1596–9.
34. Jefferson G. The tentorial pressure cone. Arch Neurol Psychiatry 1938;40: 857–76.
35. Hasbun R, Abrahams J, Jekel J, et al. Computed tomography of the head before lumbar puncture in adults with suspected meningitis. N Engl J Med 2001;345: 1727–33.
36. Rotbart HA, et al. Enteroviruses. In: Murray PR, Baron EJ, Pfaller MA, et al, editors. Manual of clinical microbiology. Washington, DC: ASM Press; 1999. p. 990–8.
37. Sawyer MH, Holland D, Aintablian N. Diagnosis of enteroviral central nervous system infection by polymerase chain reaction during a large community outbreak. Pediatr Infect Dis J 1994;3:177–82.
38. Nigrovic LE, Kupperman N, Macias CG, et al, Pediatric Emergency Medicine Collaborative Research Committee of the American Academy of Pediatrics. Clinical prediction rule for identifying children with cerebrospinal fluid pleocytosis at very low risk for bacterial meningitis. JAMA 2007;297(1):52–60.
39. Dubos F, Martinot A, Gendrel D, et al. Clinical decision rules for evaluating meningitis in children. Curr Opin Neurol 2009;22(3):288–93.
40. Rotbart HA, Webster AD, Pleconaril Treatment Registry Group. Treatment of potentially life-threatening enterovirus infections with pleconaril. Clin Infect Dis 2001;22:335–41.
41. Thomson J, Shah S. Viral meningitis. In: The nervous system. Bope E, Kellerman R; Conn's current therapy 2013. 1st edition. Philadelphia: Saunders, an imprint of Elsevier; 2013. p. 670–3.

42. Bamberger D. Diagnosis, initial management and prevention of meningitis. Am Fam Physician 2010;82(12):1491–8.
43. Rotbart HA, Brennan PJ, Fife KH, et al. Enterovirus meningitis in adults. Clin Infect Dis 1998;27:896–8.
44. Parasuraman TV, Frenia K, Romero J. Enteroviral meningitis. Cost of illness and considerations for the economic evaluations of potential therapies. Pharmacoeconomics 2001;19:3–12.
45. Thigpen MC, Whitney CG, Messonier NE, et al. Bacterial meningitis in the United States, 1998-2007. N Engl J Med 2011;364:2016–25.
46. Schlech WF III, Ward JI, Band JD, et al. Bacterial meningitis in the United States, 1978 through 1981. The National Bacterial Meningitis Surveillance Study. JAMA 1985;253:1749–54.
47. Wenger JD, Hightower AW, Facklam RR, et al. Bacterial meningitis in the United States, 1986: report of a multistate surveillance study. The Bacterial Meningitis Study Group. J Infect Dis 1990;162:1316.
48. Dery MA, Hasbun R. Changing epidemiology of bacterial meningitis. Curr Infect Dis Rep 2007;9:301–7.
49. Schuchat A. Epidemiology of group B streptococcal disease in the United States: shifting paradigms. Clin Microbiol Rev 1998;11:497–513.
50. Cochi SL, Broome CV. Vaccine prevention of *Haemophilus influenzae* type b disease: past, present and future. Pediatr Infect Dis 1986;5:12.
51. Centers for Disease Control and Prevention (CDC). Progress toward eliminating *Haemophilus influenzae* type b disease among infants and children—United States, 1987-1997. MMWR Morb Mortal Wkly Rep 1998;47:993.
52. Fijen CA, Kuijper EJ, Tjia HG, et al. Complement deficiency predisposes for meningitis due to nongroupable meningococci and *Neisseria*-related bacteria. Clin Infect Dis 1994;18:780–4.
53. McClelland S III, Hall WA. Postoperative central nervous system infection: incidence and associated factors in 2111 neurosurgical procedures. Clin Infect Dis 2007;45:55–9.
54. Kim KS. Mechanisms of microbial traversal of the blood-brain barrier. Nat Rev Microbiol 2008;6:625–34.
55. van de Beek D, de Gans J, Spanjaard L, et al. Clinical features and prognostic factors in adults with bacterial meningitis. N Engl J Med 2004;351:1849–59.
56. Marx GE, Chan ED. Tuberculous meningitis: diagnosis and treatment overview. Tuberc Res Treat 2011;2011:798764. http://dx.doi.org/10.1155/2011/798764.
57. Reik L. Neurologic abnormalities of Lyme disease. Medicine 1979;58:281–94.
58. Saravolatz LD, Manzor O, VanderVelde N, et al. Broad-range bacterial polymerase chain reaction for early detection of bacterial meningitis. Clin Infect Dis 2003;36:40–5.
59. de Gans J, van de Beek D. Dexamethasone in adults with bacterial meningitis. N Engl J Med 2002;347:1549–56.
60. Van de Beek D, de Gans J, Tunkel AR. Community acquired bacterial meningitis in adults. N Engl J Med 2006;354:44–53.
61. Purcell B, Samuellsson S, Hahne SJ. Effectiveness of antibiotics in preventing meningococcal disease after a case: systematic review. BMJ 2004;328:1339.
62. American Academy of Pediatrics. *Haemophilus influenzae* infections and meningococcal infections. In: Pickering LK, Baker CJ, Kimberlin DW, et al, editors. Red book 2012 report of the Committee on Infectious Diseases. Elk Grove Village (IL): American Academy of Pediatrics; 2012. p. 348.503–4.

Acute Gastroenteritis

Nancy S. Graves, MD

KEYWORDS

- Gastroenteritis • Infectious • Vomiting • Diarrhea • Abdominal pain

KEY POINTS

- Acute gastroenteritis is a common infectious disease syndrome, causing a combination of nausea, vomiting, diarrhea, and abdominal pain. The Centers for Disease Control and Prevention (CDC) estimate there are more than 350 million cases of acute gastroenteritis in the United States annually, and 48 million of these cases are caused by foodborne bacteria.
- Traveler's diarrhea affects more than half of people traveling from developed countries to developing countries. Prevention can be summarized by the caution, "boil it, cook it, peel it, or forget it."
- Except in cases of fever, bloody diarrhea, immunocompromised patients, or patients with significant comorbidities, identifying a specific pathogen is rarely indicated in acute bacterial gastroenteritis because illness is usually self-limited.
- In both adult and pediatric patients, the prevalence of *Clostridium difficile* is increasing in the United States. Contact precautions, public health education, and prudent use of antibiotics are still necessary goals. Complicating these efforts are that there is increasing antibiotic resistance to *C difficile* and a new strain, NAP1/027/III, has been emerging since the early 2000s. This new strain has a high association with community onset and has been linked to increasing frequency and severity of illness. There is research into the possibility that the community onset may be related to animals and to retail meat, where the new strain has been detected.
- Preventing dehydration or providing appropriate rehydration is the primary supportive treatment of acute gastroenteritis.

INTRODUCTION
Definition

Gastroenteritis is inflammation of the stomach, small intestine, or large intestine, leading to a combination of abdominal pain, cramping, nausea, vomiting, and diarrhea. Acute gastroenteritis usually lasts fewer than 14 days. This is in contrast to persistent gastroenteritis, which lasts between 14 and 30 days, and chronic gastroenteritis, which lasts more than 30 days.[1]

Department of Family and Community Medicine, Milton S. Hershey Medical Center, Penn State Hershey, 500 University Drive, Hershey, PA 17033, USA
E-mail address: ngraves@hmc.psu.edu

Prim Care Clin Office Pract 40 (2013) 727–741
http://dx.doi.org/10.1016/j.pop.2013.05.006   **primarycare.theclinics.com**
0095-4543/13/$ – see front matter © 2013 Elsevier Inc. All rights reserved.

Epidemiology

In the United States, acute gastroenteritis is often viewed as a nuisance rather than the life-threatening illness it can be in developing countries. Although significant morbidity and mortality have been attributed to acute diarrheal illnesses in the United States, epidemiologic studies in this country have not been as comprehensive as those conducted in developing nations. The CDC, however, estimate that there are more than 350 million cases of acute diarrheal illnesses in the United States annually. Acute gastroenteritis compares with upper respiratory illnesses as the most common infectious disease syndrome.[2,3]

Using data from the National Center for Health Statistics, the CDC recently reported that deaths from all-cause gastroenteritis increased from approximately 7000 to more than 17,000 per year from 1999 to 2007. Adults over 65 years old made up 83% of these deaths and *C difficile* accounted for two-thirds of these deaths, reflecting that the most significant morbidity and mortality are experienced by the extremes of age.[4]

Etiology

Etiology of acute gastroenteritis

Acute gastroenteritis is caused by many infectious agents as listed in **Table 1**.

Assessing the precise incidence and cause of acute infectious gastroenteritis is made difficult because not everyone reports their symptoms or seeks medical care. In addition, stool cultures, which are used to identify bacterial causes of gastroenteritis, are only positive in 1.5% to 5.6% of cases.[5]

Viral causes of acute gastroenteritis are dominated by rotavirus and norovirus. In the United States, it is estimated that 15 to 25 million episodes of viral gastroenteritis occur each year, leading to 3 to 5 million office visits and 200,000 hospitalizations.[6,7]

Rotavirus causes a particularly severe dehydrating gastroenteritis that affects young children. The severity of the infection is made worse by malnourishment, making rotavirus a significant cause of mortality in children worldwide, responsible for approximately 500,000 deaths annually.[8,9] The introduction of the rotavirus vaccine in the United States and Europe has been effective at reducing rotavirus gastroenteritis. There has been a 67% decrease in positive laboratory diagnosis attributed to vaccination.[10]

Norovirus, however, causes the most outbreaks of nonbacterial acute gastroenteritis in all age groups. It often occurs in epidemic outbreaks in schools, nursing homes, cruise ships, prisons, and other group settings. Symptoms of severe vomiting are usually self-limited, lasting 12 to 60 hours. Transmission of this stable virus is through the fecal-oral route, with viral shredding lasting on average 10 to 14 days after onset of symptoms.[11]

Table 1 Infectious causes of acute gastroenteritis		
Viral: 50%–70%	**Bacterial: 15%–20%**	**Parasitic: 10%–15%**
Norovirus	Shigella	Giardia
Rotavirus	Salmonella	Amebiasis
Enteric adenovirus types 40 and 41	Campylobacter	Cryptosporidium
Astrovirus	*E coli*	Isospora
Coronavirus	Vibrio	Cyclospora
Some picornaviruses	Yersinia	Microsporidium
	C difficile	

Rotavirus and enteric adenovirus can be detected by rapid assays for the viral antigen in stool. Norovirus is best detected by reverse transcriptase–polymerase chain reaction.

Medications and toxic ingestions that cause acute diarrhea or gastroenteritis include those listed in **Table 2**.

Etiology of chronic gastroenteritis

Causes of persistent or chronic gastroenteritis include parasitic infections, medications, inflammatory bowel disease (ulcerative colitis, Crohn disease, collagenous colitis, and microscopic colitis), irritable bowel syndrome, eosinophilic gastroenteritis, celiac disease, lactose intolerance, colorectal cancer, bowel obstruction, malabsorption, and ischemic bowel.

Immunocompromised hosts are most vulnerable to chronic gastroenteritis infections. *Crytosporidium* has been a cause of chronic diarrhea in persons with AIDS. It is also responsible for large outbreaks in day care centers and public swimming pools and has contaminated public water supplies. One of the reasons for these outbreaks is that the oocytes are resistant to bleach or other disinfectants, making them easily transmittable by contact with contaminated surfaces or by person-to-person contact. *Giardia* is another common cause of chronic gastroenteritis. It is found in contaminated streams but is also common in day care centers and swimming pools. *Giardia* causes bloating, flatulence, and explosive, pale, foul-smelling diarrhea.

TYPES OF ACUTE GASTROENTERITIS

The remainder of this article focuses on acute bacterial gastroenteritis, reviewing the common pathogens that cause traveler's gastroenteritis, foodborne gastroenteritis, and antibiotic-associated gastroenteritis. Each section addresses transmission, pathophysiology, the incubation period, symptoms, symptom duration, management, and prevention.

Traveler's Diarrhea

Travelers to developing countries often present to their primary care providers with concerns about traveler's diarrhea and how to avoid or treat this problem should it occur; 40% to 60% of travelers to developing countries acquire this problem. It should also be considered if diarrhea develops within 10 days of their return home.

For epidemiologic reasons, traveler's diarrhea is divided into classic, moderate, and mild forms.

Table 2
Medications and toxic ingestions that cause acute diarrhea or gastroenteritis

Medications	Toxic Ingestions
Antibiotics	Organophosphates
Laxative abuse	Poisonous mushrooms
Sorbitol	Arsenic
Colchicine	Ciguatera or scombroid
Cardiac antidysrhythmics	
Nonsteroidal anti-inflammatory drugs[12]	
Chemotherapeutics	
Antacids	

- Classic: 3 of more unformed bowel movements per 24 hours plus 1 of the following: nausea, vomiting, fever, abdominal pain, and blood in the stool
- Moderate: 1 to 2 unformed bowel movements per 24 hours plus 1 of the above symptoms OR more than 2 unformed bowel movements
- Mild: 1 to 2 unformed bowel movements

Transmission
Traveler's diarrhea is usually transmitted by contaminated food or water. It can be caused by bacteria, viruses, or parasites. Bacteria cause the majority of cases of traveler's diarrhea. The most common are enterotoxigenic E coli (ETEC), followed by Salmonella, Campylobacter jejuni, and Shigella. In 1 study of 322 patients, ETEC caused 12% of bacterial traveler's diarrhea, Salmonella 8%, Campylobacter jejuni 6%, and Shigella less than 1%. In another study of 636 travelers, ETEC caused 30% and enteroaggregative E coli caused 26% of cases.[13,14]

Coinfection with an additional pathogen was found in 20% of travelers.[14]

Areas of the world with the highest risk are countries in Asia, outside of Singapore, on the African continent, outside of South Africa, and in Central and South America.

Pathogenesis
Pathogenesis is discussed in detail for each bacterial cause.

Incubation
Incubation is 4 to 14 days after arrival in a developing nation.

Symptoms
Common symptoms include malaise, anorexia, abdominal pain and cramping, watery diarrhea, nausea and vomiting, and low-grade fever. If caused by Campylobacter jejuni or Shigella, symptoms may progress to colitis, bloody diarrhea, and tenesmus.

Duration
Duration is 1 to 5 days and generally self-limited, but, in 8% to 15% of cases, symptoms last longer than 1 week.[15] If bloating, nausea, or other gastrointestinal symptoms persist for more than 14 days, consider alternative diagnoses, such as parasitic infection.

Diagnosis
The diagnosis is often clinical and confirmation is usually not pursued because traveler's diarrhea is self-limited. Stool cultures may be useful in patients with severe symptoms, prolonged illness, bloody diarrhea, and fever. Stool cultures, however, do not differentiate between nonpathogenic E coli and ETEC or enteroaggregative E coli.

Treatment

- Fluid replacement is the mainstay of symptomatic treatment, plus or minus diet restrictions. There is limited information about whether a clear liquid diet versus an unrestricted diet significantly changes the duration or severity of symptoms because traveler's diarrhea is usually self-limited, lasting 3 to 5 days. Oral rehydration is ideal, but intravenous hydration may be necessary in the setting of dehydration.
- Antibiotics may shorten the course by 1 to 2 days. Travelers often request a prescription for antibiotics that may be taken at the onset of symptoms. Ciprofloxacin (500 mg as a single dose or twice a day for 1–2 days) is commonly sufficient, although resistance to quinolones is increasing, especially for Campylobacter jejuni. Quinolones are not Food and Drug Administration approved for pregnancy

or for treating traveler's diarrhea in children. Azithromycin is appropriate in these groups. In adults, a single 1-g dose is effective. In children, recommended dosing is 10 mg/kg as a single dose, not to exceed 1 g. Rifaximin (200 mg 3 times a day) has been shown effective and, with increasing quinolone resistance, it is increasingly used.[16]

- Antimotility agents, such as loperamide or diphenoxylate, can decrease stool frequency but do not alter the course of the infection. Their use should be avoided in cases of fever or rectal bleeding.
- *Lactobacillus GG*, a specific probiotic, has been shown to decrease diarrhea caused by the pathogens that typically cause traveler's gastroenteritis. Other *Lactobacillus* preparations, however, using nonviable probiotics, have not.[17,18]

Prevention

In 2001, the Infectious Diseases Society of America (IDSA) published guidelines to assist travelers in decreasing their chances of contracting traveler's diarrhea:

- Water must be boiled for 3 minutes to kill pathogens. Two drops of bleach or 5 drops of iodine kill pathogens in water within 30 minutes.
- Freezing does not kill pathogens. Avoid ice, request bottled beverages, and use a straw versus a glass.
- Fruit that must be peeled is safe. Fruit that is not peeled or raw vegetables should be avoided.
- Steam table buffets pose a high risk of contracting traveler's gastroenteritis.
- Communal condiments are frequently contaminated and should be avoided.

Medications, such as H_2 blockers and proton pump inhibitors, can increase susceptibility to traveler's diarrhea. These medications lower gastric acidity and can increase the chance of contracting traveler's diarrhea by allowing more pathogens to survive transit to the small bowel. Similarly, conditions or medications that slow gastric motility allow the number of pathogens to accumulate.

Foodborne Acute Gastroenteritis

The CDC estimate that 48 million cases of foodborne bacterial gastroenteritis occur annually in the United States, leading to 125,000 hospitalizations, 3000 deaths, and costs greater than $150 billion.[2] The Foodborne Disease Active Surveillance Network (or Food-Net program) was established in 1996 by the CDC to track foodborne gastrointestinal illnesses in the United States. Data from this 10-site study that covers 46 million cases suggests that 1 in 5 episodes of gastroenteritis are caused by foodborne pathogens. Data from 2010 show little significant overall change in the known foodborne causes of acute gastroenteritis over the past 4 years. The data did, however, show a decline in Shiga toxin–producing *E coli* O157:H7 and *Shigella*. *Vibrio* gastroenteritis increased over this time period and Salmonella incidence was unchanged, despite increasing awareness and efforts to decrease these infections. In general, treatment of foodborne gastroenteritis can range in cost from $78 in Montana to $162 in New Jersey. The total cost per case, including productivity losses, can be as high as $1506, as noted in Connecticut.[3] There is also research suggesting, however, a significant presence of unspecified agents causing 38.4 million cases of foodborne acute gastroenteritis.[19] Reasons for this include a limited amount of data because not all cases of foodborne gastroenteritis are reported nor is a specific etiology identified; other microbes or chemicals in food could cause or contribute to illness; and, finally, new causes being discovered and known causes, such as *C difficile*, not thought to be transmitted by food, have been detected in retail meat products,[19] suggesting a new route of transmission.

Pathogenesis

The pathogenesis of foodborne gastroenteritis can be broken down into 3 mechanisms:

1. Pathogens that make a toxin in the food before it is consumed (preformed toxin)
2. Pathogens that make a toxin in the gastrointestinal tract, after the food is ingested
3. Pathogens that invade the bowel wall and directly break down the epithelial lining, releasing factors that cause an inflammatory diarrhea.

1. Preformed toxins: *Staphylococcus aureus* and *Bacillus cereus* produce heat-stable enterotoxins in the food before it is consumed.

> Transmission: These pathogens are usually transmitted by a food handler and often found in summer picnic foods.
> *S aureus*: grows well in dairy, meat, eggs, and salads
> *Bacillus cereus*: grows in starchy foods, such as rice, but is also found in beef, pork, and vegetables
> Incubation: 1–6 hours. Ingestion of preformed toxins leads to rapid onset of symptoms.
> Pathophysiology: These bacteria usually affect the small intestine, causing nausea, profuse vomiting, and abdominal pain/cramping. The emetic enterotoxin can be found in vomitus and the food. Testing is rarely conducted, however, because illnesses are self-limited. In cases of preformed toxins, there is no risk of person-to-person spread.
> Symptoms: Sudden onset of nausea and vomiting after eating suggests ingestion of a preformed toxin.
> Diagnosis: Stool studies are not contributory. Diagnosis is usually made based on history and food diary.
> Treatment: No antibiotics needed because it is a preformed enterotoxin.
> Supportive care and parenteral antiemetics help control vomiting.
> Prognosis: Rapid spontaneous recovery in 1 day is typical.

2. Pathogens that transmit illness by making a toxin after consumption

a. *C perfringens*

> Transmission: ingestion of spores that have germinated in food products, such as beef, pork, home canned foods, and poultry[1]
> Pathophysiology: Once spores reach the small intestine, they produce an enterotoxin, leading to watery diarrhea.
> Incubation: 6–48 hours
> Symptoms: frequent watery stools and abdominal cramping; rarely, fever, nausea, and vomiting
> Duration: usually less than 24 hours
> Treatment: Rarely does a patient need intravenous fluids. Antibiotics are of no use given the short duration of symptoms.
> Diagnosis: Usually unnecessary given the short lived nature of this illness, but fecal leukocytes are present because this is an inflammatory gastroenteritis.
> Prognosis: Self-limited, rarely lasting more than 24 hours. Ingestion of type C strain of these bacteria, however, can lead to a serious illness, enteritis necroticans (pigbel). Symptoms include severe abdominal pain, vomiting, diarrhea, and possible shock and can be rapidly fatal.
> Prevention: Do not keep foods that have already been cooked warm for long periods of time.

b. ETEC

> Transmission: ingestion of food or water contaminated by infected fecal matter

Pathophysiology: Bacteria attach to the wall of the small bowel and enterotoxins are released, drawing fluid and electrolytes from the mucosa into the lumen, causing profuse watery diarrhea.

Incubation: 24–72 hours after ingestion

Symptoms: wide-ranging, from mild to severe diarrhea

Duration: 48–72 hours

Treatment: hydration plus ciprofloxacin (500 mg twice daily × 3 days) or Bactrim DS (twice daily × 3 days)

Prevention: safe preparation of food and the avoidance of keeping foods that have already been cooked warm for long periods of time

3. Pathogens that directly invade the bowel wall causing inflammatory diarrhea

a. Enterohemorrhagic *E coli* (EHEC) (Shiga toxin producing)

E coli O157:H7 is 1 of at least 30 serotypes of *E coli* that make shiga-like toxin. It was discovered in 1982, after 2 outbreaks traced to undercooked beef. In May 2011, another serotype, O104:H4, was discovered in Germany.[20] The CDC estimate 110,000 cases and 2100 hospitalizations annually in the United States.[1]

Transmission: These bacteria are present in the intestines of cows and transferred initially through processing and then ingested through undercooked animal food products. Transmission can also occur through contaminated water, raw milk, unpasteurized apple cider, petting zoos, and day care centers.[1]

Pathophysiology: Bacteria attack epithelial cells of the cecum and the large bowel. The shiga-like toxins, called verotoxins, destroy the cells, leading to hemorrhagic colitis.

Incubation: 1–9 days, with 3–4 days typical

Symptoms: Watery diarrhea develops that quickly becomes bloody. Elevated white cell count, abdominal pain, cramping, and vomiting are also commonly seen. The absence of fever (or only a low-grade fever) helps differentiate EHEC from other bacterial causes of bloody acute gastroenteritis.

Duration: 1 week for uncomplicated EHEC infection

Diagnosis: The CDC recommend all stool cultures be screened for *E coli* O157:H and certainly all bloody stool samples. Fecal leukocytes are present in 50% of cases. *E coli* O157:H7 can be screened for using a sorbitol MacConkey agar. Both stool cultures and toxin assays are recommended.

Complications: Hemolytic uremic syndrome (HUS) is associated with Shiga toxin 2 and is a complication seen in 6% to 9% of EHEC causes of acute gastroenteritis.[21] The CDC estimate that greater than 90% of HUS is associated with *E coli* O157:H7. HUS is often seen in children younger than 4 years old and the elderly. There is some concern that empiric antibiotic use may increase the risk of developing HUS.[22] Long-term sequelae caused by this complication include, hypertension, proteinuria, decreased glomerular filtration rate, and, less commonly, seizure, coma, or motor deficits.[23]

Thrombotic thrombocytopenia purpura, which shares many similar features with HUS, presents with prominent neurologic findings rather than renal failure. Rarely, pseudomembranous colitis is associated with *E coli* O157:H7.

Treatment: Treatment is largely supportive. Antibiotics do not shorten the duration of illness and should be avoided. There is some thought that empiric antibiotics or antiperistaltics may increase the chance of developing complications.[24]

Prognosis: Uncomplicated cases resolve spontaneously in 7 to 10 days. A carrier state may last an additional 1 to 2 weeks. Hospitalization is required for 23% to 47% of patients, median length of stay 6 to 14 days. Mortality rate is 1% to 2% and is highest in the elderly population.[1]

Prevention: The best prevention is practicing good hand hygiene and fully cooking meat. In addition, the Department of Agriculture has been improving and continues to improve the slaughter process.

b. Salmonella

Transmission: Salmonella is transmitted through the consumption of contaminated raw or undercooked eggs, meats, raw milk, ice cream, peanuts, fruits, and vegetables. Transmission also occurs through contact with infected animals, such as turtles and pet ducklings.[11]

Pathophysiology: bacteria that survive the acidity of the stomach, colonize the intestine, and move across the intestinal epithelium, either by direct invasion of enterocytes or through dendritic cells inserted into epithelial cells. Once present, the inflammatory process begins releasing cytokines, neutrophils, macrophages, and T cells and B cells. This inflammatory response decreases normal intestinal flora and allows the pathogen to proliferate. The nontyphoid Salmonella produce a more localized response and the typhi serotype (the cause of typhoid fever) tends to be more invasive and more often results in bacteremia.[25]

Incubation: 6–48 hours[11]

Duration: 1–7 days

Symptoms: nausea, vomiting, fever, cramping abdominal pain, possibly bloody diarrhea

Treatment: not usually recommended. Exceptions include severe illness, extremes of age, valvular heart disease, uremia, or malignancy. In the case of these exceptions, a third-generation cephalosporin or fluoroquinolone for 5 to 7 days is indicated.

Complications: Antibiotic use can increase carrier state. Additional complications include transient reactive arthritis, which can be seen in up to 30% of adult patients, and Reiter syndrome, which occurs in 2% of patients.

Prognosis: Most patients recover in 2 to 5 days. Sustained or intermittent bacteremia may occur in immunocompromised patients.

c. *Campylobacter jejuni*

Population: usually under 5 years of age

Transmission: handling or eating raw or undercooked poultry or raw milk or cheeses, by contaminated drinking water, or by handling infected animals[1]

Pathophysiology: direct invasion of epithelial cells of the colon inducing inflammation

Incubation: 1 to 10 days

Duration: 5 to 14 days

Symptoms: Usually rapid onset with fever, chills, headache, and malaise followed by abdominal pain, nausea, vomiting, and diarrhea. Diarrhea may be grossly bloody or melanotic in 60% to 90% of patients.

Treatment: Empiric antibiotics are not recommended in healthy patients. Stool culture is appropriate. Antibiotics shorten the illness by 1 to 1.5 days. Erythromycin or azithromycin × 5 days (resistance to fluoroquinolones).

Complications: *Campylobacter jejuni* gastroenteritis is associated with postinfectious Guillain-Barré syndrome, incidence 1 per 1000. In cases of more severe symptoms, this can be less reversible.[26]

Prognosis: Most patients recover within 1 week. Relapses are common but tend to be milder than the original infection. Fatalities are rare.

d. *Vibrio parahaemolyticus*

It is not common in the United States, but worldwide this pathogen is the most common cause of bacterial gastroenteritis.[1]

Transmission: eating contaminated seafood, crabs, oysters, or clams or by exposure of an open wound to contaminated seawater (Gulf of Mexico). It has been transmitted through airline food.

Pathophysiology: production of a heat-stable enterotoxin, inducing a secretory diarrhea and hemolysis

Incubation: 6 hours to 4 days

Duration: self-limited up to 3 days, commonly 24 to 48 hours

Symptoms: abrupt onset of severe watery diarrhea, abdominal cramping, nausea, and vomiting are common symptoms. Fever occurs less commonly.

Diagnosis: can be cultured on thiosulfate citrate–bile salts sucrose if ingestion of contaminated seafood within 3 days before testing[1]

Treatment: tetracycline × 3 days, ciprofloxacin × 1 dose, or chloramphenicol

e. Shigella

Population: usually has an impact on children less than 5 years of age. It is rare in the United States.

Transmission: consumption of contaminated food or water or by person-to-person or fecal-oral route

Pathophysiology: invades colonic epithelia cells; Shiga toxin causes inflammation and results in hemorrhagic colitis.[1]

Incubation: 1 to 6 days

Duration: self-limiting, lasting 2 to 5 days

Symptoms: Fever, cramping abdominal pain, and diarrhea that is often bloody. Infants may not have bloody diarrhea.

Treatment: ciprofloxacin (500 mg twice a day × 3–5 days), trimethoprim/sulfamethoxazole (160 mg twice a day × 3–5 days), or azithromycin (500 mg once daily for 3 days).

Prognosis: Most patients recover in 1 week. Untreated patients shed bacteria in stool for 2 weeks. Relapse occurs in 10% of patients if not treated with antibiotics.

Antibiotic-Associated Diarrhea

Antibiotic-associated diarrhea is also called *C difficile* colitis. This infection often occurs in hospitalized patients, with increasing risk correlating with length of hospital stay. The use of multiple antibiotics and duration of antibiotic are associated with an increased risk of *C difficile* infection. Patients older than 65 years of age and those who are immunocompromised are at an increased risk of developing *C difficile* colitis, likely related to comorbid conditions.[27] The prevalence of *C difficile* associated colitis is increasing in the United States, both in pediatric and adult admissions. From 2001 to 2006, pediatric *C difficile* admissions increased from 2.6 to 4 cases per 1000.[28] The National Hospital Discharge Survey found the rate for *C difficile* colitis increased from 31 per 100,000 in 1996 to 61 per 100,000 in 2003.[29]

Antibiotics most often associated with *C difficile* infection are flouroquinolones, clindamycin, cephalosporins, and penicillins. Those least associated with *C difficile* infection include doxycycline, aminoglycosides, vancomycin, and metronidazole. Proton pump inhibitors have also been associated with increased susceptibility to *C difficile* infection. Studies found that the use proton pump inhibitors increased the risk 1.4 to 2.75 times compared with those without proton pump inhibitor use.[30]

Transmission
Transmission occurs by fecal-oral route and colonization occurs because antibiotic use has disturbed the normal flora of the intestinal tract.

Pathophysiology
C difficile is an anaerobic bacterium that forms spores capable of producing exotoxins. The spores are heat resistant, acid resistant, and antibiotic resistant. They are also resistant to alcohol-based hand sanitizer, so caregivers must wash their hands in soap and water. Once in the colon, the bacteria become functional and produce toxin A (enterotoxin) and toxin B (cytotoxin). Both toxins lead to inflammation, mucosal injury, and secretory diarrhea.[31] Although toxin B is more virulent than toxin A, they both inactivate regulatory pathways, causing cell apoptosis, mucosal ulceration, and neutrophil chemotaxis to produce the pseudomembranes, common in this infection.[32] Pseudomenbranes are composed of neutrophils, fibrin, epithelial debris, and mucin. Pseudomembranes are not found in all patients, for example, those with ulcerative colitis or who are on immunosuppressive agents, such as steroids or cyclosporine.[33] The hypothesized reason for this is that pseudomembranes develop because of the host immunoreactions.[33]

A new strain of C difficile, hypervirulent North American pulsed-field type 1 (NAP1/027/III), has been suspected in epidemic outbreaks since the early 2000s. It produces a binary toxin in addition to larger quantities of toxin A and toxin B and is associated with increasing incidence and severity of illness. It is resistant to fluoroquinolones.[1] It is associated with community onset and there is concern for transmission via animals and retail meat.[34]

Incubation and duration
Symptom onset may start during use of antibiotics or up to 3 to 4 weeks after antibiotic completion. Symptoms can resolve after stopping the offending antibiotic or follow a complicated and prolonged course.

Symptoms
Patients can present with abdominal pain and mild to moderate watery diarrhea. C difficile can also present with fever, nausea, severe abdominal pain, profuse diarrhea, and, possibly, bloody diarrhea.

Diagnosis
C difficile toxin assay is widely used and available. It must be done on liquid or unformed stool. Stool cultures are sensitive but not clinically useful because results are not rapid. Also, C difficile is present in stool of healthy people and infants. Fecal leukocyte testing is not diagnostic. Sigmoidoscopy and colonoscopy is occasionally used but the risk of perforation is possible. A complete blood cell count to identify leukocytosis and thrombocytosis, albumin level, and lactate may also be useful.

Treatment
Discontinuation of the offending antibiotic is one of the first steps in treatment. According to IDSA treatment guidelines, mild to moderate disease should be treated with metronidazole (500 mg 3 times daily × 10–14 days) and severe disease should be treated with vancomycin (125 mg 4 times daily for 10–14 days). For a first recurrence, treat the same as the initial episode. For a second recurrence, however, use of vancomycin in a tapered or pulsed dose is recommended.

A Cochrane review from 2008 concluded that there is inconclusive evidence supporting the benefit of probiotics in the treatment of *C difficile*. Stool transplantation in patients with recurrent or refractory *C difficile* colitis may be useful.[35] Antiperistaltic medications should be avoided, because they increase the risk for toxic megacolon.

Complications
Complications include toxic megacolon.

Prevention
Use contact precautions—isolate patients in private rooms and gown and glove all visitors and health care workers. Mandate that everyone wash hands with soap and water (**Table 3**).

EVALUATION OF PATIENTS PRESENTING WITH SIGNS AND SYMPTOMS OF ACUTE GASTROENTERITIS, ETIOLOGY UNKNOWN
History

Important questions to consider when exploring the history of acute gastroenteritis are listed in (**Box 1**).

Physical Examination Findings

1. Abnormal vital signs: fever and/or orthostatic blood pressure, and/or tachycardia, and/or pain
2. Clinical signs of dehydration include the following: dry mucus membranes, decreased skin turgor, absent jugular vein pulsations, mental status changes

These and other physical examination findings, such as abdominal pain, have poor predictive value but contribute to the diagnosis and help with appropriate management of the illness.

Diagnostics

Test if symptoms are prolonged or severe or if the patient was recently hospitalized or has fever, bloody stool, systemic illness, recent antibiotic use, or day care center attendance. Assess serum electrolytes, serum urea nitrogen, creatinine to evaluate hydration, and acid-base status. A complete blood cell count is nonspecific but, if eosinophils are elevated, a parasitic infection should be considered.

Table 3
Onset, duration, and symptoms as caused by specific bacteria

Bacteria	Onset	Duration	Signs
Salmonella	6–48 h	1–7 d	N, V, F, P, ± blood
Campylobacter	1–10 d	5–14 d	F, H, P, N, V ± blood
Vibrio	6 h–4 d	SL (up to 3 d)	N, V, D
Shigella	1–6 d	SL (2–3 d)	F, P, D, ± blood
ETEC	1–3 d	2–3 d	D
C perfringens	8–16 h	Less than 24 h	P, D
EHEC	1–9 d	1 wk	N, P, D + blood
C difficile	4–5 d	Variable	F, N, P, D ± blood

Abbreviations: D, diarrhea; F, fever; H, headache; N, nausea; P, abdominal pain; SL, self-limiting; V, vomiting.

Box 1
Questions to consider in the evaluation of patient with signs and symptoms of acute gastroenteritis

1. Abrupt or gradual onset of symptoms. In cases of foodborne illness, how many hours after eating before symptoms onset?
2. Duration of symptoms
3. Characteristics of stool: watery, bloody, mucus, and color
4. Frequency and quantity of bowel movements.
5. Presence of fever, tenesmus, nausea, vomiting, headache, abdominal pain, malaise
6. Recent hospitalization, recent antibiotic use
7. Recent travel, pets, occupational exposures
8. Food history, specifically consumption of raw milk, cheese, undercooked beef, pork, poultry
9. Immunocompromised
10. Family members, coworkers, or other close contacts with similar symptoms
11. Evidence of dehydration: thirst, tachycardia, decreased urine output, lethargy, orthostasis

1. Fecal leukocytes and occult blood: The presence of these suggests a bacterial cause of the acute gastroenteritis. The sensitivity of fecal leukocyte testing varies tremendously. A meta-analysis reported that at 70% sensitivity, fecal leukocytes were only 50% specific for an inflammatory process.[36]
2. Fecal lactoferrin: Use when an inflammatory process is considered or when there is fever, tenesmus, or bloody stool. It is a more sensitive test for fecal leukocytes, because lactoferrin is a marker for fecal leukocytes, with sensitivity and specificity between 90% and 100%. Test is not readily available.[5]
3. Stool cultures: The IDSA published guidelines for diagnosis and management of infectious gastroenteritis in 2001, but controversy remains as to when stool cultures are most useful. This controversy is not helped by the low rate of positive stool cultures.[1]
   o According to IDSA recommendations, stool cultures are appropriate if symptoms do not quickly resolve, if fever or bloody stool are present, if patients' comorbidities put them at risk for complications, or if patients are immunocompromised. Culture for Salmonella, shigella, campylobacter, E coli O157:H7 (also do Shiga toxin assay if blood in stool).
   o Food handlers may require negative cultures to return to work.
4. C difficile assay: if hospitalized or if recent antibiotics or chemotherapy
5. Stool ova and parasites: Generally, testing stool for ova and parasites is low yield and not cost effective. It is appropriate if symptoms and exposure history support a parasitic or protozoal etiology, bloody diarrhea without fecal leukocytes, or persistent diarrhea in day care centers or aer associated with a community waterborne outbreak. In these cases, 3 samples, taken on 3 consecutive days, should be sent to catch parasite excretion.

Treatment

General recommendations
Guidelines emphasize hydration or rehydration plus diet changes and bowel rest. Oral rehydration is best, if possible, and is often underutilized in the United States. In

> **Box 2**
> **WHO rehydration recommendations**
>
> *Manufactured 1-L solutions contain*
>
> - 3.5 g Sodium chloride
> - 2.5 g Sodium bicarbonate
> - 1.5 g Potassium chloride
> - 20 g Glucose
>
> *Home 1-L solutions contain[37]*
>
> - ½ Teaspoon salt
> - ½ Teaspoon baking soda
> - 4 Teaspoons sugar

diarrheal illnesses that involve the small intestine, oral rehydration is effective because the small bowel can still absorb water but requires sodium-glucose cotransport. To provide the glucose and electrolytes, the World Health Organization recommends rehydration with water containing salt, sodium bicarbonate, and glucose. Gatorade and other sports drinks do not contain sufficient salt (**Box 2**).

Antibiotics
Empiric antibiotics should be used with caution. IDSA treatment guidelines from 2001 suggest empiric treatment of moderate to severe traveler's gastroenteritis; those with more than 8 stools per day, dehydration, symptoms more than a week; or immuno-compromised patients. Empiric treatment can also be considered with the presence of fever and bloody stools. Empiric treatments include ciprofloxacin (500 mg twice a day for 3 to 5 days), norfloxacin (400 mg twice a day for 3–5 days), or levofloxacin (500 mg daily for 3–5 days). In areas where fluoroquinolone resistance is a problem, azithromycin (500 mg daily for 3 days) is recommended. Specific treatments of other pathogens are discussed previously. These treatment guidelines, however, are for immunocompetent patients. For immunocompromised hosts, antibiotic treatment should be extended for 7 to 10 days and may be considered when not recommended for immunocompetent patients and there is a lower threshold for hospitalization.

Dietary modifications
A short period of clear liquids with adequate electrolyte replacement is generally ideal. In patients with watery diarrhea, boiled rice, potato, noodles or oats with salt, soup, crackers, or bananas are recommended. This is often referred to as the BRAT diet—bananas, rice, applesauce, and toast. Avoid high-fat foods until normal bowel function returns. Secondary lactose malabsorption or intolerance occurs after infectious gastroenteritis and may last for several weeks, so avoiding lactose-containing foods during this time is appropriate.[38]

REFERENCES

1. Craig S, Zich DK. Gastroenteritis. In: Marx JA, editor. Rosen's emergency medicine. 7th edition. 2009; p. 1200.
2. Mead PS, Slutsker L, Dietz V, et al. Food-related illness and death in the United States. Emerg Infect Dis 1999;5:607.

3. Scharff RL. Health-related costs from foodborne illness and death in the United States. The Produce Safety Project at Georgetown University. Available at: www.producesafetyproject.org. Accessed March, 2013.

4. CDC Division of News and Electronic Media. Deaths from gastroenteritis double. Available at: www.cdc.gov. Accessed March 14, 2012.

5. Guerrant RL, Van Gilder T, Steiner TS, et al. Practice guidelines for the management of infectious diarrhea. Clin Infect Dis 2001;32:337–8.

6. Matson DO, Estes MK. Impact of rotavirus infection at a large pediatric hospital. J Infect Dis 1990;162:598.

7. Tucker AW, Haddix AC, Bresee JS, et al. Cost-effectiveness analysis of a rotavirus immunization program for the United States. JAMA 1998;279:1371.

8. Grimwood K, Buttery JP. Clinical update: rotavirus gastroenteritis and its prevention. Lancet 2007;370:302.

9. Parashar UD, Burton A, Lanata C, et al. Global mortality associated with rotavirus disease among children 2004. J Infect Dis 2009;200(Suppl 1):S9.

10. Parashar UD, Glass RI. Rotavirus vaccines—early success, remaining questions. N Engl J Med 2009;360:1063.

11. Getto L, Zeserson E, Breyer M. Vomitting, diarrhea, constipation and gastroenteritis. Emerg Med Clin North Am 2011;29:224.

12. Etienney I, Beaugerie L, Viboud C, et al. Non-steroidal anti-inflammatory drugs as a risk factor for acute diarrhea: case crossover study. Gut 2003;52(2):260–3.

13. Steffen R, Collard F, Tornieporth N, et al. Epidemiology, etiology and impact of travelers' diarrhea in Jamaica. JAMA 1999;281:811.

14. Adachi JA, Jiang ZD, Mathewson JJ, et al. Enteroaggregative Escherichia coli as a major etiologic agent in traveler's diarrhea in 3 regions of the world. Clin Infect Dis 2001;32:1706.

15. Rendi-Wagner P, Kollaritsch H. Drug prophylaxis for travelers' diarrhea. Clin Infect Dis 2002;34:628.

16. Steffen R, Sack DA, Riopel L, et al. Therapy of travelers' diarrhea with rifaximin on various continents. Am J Gastroenterol 2003;98:1073.

17. Hilton E, Kolakowski P, Singer C, et al. Efficacy of Latobacillis GG as a diarrheal prevention in travelers. J Travel Med 1997;4:41.

18. Briand V, Buffet P, Genty S, et al. Absence of efficacy of nonviable Lactobacillus acidophilus for thr prevention of treavelers' diarrhea: a randomized, double-blind, controlled study. Clin Infect Dis 2006;43:1170.

19. Scallan E, Griffin PM, Angulo F, et al. Foodborne illness acquired in the United States-unspecified agents. Emerg Infect Dis 2011;17(1). Available at: www.cdc.gov/eid. Accessed March 2013.

20. Frank C, Weber D, Cramer JP, et al. Eipdemic profile of Shiga-toxin-producing Escherichia coli O104:H4 outbreak in Germany. N Engl J Med 2011;365:1771.

21. Tarr PI, Gordon CA, Chandler WL. Shiga-toxin-producing Escherichia coli and haemolytic uraemic syndrome. Lancet 2005;365:1073.

22. Wong CS, Jelacic S, Habeeb RL, et al. The risk of the hemolytic-uremic syndrome after antibiotic treatment of Escherichia coli O157:H7 infections. N Engl J Med 2000;342:1930.

23. Rosales A, Hofer J, Zimmerhackl LB, et al. Need for long-term follow-up in enterhemorrhagic Escherchia coli-associated hemolytic uremic syndrome due to late-emerging sequelae. Clin Infect Dis 2012;54:1413.

24. Nelson JM, Griffin PM, Jones TF, et al. Antimicrobial and antimotility agent use in persons with shiga toxin-producing Escherichia coli O157:H7 infection in FoodNet Sites. Clin Infect Dis 2011;52:1130.

25. Giannella RA. Salmonella. In: Baron S, editor. Medical microbiology. 4th edition. Galveston (TX). Chapter 21. Available at: www.ncbi.nlm.nih.gov/books/NBK8435. Accessed March 2013.
26. Nachamkin I, Allos BM, Ho T. Campylobacter species and Guillain-Barre syndrome. Clin Microbiol Rev 1998;11:555.
27. Campbell RR, Beere D, Wilcock GK, et al. Clostridium difficile in acute and long-stay elderly patients. Age Ageing 1988;17:333.
28. Kim J, Smathers SA, Prasad P, et al. Epidemiological features of Clostridium difficile-associated disease among inpatients at children's hospitals in the United States, 2001-2006. Pediatrics 2008;122(6):1266–70.
29. MacDonald CL, Owings M, Jernigan DB. Clostridium difficile infection in patients discharged from US short-stay hospitals, 1996-2003. Emerg Infect Dis 2006; 12(3):409–14.
30. Dial S, Delaney JA, BArkun AN, et al. Use of gastric acid-suppressive agents and the risk of community-acquired Clostridium difficile-associated disease. JAMA 2005;294:2989.
31. Sears CL, Kaper JB. Enteric bacterial toxins: mechanisms of action and likage to intestinal secretion. Microbiol Rev 1996;60:167.
32. Kuehne SA, Cartman ST, Heap JT, et al. The role of toxin A and toxin B in Clostridium difficile infection. Nature 2010;467:711.
33. Nomura K, Fujimotos Y, Yamashta M, et al. Absence of pseudomembranes in Clostridium difficile-associated diarrhea in patients using immunosuppression agents. Scand J Gastroenterol 2009;44:74–8.
34. Mulvey MR, Boyd DA, Gravel D, et al. Hypervirulent Clostridium difficile strains in hospitalized patients, Canada. Emerg Infect Dis 2010;16(4):678–81 (sited May 13, 2013). Available at: http://wwwnc.cdc.gov/eid/article/16/4/09-1152.htm. Accessed March 2013.
35. van Nood E, Vrieze A, Nieuwdorp M, et al. Duodenal infusion of donor feces for recurrent Clostridium difficile. N Engl J Med 2013;368(5):407.
36. Huicho L, Sanchez D, Contreras M, et al. Occult blood and fecal leukocytes as screening tests in childhood infectious diarrhea:an old problem revisited. Pediatr Infect Dis J 1993;12:474.
37. de Zoysa I, Kirkwood B, Feachem R, et al. Preparation of sugar-salt solutions. Trans R Soc Trop Med Hyg 1984;78:260.
38. DuPont HL. Guidelines on acute infectious diarrhea in adults. The Practice Parameters Committee of the American College of Gastroenterology. Am J Gastroenterol 1997;92:1962.

Tuberculosis: An Overview

Wanda Cruz-Knight, MD, MBA*, Lyla Blake-Gumbs, MD, MPH

KEYWORDS

- Latent tuberculosis infection • Clinical presentations tuberculosis
- Treatment of tuberculosis • Genital tuberculosis • Transmission of tuberculosis

KEY POINTS

- Tuberculosis (TB) is still a public health issue. TB continues to reign as one of the world's deadliest diseases. One-third of the world's population has been infected with TB. Identified cases of mycobacterium must be notified in an attempt to reduce the public health impact of TB on the population.
- The principal cause of tissue destruction from *Mycobacterium tuberculosis* (MTB) infection is related to an organism's ability to incite intense host immune reactions to antigenic cell wall proteins.
- TB transmission occurs via inhalation of droplet nuclei. Person-to-person transmission continues to present significant public health issues as work continues toward decreasing the spread of TB.
- The Centers for Disease Control and Prevention (CDC) recommends that high-risk populations in the United States be screened for latent infection, including HIV patients, intravenous (IV) drug users, health care workers who serve high-risk populations, and contacts of individuals with pulmonary TB.
- The most common site for the development of TB is the lungs; 85% of patients with TB present with pulmonary complaints. Extrapulmonary TB may present with primary infection or can be accompanied by reactivation.
- Tuberculin skin test (TST) and interferon-γ release assay (IGRA) are the standard methods for identifying persons infected with the mycobacterium.
- TB may clinically manifest as primary TB, reactivation TB, laryngeal TB, endobronchial TB, lower lung field TB infection, and tuberculoma. Clinical manifestations of TB vary according to site of mycobacterial proliferation.
- Primary pulmonary TB is often accompanied by a normal chest radiograph. Hilar adenopathy is the most common chest abnormality.
- Treatment of TB depends on whether latent TB infection (LTBI) or active TB is treated. Initial empiric treatment of MTB consists of a 4-drug regimen: isoniazid, rifampin, pyrazinamide, and either ethambutol or streptomycin. Once the MTB isolate is known to be fully susceptible, ethambutol (or streptomycin, if it is used as a fourth drug) can be discontinued. Patients diagnosed with active MTB should undergo sputum analysis for MTB weekly until sputum conversion is documented. Treatment duration is typically 6 to 9 months.

Department of Family Medicine and Community Health, University Hospitals Case Medical Center, Case Western Reserve University School of Medicine, 11100 Euclid Avenue, Cleveland, OH 44118, USA
* Corresponding author.
E-mail address: Wanda.Cruz-Knight@UHhospitals.org

Prim Care Clin Office Pract 40 (2013) 743–756
http://dx.doi.org/10.1016/j.pop.2013.06.003
0095-4543/13/$ – see front matter © 2013 Elsevier Inc. All rights reserved.

INTRODUCTION

TB is an infectious disease caused by MTB. Mycobacterium commonly affects the lungs but may affect almost any organ system, including the lymph nodes, central nervous system, liver, bones, genitourinary tract, and gastrointestinal tract. TB is highly transmissible through respiratory droplets. Identified cases of mycobacterium must be notified in an attempt to reduce the public health impact of TB on the population.

MYCOBACTERIUM TUBERCULOSIS

MBT is large nonmotile rod-shaped obligate aerobic bacterium requiring oxygen for survival. Commonly introduced to the body through inhalation of droplet nuclei, MTB is usually found in well-aerated upper lobes of the longs.[1] As a facultative intracellular parasite, the bacterium inhabits macrophages, multiplying within the macrophages. As the bacterium proliferates, they are released from dying macrophages into the alveolar environment. The fate of the mycobacterium is dependent on the host's immune system. A healthy immune system may clear the bacterium whereas exposure may also lead to LTBI or progress to primary TB.

The cellular immune system leads to successful containment of TB. This response is mediated by helper T cells. The ability of T cells and macrophages to block the proliferating bacterium, by forming a granuloma consisting of a caseous center (necrotic cells) surrounded by macrophages and lymphocytes, prevents the growth and spread of mycobacterium. This is the basis for LTBI, where a person infected with MTB does not currently have active TB disease.[2] Unfortunately, 5% to 10% of persons with LTBI are at risk of progressing to active TB; therefore, the authors most actively identify individuals with LTBI and treat to prevent progression to active TB. Individuals with LTBI are noninfectious. Immunocompromised individuals, such as those with HIV infection, cancer, or patients on immunosuppressing medications, are at higher risk of progression to active TB from primary infection or reactivation.

PATHOPHYSIOLOGY

Transmission occurs when inhaled droplet nuclei are deposited within the terminal airspaces of the lung. A cellular immune response that can be detected by a reaction to the TST occurs when tuberculi numbers reach 1000 to 10,000. This usually occurs within 2 to 12 weeks after infection.[3]

MTB have multiple cell wall constituents consisting of glycoproteins, phopholipids, and wax D.[1] These constituents activate Langerhans cells, lymphocytes, and polymorphonuclear leukocytes. Their antigenicity promotes a vigorous, nonspecific immune response. Infection MTB does not always lead to actual TB. The infection may be cleared by the host immune system or suppressed into an inactive form, LTBI, with resistant hosts controlling mycobacterial growth at distant foci before the development of disease. Patients with LTBI cannot spread TB.

The most common site for the development of TB is the lungs; 85% of patients with TB present with pulmonary complaints. Extrapulmonary TB may present with primary infection or can be accompanied by reactivation.

Common extrapulmonary sites are as follows:

- Mediastinal, retroperitoneal, and cervical (scrofula) lymph nodes—the most common site of tuberculous lymphadenitis (scrofula) is in the neck, along the sternocleidomastoid muscle; it is usually unilateral and causes little or no pain; advanced cases of tuberculous lymphadenitis may suppurate and form a draining sinus

- Vertebral bodies
- Adrenals
- Meninges
- Gastrointestinal tract

The principal cause of tissue destruction from MTB infection is related to an organism's ability to incite intense host immune reactions to antigenic cell wall proteins. Mycoplasm forms spherical tubercles consisting of up to 3-mm nodules with approximately 4 cellular zones. The lesions are epithelioid granulomas with central caseation necrosis. The primary lesion is usually found within alveolar macrophages in subpleural regions of the lung; local proliferation of bacilli occurs and spread through the lymphatics to a hilar node, forming the Ghon complex.

Tuberculi nodules consist of

- A central caseation necrosis
- An inner cellular zone of epithelioid macrophages and Langerhans giant cells admixed with lymphocytes
- An outer cellular zone of lymphocytes, plasma cells, and immature macrophages
- A rim of fibrosis (in healing lesions)

Healing of tuberculin lesions may take various forms and stages. Initial lesions may heal and the infection become latent before symptomatic disease occurs. Smaller tubercles may resolve completely. Fibrosis occurs when hydrolytic enzymes dissolve tubercles and larger lesions are surrounded by a fibrous capsule. Such fibrocaseous nodules usually contain viable mycobacteria and are potential lifelong foci for reactivation or cavitation. Some nodules calcify or ossify and are seen easily on chest radiographs.

Tissues within areas of caseation necrosis have high levels of fatty acids, low pH, and low oxygen tension, all of which inhibit growth of the tubercle bacillus.[1] The body's immune responses ability to manage this initial infection and the proliferation of mycoplasm prevent development of primary TB. Otherwise, purulent exudates with large numbers of acid-fast bacilli (AFB) become present in sputum and tissue. Subserosal granulomas may rupture into the pleural or pericardial spaces and create serous inflammation and effusions. The immune systems response to the mycobacteria may lead to either proliferative or exudative lesions. Both types of lesions can develop in the same host, because infective dose and local immunity vary from site to site.

Proliferative lesions occur when there is a small bacillary load and the host cellular immune responses dominate. Tubercles are compact, with admixed activated macrophages admixed surrounded by proliferating lymphocytes, plasma cells, and an outer rim of fibrosis. Intracellular killing of mycobacteria is effective, and the bacillary load remains low. When large numbers of bacilli are present and host defenses are weak, then exudative lesions predominate. These loose aggregates of immature macrophages, neutrophils, fibrin, and caseation necrosis are sites of mycobacterial growth. Untreated, these lesions progress and infection spreads.

EPIDEMIOLOGY

TB continues to reign as one of the world's deadliest diseases. One-third of the world's population has been infected with TB.[3,4] In the United States, there are an estimated 9 million people with LTBI.[5,6] Worldwide in 2011, there were approximately 1.4 million TB-related deaths. Among HIV-infected individuals, TB is the leading cause of death. Foreign-born individuals are 10 times more likely to be infected with TB than those born in the United States. In the United States, the rate of TB is declining.[4]

TRANSMISSION

TB transmission occurs via inhalation of droplet nuclei. Person-to-person transmission continues to present significant public health issues as work continues toward decreasing the spread of TB. Individuals with undiagnosed active untreated pulmonary or laryngeal disease are contagious, particularly when cavitary disease is present or when the sputum is AFB smear positive.[7] Likewise, patients with sputum smear-negative, culture-positive pulmonary TB can also transmit infection. In immonocompetent individuals, TB can remain in an inactive (dormant) state for years without causing symptoms or spreading to other people.[8] Only individuals with active TB can spread the disease. Isolated extrapulmonary TB is not contagious, although such patients require careful evaluation for pulmonary or laryngeal TB.[9] Immunocompromised patients with extrapulmonary TB should be presumed to have pulmonary TB until proved otherwise with negative sputum samples, even if chest radiography is normal.[10]

SCREENING/DIAGNOSES

The CDC recommends that high-risk populations in the United States are screened for latent infection, including HIV patients, IV drug users, health care workers who serve high-risk populations, and contacts of individuals with pulmonary TB.[11] The US Preventive Services Task Force recommends routine screening for TB in high-risk populations.[12] The goal of this recommendation is to identify persons at significant risk for progressing to active disease. A validated risk-assessment questionnaire may be used to identify children who are likely to benefit from screening. Screening persons other than high-risk populations places a burden on resources and is, therefore, not recommended.[13]

TST and IGRA are the standard methods for identifying persons infected with the mycobacterium.[14] All individuals with positive screens and suspicious for active infection should have a chest radiograph, 3 sputum samples obtained for AFB, nucleic acid amplification test (NAAT), complete blood cell count, and electrolytes (eg, sodium). If a patient is unable to spontaneously produce sputum, it should be induced (with appropriate precautions to prevent transmission) or obtained via a gastric aspirate. Stained smears should be made from sputum specimens to identify AFB, because this is the first bacteriologic evidence of infection and gives an estimate of how infectious a patient is.[15] If AFBs are seen on smear, therapy should be started and patients maintained in isolation.

Sputum culture may also be used for diagnosis of TB. It is more sensitive than smear staining, facilitates identification of the mycobacterium species by nucleic acid hybridization or amplification, and evaluates drug sensitivity. Limitations of sputum culture are dependent on the medium used to culture mycobacterium. Cultures may take 4 to 8 weeks to get results.

NAAT performed on at least one respiratory specimen may also be used as a diagnostic tool.[14] NAAT may speed the diagnosis in smear-negative cases or in patients with other strains of mycobacterium. Genotyping is expensive and best used when there are TB outbreaks. Finally, patients with positive TB tests should also be tested for HIV within 2 months of diagnosis.

One of the diagnostic challenges is secondary to accurate testing; 40% to 50% of TB cases are AFB smear negative and 15% to 20% have negative cultures. If there is a strong clinical suspicion of active TB, especially when accompanied by a positive skin test, empiric TB therapy may be tried before laboratory confirmation of infection. In patients with low suspicion for active TB and smears negative for AFB, it is acceptable to wait for the results of AFB culture or repeat chest radiograph before starting treatment.

The TST or IGRA helps diagnose LTBI in a person exposed to MTB but without signs of active TB.[16] The TST and IGRA measure the response of T cells to TB antigens. Because false-negative results occur in 20% to 25% of patients with active pulmonary TB, these tests should not be used alone to exclude a diagnosis of active TB.[17] Immunocompetence and vaccination status may affect interpretation of the TST. Induration of greater than or equal to 15 mm in diameter is a positive test in an immunocompetent person.[18] Immunocompromised individuals may require a 2-step testing approach at least 2 weeks apart to prime the immune system. In this subset of patients, induration of greater than or equal to 10 mm is considered a positive test. In individuals with a history of bacille Calmette-Guérin, vaccination and IGRA are preferred due to superior specificity. IGRA is also used for patient subsets at high risk of TB but low adherence with TB testing, requiring a 48- to 72-hour confirmatory reading, as in the case of the TST.[13]

The CDC and American Thoracic Society recommend targeted testing for LTBI in high-risk groups, such as people with HIV, IV drug users, health care workers who serve high-risk populations, and contacts of individuals with pulmonary TB. Patients receiving tumor necrosis factor α antagonist should be tested before initiation of therapy.

CLINICAL MANIFESTATION

TB may clinically manifest as primary TB, reactivation TB, laryngeal TB, endobronchial TB, lower lung field TB infection, and tuberculoma. Clinical manifestations of TB vary according to site of mycobacterial proliferation.[13] The most common route of entry of MTB is through the bronchial system. Patients with pleural TB may present with a chronic cough, night sweat, pleurisy, blood-tinged sputum, and weight loss.[19,20] TB initial presentation may mimic other medical conditions. The table below highlights the common clinical presentations of TB.

Clinical Presentations of Tuberculosis	
Site of Organism Proliferation	Clinical Symptoms
Pleural TB	Blood-tinged sputum producing chronic cough, pleurisy, chest pain
TB lymphadenitis	Enlarged cervical or supraclavicular lymphnodes
Tuberculous meningits	Persistent or intermittent headach for 2–3 weeks. Mental status changes, coma
Skeletal TB	Spine is most common site (Pott disease). Back pain, stiffness, lower extremity paralysis (50%) occurrence
Tuberculous arthritis	Involves on joint. Hips and knees more commonly affected. Pain precedes radiographic changes
Genitourinary TB	Flank pain, dysuria, and frequent urination. Men may present with painful scrotal mass, prostatitis, orchitis, or epididymitis. In women, condition may mimic pelvic inflammatory disease. 10% of sterility in women worldwide and 1% of women in industrialized countries
Gastrointestinal TB	TB may infect any site along the gastrointestinal tract. TB can manifest as nonhealing ulcers of the mouth or anus, difficulty swallowing, abdominal pain (peptic ulcer like), malabsorption, pain diarrhea, or hematochezia

Patients with TB lymphadenitis most commonly present with enlarged lymph nodes in the cervical and supraclavicular areas.[21] There can be unilateral or bilateral involvement. In patients suspected of having TB with superficial lymphadenitis, the first diagnostic test should be fine-needle aspiration. For questionable diagnosis, lymph node excisional biopsy should be obtained. In patients with skeletal TB, approximately 70% have a positive tuberculin skin test.[22] In skeletal TB, pain of the involved area is the most common complaint with absent constitutional symptoms. Because onset of symptoms is gradual, diagnosis is frequently delayed. Patients may present with lower extremity paralysis or limited movement with local swelling. Patients may also present with a nontender abscess. When a diagnosis of TB arthritis/skeletal TB is in question, then synovial biopsy or tissue biopsy is the diagnostic modality. Although fluid/tissue cultures may be positive in up to 80% of cases, AFB smear is a poor diagnostic modality.[23]

Patients with central nervous system TB and meningitis or intracranial tuberculomas (rounded mass lesions can develop during primary infection or when a focus of reactivation TB becomes encapsulated) may present with headache, neck stiffness, altered mental status, and cranial nerve abnormalities.[24] Cerebrospinal fluid examination is essential for diagnosis of TB meningitis. Rapid diagnosis leads to improved outcomes but depends on a high level of suspicion, especially in industrialized medicine.[25] AFB culture of cerebrospinal fluid is definitive modality for diagnosis, whereas cerebrospinal fluid analysis is usually normal. Because awaiting cultures may present a delay in cure, treatment is initiated presumptively based on clinical suspicion, risk factors, and cerebrospinal fluid results. Approximately 50% of patients with central nervous system TB have chest radiograph abnormalities consistent with pulmonary TB; head CT or MRI may show tuberculomas or signs of intracranial pressure.[26]

In abdominal TB, the TST is positive 70% of the time with radiographic evidence of LTBI.[27] Patients may present with abdominal swelling (ascites), abdominal pain, fever, and/or change in bowel habits. Diagnosis is based on culture growth from ascetic fluid or biopsy. TB enteritis presents most commonly with ileocecum involvement, followed by ileum, cecum, and ascending colon. Patients most commonly present with chronic abdominal pain. Changes in bowel habits are usually present along with heme-positive stool. Emergency clinical presentations may be due to small bowel obstruction or a right lower quadrant mass. Peritoneal fluid culture is 92% sensitive but results may take up to 8 weeks. Peritoneal biopsy may reveal military nodules over the peritoneum and lead to presumptive diagnosis in 80% to 95% of patients. TB enteritis is best diagnosed by colonoscopy and biopsy, which may reveal ulcers, pseudopolyps, or nodules.

Genitourinary TB may present as dysuria, hematuria, and urinary frequency.[28] Although symptoms may be absent in up to 30% of patients, men may present with a scrotal mass and women may present with pelvic inflammatory disease–like symptoms.[29,30] Constitutional symptoms are rare. Diagnosis is often delayed, leading to kidney involvement. Chest radiograph is abnormal in 40% to 75% of patients, with positive skin test in up to 90% of patients.[31] Diagnosis depends on culturing TB from morning urine samples (3 are recommended) or biopsy of a lesion seen on cystoscope or other imaging modalities. Urine culture for TB may be positive in 80% of patients; 3 samples for culture improve sensitivity; this requires a high level of suspicion. The classic finding of sterile pyuria is neither sensitive nor specific. Definitive diagnosis of genital TB is based on tissue biopsy.[32]

Pericardial TB is rare but may present with chest or pleurisy and cardiac effusion on imaging. Chest radiograph shows cardiomegaly (up to 95% of cases) and pleural effusion (approximately 50%) with low-voltage ECG occurring 25% of the time. T-wave inversion is common in approximately 90% of patients. Diagnosis requires pericardial fluid or biopsy. AFB smear is commonly negative; cultures are positive only 50% of the time; biopsy leads to a higher diagnostic yield.

Patients presenting with full-blown constitutional symptoms and a diagnosis of TB should be evaluated for disseminated TB.[33] The diagnosis is based on the number of organs involved. The most common organs are lungs, liver, spleen, kidneys, and bone marrow. Chest radiograph (if nondiagnostic, consider a chest CT), sputum for AFB smear and culture, blood culture for mycobacteria, and first morning void urine for AFB should be obtained.[34] Lumber puncture and biopsy of superficial lymph nodes may be done based on clinical presentation. Sputum smear is positive in one-third of patients, with culture positive in approximately 60%. TST is positive in only 45% of patients with disseminated disease. Prompt diagnosis of disseminated TB is necessary to improve clinical outcome.

Elderly individuals with TB may not display typical signs and symptoms of TB infection due to poor immunogenicity. Active TB infection in this age group may manifest as nonresolving pneumonitis. Likewise, signs and symptoms of extrapulmonary TB may be nonspecific and include leukocytosis, anemia, and hyponatremia due to the release of antidiuretic hormone–like hormone from affected lung tissue.

RADIOGRAPHIC MANIFESTATION

Primary pulmonary TB is often accompanied by a normal chest radiograph. Hilar adenopathy is the most common chest abnormality. There are studies showing a 65% occurrence of cases.[35] Hilar changes can occur within a week after skin test conversion or in the span of 2 months. In most cases, these findings often resolve within the first year of detecting a positive skin test for primary TB.

Another study showed one-third of the 517 converters developed pleural effusions, within the first 3 to 4 months after infection but occasionally as late as 1 year.[36] Pulmonary infiltrates were documented in 27% of patients.[37] Perihilar and right-sided infiltrates were the most common, and ipsilateral hilar enlargement was the rule. Although contralateral hilar changes sometimes were present, only 2% of patients had bilateral infiltrates. Lower and upper lobe infiltrates were observed in 33% and 13% of adults, respectively; 43% of adults with infiltrates also had effusions. Most infiltrates resolved over months to years. In 20 patients (15% of cases), however, the infiltrates progressed within the first year after skin test conversion, so-called progressive primary TB. The majority of these patients had progression of disease at the original site, and 4 developed cavitation.[38]

In studies looking at culture positive, the most common radiologic finding was hilar lymphadenopathy, present in 67% of cases.[39] Right middle lobe collapse may complicate the adenopathy but usually resolves with therapy.

Several factors probably favor involvement of the right middle lobe[39]:

• Dense lymph nodes
• Longer length and smaller internal caliber
• Sharper branching angle

Pleural effusions are also common in active TB infection. A Canadian retrospective study demonstrated pulmonary infiltrates in 63% of patients, and 85% of infiltrates were in the midlung to lower lung fields.[40] Two patients had cavitation and 2 others evidence of endobronchial spread. A majority of patients with reactivation TB have abnormalities on chest radiography. Reactivation TB typically involves the apical-posterior segments of the upper lobes (80%–90% of patients), followed in frequency by the superior segment of the lower lobes and the anterior segment of the upper lobes.[41]

Atypical radiographic patterns may occur in up to 30% adults with reactivation TB. Findings may include hilar adenopathy, infiltrates or cavities in the middle or lower lung zones, pleural effusions, and solitary nodules. Atypical findings are seen more often in the setting of primary TB. Ironically, approximately 5% of patients with active TB present with upper lobe fibrocalcific changes thought to be indicative of healed primary TB. In the setting of pulmonary symptoms, these patients should be evaluated for active TB. A normal chest radiograph is also possible even in active pulmonary TB.

CT scanning of chest is more sensitive than plain chest films for diagnosis, with higher sensitivity for smaller lesions located in the apex of the lung.[42] CT scan may demonstrate a cavity or apicoposterior infiltrates, cavities, pleural effusions, fibrotic lesions causing distortion of lung parenchyma, elevation of fissures and hila, pleural adhesions, and formation of traction bronchiectasis. To detect early bronchogenic spread, high-resolution CT is the imaging technique of choice. The most common findings consist of centrilobular 2-mm to 4-mm nodules or branching linear lesions representing intra-bronchiolar and peribronchiolar caseation necrosis. MRI detects intrathoracic lymph-adenopathy, pericardial thickening, and pericardial and pleural effusions.

Currently, there is no role for routine use of positron emission tomography (PET) for evaluation of TB. PET uptake of fludeoxyglucose F 18 (FDG) does not differentiate infection from tumor, but the macrophages in active TB do not proliferate and do not need choline C 11, resulting in low choline C 11 uptake; this in contrast to the macrophages in malignancy. Therefore, the combination of a high FDG and low choline C 11 uptake on PET may be useful but not diagnostic of TB.

Tuberculous infection of the tracheobronchial tree can develop from direct extension to the bronchi from a parencymal focus. This happens from infected sputum that leads to spread of MTB. The lesions are seen in the main and upper bronchi. Five percent of the time the lower trachea is involved. Endobronchial TB has been described in 10% to 40% of patients with active pulmonary TB. Bronchial stenosis is observed in 90% of cases not receiving early diagnosis to prevent development of fibrosis.

TREATMENT

Treatment of TB depends on whether LTBI or active TB is treated. If a patient has had recent close contact with a person with active TB but is still in the 12-week window where TST may be negative, immediate LTBI treatment should be considered if the patient is at high risk of progression to active TB or has increased susceptibility to disease.[43] In patients with significant exposure with active TB repeat, TST should be performed 12 weeks after contact has ended, and treatment should be continued if the TST result is positive or discontinued if the result is negative. The exception to this recommendation is that persons who are immunocompromised, including those with HIV infection, who had contact with individuals with active TB should continue treatment of LTBI, even if repeat TST is negative.

Initial empiric treatment of MTB consists of a 4-drug regimen: isoniazid, rifampin, pyrazinamide, and either ethambutol or streptomycin.[44] Once the MTB isolate is known to be fully susceptible, ethambutol (or streptomycin, if it is used as a fourth drug) can be discontinued.[45] Patients diagnosed with active MTB should undergo sputum analysis for MTB weekly until sputum conversion is documented. Treatment duration is typically 6 to 9 months.

Pyrazinamide may be stopped after 2 months of treatment of a proved susceptible isolate. Isoniazid plus rifampin must be continued for an additional 4 months. If isolated isoniazid resistance is proved, isoniazid should be stopped and rifampin, pyrazinamide, and ethambutol should be continued for the entire 6 months. It is necessary to extend therapy if the patient has cavitary disease and/or remains culture-positive after the first 2 months of treatment.

Patients receiving pyrazinamide should undergo baseline and periodic serum uric acid assessments, and those receiving long-term ethambutol therapy should undergo baseline and periodic visual acuity and red-green color perception testing (ie, the Ishihara test for color blindness). Monitoring for toxicity includes baseline and periodic liver enzymes, complete blood cell count, and serum creatinine.

The development of drug resistance to 1 or more drugs by MTB is a major concern worldwide. Typically, drug resistance results from spontaneous mutations within the MTB DNA. Strains of drug-resistant MTB (DR-MTB) were first demonstrated after streptomycin was introduced as a treatment in 1944.[46] Rates of drug resistance are highest in cases where previous treatment has occurred, especially when treatment has been incomplete due to either poor adherence or inadequate therapeutic regimen.

Currently, 17% of newly diagnosed MTB cases are resistant to 1 or more first-line agents. Isoniazid is the drug most commonly associated with resistance (10%), but MTB strains can develop resistance to any medication or combination of medications.[47] Strains resistant to both isoniazid and rifampin, the 2 most effective currently available drugs, and possibly resistant to other drugs are called multidrug resistant (MDR) and were first reported on in the early 1980s. MDR cases are now found worldwide. In 2009, WHO estimated that there were 440,000 new MDR-TB cases or 3.3% of new TB cases were MDR.[49] Annual mortality from MDR-TB was estimated to be

---

Box 1
High-risk populations needing targeted tuberculin testing and treatment of latent infection

Persons at high risk of exposure to and infection with MBT

Persons in close contact with someone who has confirmed active TB

Foreign-born persons from endemic countries who have been living in the United States for 5 years or less (especially children younger than 4 years)

Residents and employees of congregate settings (eg, correctional facilities, long-term care facilities, and homeless shelters)

Health care workers with high-risk patients

Medically underserved, low-income populations

Infants, children, and adolescents exposed to adults in high-risk categories

Persons at high risk of progression from LTBI to active disease

Persons with HIV infection

Persons recently (within the past 2 years) infected with MTB

Children younger than 4 years

Patients who are immunosuppressed (eg, those with diabetes, chronic or end-stage renal disease, silicosis, cancer, malnutrition, prolonged steroid use, or organ transplants; those taking tumor necrosis factor α inhibitors)

Data from Potter B, Rindfleisch K, Kraus CK. Management of active tuberculosis. Am Fam Physician 2005;72(11):2225–32.

Table 1
Currently available antituberculosis drugs

Group 1: first-line oral anti-TB drugs	Isoniazid (H) Rifampin or rifampicin (R) Ethambutol (E)
Group 2: injectables	Pyrazinamide (Z) rifabutin (Rfb) Kanamycin amikacin Capreomycin streptomycin[a]
Group 3: fluoroquinolones	Levofloxacin moxifloxacin Ofloxacin Gatifloxacin
Group 4: oral bacteriostatic second-line drugs	Ethionamide Protionamide Cycloserine terizidone
Group 5: anti-TB drugs with unclear efficacy or role	p-Aminosalicylic acid clofazimine linezolid Amoxicillin/clavulanate thioacetazone Clarithromycin imipenem

[a] Considered a first-line drug.

150,000 worldwide.[48] Inadequate treatment of MDR-TB leads to treatment failure, increased mortality, and the creation of MTB strains with an even more complex resistance profile.

Directly observed therapy short-term (DOTS) programs increase the likelihood of adherence and treatment completion and reduce the risk of the development of DR-MTB and extensively drug-resistant TB (XDR-TB).[49] DOTS is recommended for all patients diagnosed with MTB, whether drug-resistant or susceptible. With DOTS, patients on the regimens (discussed previously) can be placed on 2- to 3-times per week dosing after an initial 2 weeks of daily dosing. Patients on twice-weekly dosing may not miss any doses. Prescribe daily therapy for patients on self-administered medication.

Treatment recommendations for MDR-TB consist of an intensive 8 months of treatment that includes pyrazinamide and a minimum of 4 additional effective second-line drugs, including a fluoroquinolone (not to include ciprofloxacin), an injectable antibiotic (either kanamycin, amikacin, capreomycin, or viomycin, but not streptomycin, which is considered a first-line drug), a thioamide (either ethionamide or prothionamide), and

Table 2
Treatment options for latent tuberculosis infection

Drug	Daily Dosage (Maximum)	Adult Intermittent Dosage (Maximum)	Duration
Isoniazid	5 mg per kg (300 mg)	15 mg per kg (900 mg per dose) twice per week	Nine months in adults and children (6 mo may be an alternative treatment duration in adults)
Rifampin (Rifadin)	10 mg per kg (600 mg)	10 mg per kg (600 mg per dose); daily dosing required when used alone	Four months in adults; 6 mo in children

Note: Rifampin plus pyrazinamide is no longer recommended for the treatment of LTBI.
Rifampin plus isoniazid (same dosing) for 3 months may be an alternative treatment option in select patients, but risk of hepatotoxicity may increase.
Data from World Health Organization. Treatment of tuberculosis: guidelines for national programmes. 4th edition. 2010. Available at: http://www.who.int. Accessed January 24, 2013.

Table 3
Adverse effects of antituberculin drugs

Drug	Main Adverse Effects	Monitoring Parameters
Isoniazid	Hepatotoxicity Lupus-like syndrome Peripheral neuropathy	Monitor LFTs and for flushing and decreased sensation in extremities LFTs should be monitored monthly in patients who are at a higher risk of hepatotoxicity, have preexisting liver disease, or develop abnormal LFT results. LFTs should also be checked in patients who develop clinical symptoms of hepatitis; isoniazid should be discontinued if findings on LFTs increase by more than 5 times the upper limits of normal in patients without symptoms of hepatotoxicity and by more than 3 times the upper limits of normal in patients with symptoms.
	Monoamine toxicity	If flushing occurs, patients should be counseled to avoid foods with high concentrations of monoamines (eg, aged cheeses, wine).
Rifampin (Rifadin)	Drug interactions Hepatotoxicity Immunologic reactions Orange discoloration of body fluids	Baseline laboratory tests (including complete blood cell count and serum creatinine measurements) and monthly; every-other-month; or 1-, 3-, or 6-mo monitoring of LFTs and clinical symptoms are acceptable for most patients but not required. LFTs should be monitored monthly or twice monthly in patients who are at a higher risk of hepatotoxicity, have preexisting liver disease, or develop abnormal LFT results. Acute renal failure Influenza-like symptoms Hemolytic anemia, thrombocytopenia (with potential for acute renal failure) Pruritus (with or without rash) Patients should be counseled about the risk of contact lens discoloration.
Pyrazinamide	Arthralgias Gastrointestinal upset Hepatotoxicity Rash	Baseline LFTs; serum creatinine may be assessed at baseline for dosing adjustments. LFTs should be monitored monthly or twice monthly in patients who are at a higher risk of hepatotoxicity or who have underlying hepatic dysfunction.
	Hyperuricemia	Check uric acid levels if patient is symptomatic
Ethambutol (Myambutol)	Optic neuritis	Baseline and monthly testing of visual acuity and color discrimination; serum creatinine may be assessed at baseline for dosing adjustments.

Abbreviation: LFT, liver function test.
Data from Potter B, Rindfleisch K, Kraus CK. Management of active tuberculosis. Am Fam Physician 2005;72(11):2225–32.

cycloserine or teridizone.[50] Treatment should be continued for a minimum of 20 months with 4 effective medications. The injectable antibiotic may be discontinued after completion of 8 months of therapy.

XDR-TB is a rare type of MDR-TB that is resistant to isoniazid and rifampin, plus any fluoroquinolone and at least 1 of 3 injectable second-line drugs (ie, amikacin, kanamycin, or capreomycin).[43] Because XDR-TB is resistant to the most potent MTB drugs, patients are left with treatment options that are much less effective. XDR-TB is of special concern for persons with HIV infection or other conditions that can weaken the immune system. These persons are more likely to develop TB disease once they are infected and, moreover, have a higher risk of death once they develop TB. See **Box 1** and **Tables 1–3** for outline of antituberculosis drugs.

REFERENCES

1. Available at: http://textbookofbacteriology.net/themicrobialworld/tuberculosis.html. Accessed February 23, 2013.
2. Jasmer RM, Nahid P, Hopewell PC. Clinical practice. Latent tuberculosis infection. N Engl J Med 2002;347(23):1860–6.
3. World Health Organization. Global tuberculosis report 2012. 2012. Available at: http://www.who.int. Accessed March 1, 2013.
4. Khan K, Wang J, Hu W, et al. Tuberculosis infection in the United States: national trends over three decades. Am J Respir Crit Care Med 2008;177:455–60.
5. Centers for Disease Control and Prevention (CDC). Decrease in reported tuberculosis cases: United States, 2009. MMWR Morb Mortal Wkly Rep 2010;59:289–94.
6. CDC. Trends in tuberculosis—United States, 2011. Available at: http://www.cdc.gov/mmwr/preview/mmwrhtml/mm6111a2.htm?s_cid=mm6111a2_w. Accessed January 25, 2013.
7. Centers for Disease Control and Prevention (CDC). Trends in tuberculosis incidence—United States, 2006. MMWR Morb Mortal Wkly Rep 2007;56:245–50.
8. Verhagen LM, van den Hof S, van Deutekom H, et al. Mycobacterial factors relevant for transmission of tuberculosis. J Infect Dis 2011;203(9):1249–55.
9. Lienhardt C. From exposure to disease: the role of environmental factors in susceptibility to an development of tuberculosis. Epidemiol Rev 2001;23:288–301.
10. Geng E, Kreiswirth B, Burzynski J, et al. Clinical and radiographic correlates of primary and reactivation tuberculosis, a molecular epidemiology study. JAMA 2005;293:2740–5.
11. Centers for Disease Control and Prevention. Questions and answers about tuberculosis. Available at: http://www.cdc.gov/tb/publications/faqs/pdfs/qa.pdf. Accessed February 3, 2012.
12. Available at: www.uspreventiveservicestaskforce.org/recommendations.htm. Accessed January 13, 2013.
13. Richeldi L. An update on the diagnosis of tuberculosis infection. Am J Respir Crit Care Med 2006;174(7):736–42.
14. Pai M, Zwerling A, Menzies D. Systematic review: T-cell-based assays for the diagnosis of latent tuberculosis infection: an update. Ann Intern Med 2008;149:177–84.
15. Breen RA, Leonard O, Perrin FM, et al. How good are systemic symptoms and blood inflammatory markers at detecting individuals with tuberculosis? Int J Tuberc Lung Dis 2008;12:44.

16. Metcalfe JZ, Everett CK, Steingart KR, et al. Interferon-γ release assays for active pulmonary tuberculosis diagnosis in adults in low- and middle-income countries: systematic review and meta-analysis. J Infect Dis 2011;204(Suppl 4):S1120–9.

17. Centers for Disease Control and Prevention (CDC). Updated guidelines for the use of nucleic acid amplification tests in the diagnosis of tuberculosis. MMWR Morb Mortal Wkly Rep 2009;58:7–10.

18. Mazurek GH, Jereb J, Vernon A, et al. Updated guidelines for using Interferon Gamma Release Assays to detect Mycobacterium tuberculosis infection—United States, 2010. MMWR Recomm Rep 2010;59:1.

19. Low SY, Hsu A, Eng P. Interventional bronchoscopy for tuberculous tracheo-bronchial stenosis. Eur Respir J 2004;24:345.

20. Buckner CB, Walker CW. Radiologic manifestations of adult tuberculosis. J Thorac Imaging 1990;5:28.

21. Barnes PF, Verdegem TD, Vachon LA, et al. Chest roentgenogram in pulmonary tuberculosis. New data on an old test. Chest 1988;94:316.

22. Oursler KK, Moore RD, Bishai WR, et al. Survival of patients with pulmonary tuberculosis: clinical and molecular epidemiologic factors. Clin Infect Dis 2002;34:752.

23. Pott P. The chirurgical works of Percivall Pott, F.R.S., surgeon to St. Bartholomew's Hospital, a new edition, with his last corrections. 1808. Clin Orthop Relat Res 2002;(398):4–10.

24. Miller LG, Asch SM, Yu EI, et al. A population-based survey of tuberculosis symptoms: how atypical are atypical presentations? Clin Infect Dis 2000;30:293.

25. Moon MS, Kim SS, Lee BJ, et al. Spinal tuberculosis in children: retrospective analysis of 124 patients. Indian J Orthop 2012;46(2):150–8.

26. Kohli A, Kapoor R. Neurological picture. Embolic spread of tuberculomas in the brain in multidrug resistant tubercular meningitis. J Neurol Neurosurg Psychiatry 2008;79(2):198.

27. Lin YL, Fan YC, Cheng CY, et al. The case | Sterile pyuria and an abnormal abdominal film. "Autonephrectomy" of right kidney. Kidney Int 2008;73(1):131–3.

28. Jung YY, Kim JK, Cho KS. Genitourinary tuberculosis: comprehensive cross-sectional imaging. AJR Am J Roentgenol 2005;184(1):143–50.

29. Madeb R, Marshall J, Nativ O, et al. Epididymal tuberculosis: case report and review of the literature. Urology 2005;65(4):798.

30. Wise GJ, Shteynshlyuger A. An update on lower urinary tract tuberculosis. Curr Urol Rep 2008;9(4):305–13.

31. Muttarak M, ChiangMai WN, Lojanapiwat B. Tuberculosis of the genitourinary tract: imaging features with pathological correlation. Singapore Med J 2005;46(10):568–74.

32. Yapar EG, Ekici E, Karasahin E, et al. Sonographic features of tuberculous peritonitis with female genital tract tuberculosis. Ultrasound Obstet Gynecol 1995;6(2):121–5.

33. Mert A, Bilir M, Tabak F, et al. Miliary tuberculosis: clinical manifestations, diagnosis and outcome in 38 adults. Respirology 2001;6:217.

34. Optican RJ, Ost A, Ravin CE. High-resolution computed tomography in the diagnosis of miliary tuberculosis. Chest 1992;102:941.

35. Poulsen A. Some clinical features of tuberculosis. Acta Tuberc Scand 1957;33:37.

36. Steele JD. The solitary pulmonary nodule. Report of a cooperative study of re-sected asymptomatic solitary pulmonary nodules in males. J Thorac Cardiovasc Surg 1963;46:21.

37. Yencha MW, Linfesty R, Blackmon A. Laryngeal tuberculosis. Am J Otolaryngol 2000;21:122.
38. Stead WW, Kerby GR, Schlueter DP, et al. The clinical spectrum of primary tuberculosis in adults. Confusion with reinfection in the pathogenesis of chronic tuberculosis. Ann Intern Med 1968;68:731.
39. Krysl J, Korzeniewska-Kosela M, Müller NL, et al. Radiologic features of pulmonary tuberculosis: an assessment of 188 cases. Can Assoc Radiol J 1994;45:101.
40. Marciniuk DD, McNab BD, Martin WT, et al. Detection of pulmonary tuberculosis in patients with a normal chest radiograph. Chest 1999;115:445.
41. Im JG, Itoh H, Shim YS, et al. Pulmonary tuberculosis: CT findings—early active disease and sequential change with antituberculous therapy. Radiology 1993; 186:653.
42. Jones BE, Ryu R, Yang Z, et al. Chest radiographic findings in patients with tuberculosis with recent or remote infection. Am J Respir Crit Care Med 1997; 156:1270-3.
43. World Health Organization. Treatment of tuberculosis: guidelines for national programmes. 4th edition 2010. Available at: http://www.who.int. Accessed January 24, 2013.
44. Gao XF, Wang L, Liu GJ, et al. Rifampicin plus pyrazinamide versus isoniazid for treating latent tuberculosis infection: a meta-analysis. Int J Tuberc Lung Dis 2006;10(10):1080-90.
45. American Thoracic Society, CDC, Infectious Diseases Society of America. Treatment of tuberculosis [Guideline]. MMWR Recomm Rep 2003;52:1-77. Accessed May 2, 2013.
46. Gillespie S. Evolution of drug resistance in Mycobacterium tuberculosis: clinical and molecular perspective. Antimicrob Agents Chemother 2002;46:267-74.
47. World Health Organization. Anti-tuberculosis drug resistance in the world. Report no. 4. Geneva (Switzerland): WHO/IUATLD global project on anti-tuberculous drug resistance surveillance; 2008. Available at: http://whqlibdoc.who.int/hq/2008/WHO_HTM_TB_2008.394_eng.pdf. Accessed May 12, 2013.
48. Udwadia Z, Amale R, Ajbani K, et al. Totally drug-resistant tuberculosis in India. Clin Infect Dis 2012;54:579-81.
49. Moonan P, Quitugua T, Pogoda J, et al. Does directly observed therapy (DOT) reduce drug resistant tuberculosis? BMC Public Health 2011;11:19.
50. Vora A. Terizidone. J Assoc Physicians India 2010;58:267-8.

Upper Respiratory Infections

Samuel N. Grief, MD, FCFP

KEYWORDS

- Pharyngitis • Sinusitis • Upper respiratory infection

KEY POINTS

- Upper respiratory infections (URIs) are infections of the mouth, nose, throat, larynx (voice box), and trachea (windpipe). URIs include nasopharyngitis (common cold), sinusitis, pharyngitis, laryngitis, and laryngotracheitis.
- Nasopharyngitis (common cold) is a frequent cause of URIs, and most patients with this diagnosis with present with nasal congestion (80%). Nasopharyngitis rarely presents with a fever. Causes are predictably viral, and determining the exact viral pathogen is usually unnecessary. Treatment of the common cold is symptomatic, and hand washing is the best prevention.
- Sinusitis is a common diagnosis seen in primary care. The diagnosis and differentiation between bacterial and viral sinusitis is made clinically, based on the history and examination. Augmentin is the antibiotic preferred by the Infectious Diseases Society of America for empiric treatment of bacterial sinusitis. Nasal steroids are highly effective for both viral and bacterial acute sinusitis.
- Identifying the cause of pharyngitis, especially group A β-hemolytic streptococcus (GABHS), is important in preventing potential life-threatening complications. Group A streptococcal infection (GAS) pharyngitis accounts for 15% to 30% of infections in children and 5% to 15% in adults. The Centor criteria are useful prediction rules for the evaluation and management of possible GAS pharyngitis. Penicillins are the drugs class of choice for streptococcal pharyngitis.
- Acute laryngotracheobronchitis (LTB) is an infectious-induced inflammatory condition affecting the larynx, trachea, and bronchi. It occurs most often in children ages 6 months to 6 years, with the peak age at 2 years. Recommended imaging for suspected croup includes anterior-posterior views of the neck, which show edematous subglottic walls converging to create a characteristic "steeple sign." The cornerstone of medical management of LTB is nebulized epinephrine and dexamethasone.

INTRODUCTION

Upper respiratory infections (URIs) are located in the upper respiratory tract, defined as the mouth, nose, throat, larynx (voice box), and trachea (windpipe). URIs can be one of the following conditions:

- Nasopharyngitis (common cold)

Department of Family Medicine, University of Illinois at Chicago, 1919 West Taylor Street, Suite 186B, Chicago, IL 60612, USA
E-mail addresses: drsgrief@yahoo.com; sgrief@uic.edu

Prim Care Clin Office Pract 40 (2013) 757–770
http://dx.doi.org/10.1016/j.pop.2013.06.004
0095-4543/13/$ – see front matter © 2013 Elsevier Inc. All rights reserved.

primarycare.theclinics.com

- Sinusitis
- Pharyngitis
- Laryngitis
- Laryngotracheitis

NASOPHARYNGITIS (COMMON COLD)

The common cold is a frequent cause of URIs and can be defined as inflammation of the nasal passages owing to a respiratory virus. The vast majority of these infections are self-limited and resolve without treatment. Frequency of the common cold varies per age group (**Table 1**).

Although URIs can happen at any time, they are most common in the fall and winter months, from September until March, because these are the usual school months when children and adolescents spend a lot of time in groups and indoors. Furthermore, many URI viruses thrive in the low humidity of the winter. Signs and symptoms of the common cold are listed in **Table 2**.

Causes of the common cold are predictably viral, with the majority of these viruses falling into 1 of 200 virus strains from 6 main families; rhinovirus, influenza A/B/C, para-influenza, respiratory syncytial virus, coronavirus, and adenovirus.

Determining which virus is the causal agent is unnecessary in the overwhelming number of cases because symptomatic therapy and "tincture of time" usually result in a full resolution of the infection. The diagnosis of a common cold is almost always based on clinical findings. Distinguishing a common cold from a more potent viral illness, such as the influenza virus, is a matter of knowing the common symptoms and signs of the flu and comparing them with those of the common cold. In rare cases, virus is cultured from nasal washings, or identified by enzyme-linked immunosorbent assay or radioimmunoassay methods (**Table 3**).

Prevention

Hand washing is the single most important activity that can reduce the risk of URI. Numerous studies have confirmed that washing with soap or using hand sanitizer lowers the risk of transmission of URI and respiratory infections.[1,2] Alcohol-based hand rubs are the most efficacious agents for reducing the number of bacteria on the hands of hospital and health care personnel. Antiseptic soaps and detergents are the next most effective, and nonantimicrobial soaps the least effective.[3,4]

Treatment of the Common Cold:
- Rest, fluids, and symptomatic measures
- Reassurance that the usual course is 6 to 10 days
- Humidification of inspired air
- Saline nasal rinse or Neti pot

Table 1 Age-specified incidence of the common cold	
Age	**Incidence/Year**
Preschool	6–10 episodes
Elementary	7–12 episodes
Adolescents	2–4 episodes

Data from Turner RB. The common cold. In: Goldman L, Schafer AI, editors. Cecil medicine. 24th edition. Philadelphia: Saunders Elsevier; 2011. Chapter 369.

Table 2
Signs and symptoms of the common cold

Sign or Symptom	Likelihood of Having with a Cold (%)
Nasal congestion/obstruction	80–100
Sneezing	50–70
Sore or scratchy throat	50
Cough	40
Hoarseness	30
Headache	25
Fatigue/malaise	20–25
Fever	0.1

Data from Lauber B. The common cold. J Gen Intern Med 1996;11:231.

- Discontinue any tobacco or alcohol
- Raise head at night with extra pillow to allow nasal passages to drain, as needed
- For infants use bulb suction, position mattress at 45°, use saline nasal drops

Patient Education
- Reassurance
- Spread is primarily hand-to-hand transmission of contaminated nasal secretions
- Aerosolized particles (cough, sneeze) do not travel far and contain little virus
- Individual susceptibility to colds depends largely on preexisting antibodies
- Advise patients to contact you if they develop dyspnea, productive cough, or temperature >102°F (39°C)

Drugs of Choice[5,6]
- Topical decongestants: reduce edema and swelling of the nasal mucosa, promote drainage; fewer side effects than oral agents (phenylephrine: Afrin, Neosynephrine)
- Topical anticholinergics: control rhinorrhea but do not relieve congestion or sneezing (Atrovent nasal spray)

Table 3
URI versus influenza: symptom presentation

Symptom	Common Cold	Seasonal Flu
Cough	Moist and productive	Dry cough (may also be productive)
Itchy/watery eyes	Common	Uncommon
Fever	Uncommon but may occur occasionally in children	Common
Exhaustion/fatigue	Mild tiredness may occur	Very common
Headache	Common; usually due to sinus pressure	Common
Sore throat	Common, but typically mild	Uncommon
Body aches	Minor	Severe
Vomiting/diarrhea	These are not symptoms of the common cold	Uncommon, but may occur occasionally in children
Onset of symptoms	Gradual	Sudden

- Oral decongestants: longer duration of action, lack of local irritation, no risk of rhinitis medicamentosa (pseudoephedrine: Sudafed; phenylephrine: found in many over-the-counter cold and sinus remedies)
- Antihistamines: safe and effective in alleviating sneezing and rhinorrhea (diphenhydramine: Benadryl; chlorpheniramine: Chlor-Trimeton)
- Cough suppressants: useful if cough interferes with sleep or normal activities; codeine and dextromethorphan have similar efficacy (Robitussin D)
- Expectorants: commonly used but efficacy not proven (guaifenesin)
- Throat lozenges: may provide temporary relief from scratchy throat

Medication Precautions
- Oral decongestants: may increase blood pressure and glucose levels; can cause arrhythmias, headache, nervousness, sleeplessness, dizziness
- Antihistamines: nasal blockage and sinus congestion can worsen
- Cough suppressants: misuse and dependence can occur
- Expectorants: can contain high concentrations of alcohol

Alternative Drugs
- Zinc: prevents viral replication in vitro; efficacy not proven
- Vitamin C: no preventive effects and very modest symptom reduction
- Echinacea: no proven efficacy
- Probiotics: efficacy not proven

Possible Complications[7]
- Lower respiratory tract infection
- Bronchial hyperreactivity/asthma flare
- Otitis media (5%–19%)
- Acute sinusitis
- Pneumonia

ACUTE SINUSITIS

Acute (rhino)sinusitis (AS) is defined as inflammation of the nasal mucosa and sinuses.[8] AS is very common. According to a recent national health survey, approximately 1 of 7 adults are affected[9] and diagnosed per year.[10,11]

Diagnosis

Distinguishing between the common cold and AS is often a matter of symptom duration. Typical common colds are self-limited and last 7 to 10 days, whereas AS can last for up to 4 weeks. Symptoms of AS are similar to those of the common cold and include nasal congestion and discharge, facial pain over the sinuses, decreased sense of smell, and cough.[8] The waxing and waning phenomenon of symptoms sets AS apart from the common cold, usually with a mild improvement of symptoms after 5 to 7 days, followed by a worsening of symptoms, including new-onset fever, headache, and/or increased nasal discharge.[12]

A bacterial origin is generally suspected and diagnosed if the following symptoms or signs are present:

- Purulent nasal discharge
- Maxillary tooth or facial pain

- Unilateral maxillary sinus tenderness
- Worsening symptoms after initial improvement[12,13]

Diagnosis of acute bacterial sinusitis (ABS) can be made if there are 2 major or 1 major and 2 minor markers, and symptoms persist beyond 7 to 10 days, start out severe, and last at least 3 to 4 consecutive days or worsen after 5 to 7 days (**Table 4**).[12]

According to the Institute for Clinical Systems Improvement (ICSI), plain sinus radiographs and other radiographic images are usually not necessary for diagnosis of sinusitis, and provide poor sensitivity and specificity.[14] Nasal endoscopy or antral puncture and culture of secretions are ideal tests, but are not feasible for the general practitioner and should be relegated to otolaryngologists, usually in the setting of diagnosing a chronic sinusitis.

Treatment

Discriminating between bacterial and viral AS is one of the most important determinants of treatment, **Table 4** is helpful for diagnosing bacterial AS that would warrant antibiotic treatment.

Bacterial causes of AS include:

- *Streptococcus pneumoniae*
- *Haemophilus influenzae*
- *Moraxella catarrhalis*

Selecting the appropriate antibiotic will help mitigate complications. **Table 5** provides guidance.

Duration of antibiotic therapy has been studied. A meta-analysis of 12 randomized controlled trials found no statistically significant difference between long-term and short-course antibiotics for cure or improvement of symptoms.[15] Five to 7 days of treatment with the appropriate antibiotic is considered effective for patients with uncomplicated ABS.

Other treatments are listed in **Table 6**, along with their usefulness.

Additional comfort measures for treating AS include:

- Maintain adequate hydration (6–10 glasses of liquids per day)
- Apply warm facial packs (warm wash cloth, hot water bottle, or gel pack for 5–10 minutes 3 or more times a day to help with pain relief)

Table 4
Signs and symptoms of acute bacterial sinusitis

Major Markers	Minor Markers
Purulent nasal discharge	Headache
Purulent postnasal discharge	Ear pain/pressure/fullness
Nasal obstruction/congestion	Sore throat
Facial congestion/fullness	Halitosis
Focal facial pain/pressure	Dental pain
Hyposmia/anosmia	Cough
Fever (temperature 102°F [39°C])	Fever (<102°F)
	Fatigue

Modified from Chow AW, Benninger MS, Brook I, et al. IDSA clinical practice guideline for acute bacterial rhinosinusitis in children and adults. Clin Infect Dis 2012;54(8):e78.

Table 5
Antibiotic regimens for acute sinusitis

Class	Line	Notes
Penicillin/amoxicillin/augmentin	First	Amoxicillin-clavulanate is recommended by the IDSA as the preferred empiric antimicrobial therapy for acute sinusitis[12]
Doxycycline	First	Doxycycline may be used as an alternative regimen to amoxicillin-clavulanate for initial empiric antimicrobial therapy for ABRS in adults because it remains highly active against respiratory pathogens[12]
Cephalosporins	Second/third	Second- and third-generation oral cephalosporins are no longer recommended[12] for empiric monotherapy for ABRS due to variable rates of resistance among *Streptococcus pneumoniae*. Combination therapy with a third-generation oral cephalosporin (cefixime or cefpodoxime) plus clindamycin may be used as second-line therapy for children with non–type I penicillin allergy or from geographic regions with high endemic rates of PNS *S pneumoniae*[12]
Quinolone	Second/third	Levofloxacin is recommended for children older than 8 y with a history of type I hypersensitivity to penicillin[12]
Sulfa	Third	Trimethoprim-sulfamethoxazole is not recommended for empiric therapy because of high rates of resistance among both *S pneumoniae* and *Haemophilus influenzae* (~30%–40%)[12]

Abbreviations: ABRS, acute bacterial rhinosinusitis; IDSA, Infectious Diseases Society of America; PNS, penicillin-nonsusceptible.

Data from Chow AW, Benninger MS, Brook I, et al. IDSA clinical practice guideline for acute bacterial rhinosinusitis in children and adults. Clin Infect Dis 2012;54(8):e92.

- Eliminate environmental factors that could trigger allergic reactions (cigarette smoke, pollution/fumes, swimming in contaminated water, and barotraumas)
- Obtain adequate rest and sleep with head of bed elevated
- Avoid extremely cold or dry air
- Engage in fastidious and frequent hand washing[14]

PHARYNGITIS
Introduction

Pharyngitis is one of the most common conditions encountered by the family physician.[18] The optimal approach for differentiating among various causes of pharyngitis requires a problem-focused history, a physical examination, and appropriate laboratory testing. Identifying the cause of pharyngitis, especially group A β-hemolytic streptococcus (GABHS), is important in preventing potential life-threatening complications.[18]

Definition

Inflammation of the pharynx, caused by one of many different viruses and/or bacteria.

Table 6 Therapeutic options for AS		
Class of Drug/Modality	Efficacy	Notes
Intranasal steroids	Decreases nasal inflammation	Highly recommended[14]
Antihistamines	Increases viscosity of nasal secretions	Not recommended[16]
Oral decongestants	Decrease amount of nasal secretions and edema	Caution in patients with uncontrolled hypertension, hyperthyroidism, coronary artery disease, diabetes, glaucoma, and benign prostatic hypertrophy; not indicated for children <6 y old
Topical decongestants	Decrease amount of nasal secretions	Use for no more than 3 d to lessen the risk of rebound nasal congestion Found to be more effective than oral decongestants[10]
Mucolytics	Thin nasal secretions	Useful adjunctive therapy[10]
Analgesics	Decrease headache and sinus pressure	Dose per manufacturer's guidelines
Saline nasal irrigation/ humidity and Neti pot	Thin nasal secretions/improve nasal clearance	Increases comfort[10]

Data from Refs.[10,14,16,17]

Epidemiology

- Acute pharyngitis is one of the 20 most reported reasons for outpatient office visits
- Peak season is late winter and early spring
- Transmission of typical viral and Group A streptococcal (GAS) pharyngitis occurs mostly by hand contact and has an incubation period of 1 to 3 days (35% transmission)

Etiology

- Pharyngitis is most likely caused by virus or bacteria[18,19]
- Also caused by reflux, rhinitis and postnasal drip, persistent cough, and allergy NB. Consider testing for infectious mononucleosis if the patient is between 10 and 25 years old
- GAS pharyngitis accounts for 15% to 30% of infections in children and 5% to 15% in adults
- GAS is the most common cause of bacterial infection
- Physical signs of GAS include:
  o Pharyngeal erythema and swelling
  o Tonsillar exudates
  o Edematous uvula
  o Palatine petechiae
  o Anterior cervical lymphadenopathy

Determining how likely a pharyngitis is due to GAS infection has been studied. Criteria have been developed to assist the practitioner in making a clinical diagnosis (**Table 7**).

Table 7
Centor clinical prediction rules for diagnosis of group A β-hemolytic streptococcus (GABHS) in adults

Points	LR+	Pretest prevalence of GABHS (%)			
		5	10	25	50
		Posttest probability of GABHS (%)			
0	0.16	1	2	5	14
1	0.3	2	3	9	23
2	0.75	4	8	20	43
3	2.1	10	19	41	68
4	6.3	25	41	68	86

One point for each: history of fever, anterior cervical adenopathy, tonsillar exudates, absence of cough.
Abbreviation: LR+, positive likelihood ratio.
Data from Ebell MH, Smith MA, Barry HC, et al. The rational clinical examination. Does this patient have strep throat? JAMA 2000;284:2916.

- Untreated, GAS pharyngitis lasts 7 to 10 days. These patients are infective during the acute phase of the illness and for 1 additional week, and are also at risk of suppurative complications (see later discussion)
- Effective antibiotic treatment decreases the infectious period to 24 hours, decreases symptoms, and prevents most complications

Complications of GAS

- Rheumatic fever: rare in the United States
- Peritonsillar abscess: toxic appearance, fluctuant peritonsillar mass, and deviation of uvula
- Poststreptococcal glomerulonephritis
- Scarlet fever: sandpaper-like exanthem

Other Bacterial Causes of Acute Pharyngitis Include:
- Gonorrhea
- Chlamydia
- Mycoplasma
- Diphtheria

Management of GAS Pharyngitis

The Infectious Diseases Society of America (IDSA) reiterates 2 principles of management:

1. Use of clinical and epidemiologic features to distinguish who may have GAS pharyngitis (see **Table 7**)
2. Antibacterial treatment of cases confirmed with a laboratory test (culture or rapid antigen testing)

Antibiotic Therapy for GAS Pharyngitis

- GAS is universally sensitive to penicillin[20,21]
- Drug of choice: penicillin V for 10 days
  - 250 mg 3 times daily for pediatrics
  - 500 mg 2 times daily for adults
- Benzathine G PCN injection for compliance problems

- Amoxicillin
  - Suspension tastes better

Alternative therapies include:

- Erythromycin
- First-generation cephalosporins
- Clindamycin
- Macrolides: resistance ranges from 13% to 31%[21]

LARYNGOTRACHEITIS/LARYNGOTRACHEOBRONCHITIS (CROUP)
Definition

Acute laryngotracheobronchitis (LTB) is an infectious-induced inflammatory condition affecting the larynx, trachea, and bronchi.

Prevalence

- Most common in children ages 6 months to 6 years, with the peak at 2 years[22]

Symptoms

- Hoarseness of voice followed by paroxysms of nonproductive, harsh, seal-like cough that ends with a characteristic inspiratory stridor. Fever, rhinorrhea, sore throat, and cough usually precede this. Symptoms may vary in intensity and last approximately 3 to 4 days if mild.
- Anterior-posterior radiograph view of the neck shows the subglottic obstruction.

Etiology

LTB is caused mostly by viruses, primarily parainfluenza virus types I and II, although others, such as influenza type A or B, respiratory syncytial virus (RSV), and adenovirus are also implicated. H influenzae type B is now a rare cause, thanks to routine immunization. Occasionally Mycoplasma pneumoniae can cause LTB.[22]

Clinical Findings

- Patients appear apprehensive and tend to lean forward
- The child may have tachypnea and might be using accessory respiratory muscles
- Inspiratory or expiratory stridor is prominent[23]
- Pulmonary examination may reveal rhonchi, crepitations, or wheezing
- Breath sounds may be diminished if upper airway obstruction is severe and air entry is greatly decreased

Severity of attack can be determined based on the Westley Croup Scale[24]:

2 or less: mild
3 to 7: moderate
8 or more: severe
Level of consciousness: Normal, including sleep = 0; disoriented = 5
Cyanosis: None = 0; with agitation = 4; at rest = 5
Stridor: None = 0; with agitation = 1; at rest = 2
Air entry: Normal = 0; decreased = 1; markedly decreased = 2
Retractions: None = 0; mild = 1; moderate = 2; severe = 3

Laboratory Findings

- The white blood cell count may be normal or mildly elevated.
- Noninvasive pulse oximetry to monitor the oxygen saturation is recommended.[25] Arterial blood gas assessment shows hypoxemia and/or hypercapnia, depending on the severity of the disease.
- Microbiologic diagnosis can be established by serology, viral or bacterial cultures from the pharynx, or rapid antigen detection enzyme immunosorbent assays such as for RSV or influenza type A.

Imaging

Lateral neck radiographs show overdistended hypopharynx, subglottic narrowing that is wider on expiration than inspiration, thickened vocal cords, and a normal epiglottis.

Anterior-posterior views of the neck show edematous subglottic walls converging to create a characteristic "steeple sign."[26]

There may also be diffuse narrowing of the trachea and bronchi.

Differential Diagnosis

Acute epiglottitis is a major differential diagnosis to be considered when a child presents with these symptoms. Radiographs of the neck can easily help differentiate the 2 conditions. Other causes of similar symptoms include foreign-body aspiration, which can be determined by history, radiographs, or endoscopic evaluation. Membranous croup or bacterial tracheitis should also be considered if the child presents with a clinical picture similar to croup but appears more toxic and has subglottic narrowing on radiographs of the neck. In milder cases, a simple URI is more likely. If sore throat is prominent, ensure adequate visualization of the tonsils to confirm absence of peritonsillar abscess. Allergic reactions (angioedema) and airway anomalies such as trachea/laryngomalacia should also be entertained.[22,24]

Complications

Severe croup, as may occur with influenza type A, may require tracheotomy or intubation in approximately 13% of patients and have an associated mortality of 0% to 2.7%.[15] A small percentage of children with prolonged intubation or severe disease may develop subglottic stenosis. A few follow-up studies have shown an increase in hyperactive airways in children with a history of croup.

Outpatient management of croup in children is feasible, as noted in **Fig. 1**.

Treatment

The cornerstone of medical management is nebulized epinephrine and dexamethasone.[24] Racemic or L-epinephrine may be used; its onset is 1 to 5 minutes and its effects last up to 2 hours. Dexamethasone in appropriate doses partners well with epinephrine, as its onset of action is 6 hours.[17] Nebulized budesonide is also now a therapeutic option.[27]

Oxygen may be administered, along with humidification, to avoid agitation and maintain oxygen saturation higher than 92%.[28]

Some children will fail medical management and require intubation. Intubation should be done in fully equipped units and preferably via the nasotracheal route. Extubation is usually attempted in about 5 to 7 days if extubation criteria are met. Extubation criteria include decreased secretions, decreased leakage around the endotracheal tube (which indicates decreased edema), and an alert child. Failure to extubate should prompt further endoscopic evaluation.[22]

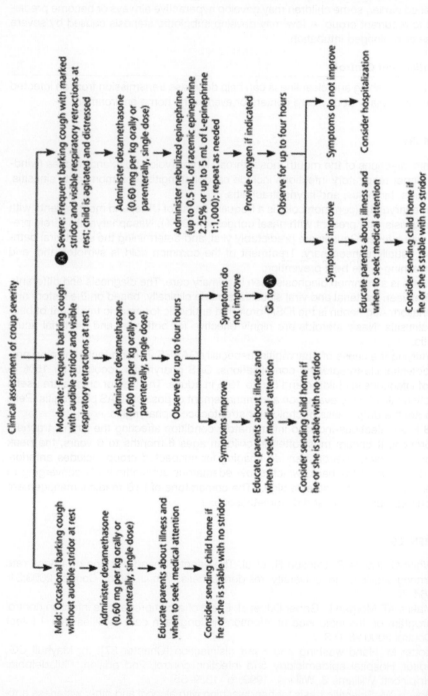

Fig. 1. Assessment and management of croup. (*From* Zoorob R, Sidani M, Murray J. Croup: an overview. Am Fam Physician 2011;83(9):1071; with permission.)

Prognosis

Croup is mostly a self-limited disease with complete uncomplicated resolution. As mentioned earlier, some children may develop hyperactive airways or become predisposed to recurrent croup. A few may develop subglottic stenosis caused by severe disease or prolonged intubation.

Prevention and Control

Good hand washing and cleanliness can help decrease transmission from an infected patient, particularly at day care centers or even in the home environment.

SUMMARY

URIs are infections of the mouth, nose, throat, larynx (voice box), and trachea (windpipe). Upper respiratory infections include nasopharyngitis (common cold), sinusitis, pharyngitis, laryngitis, and laryngotracheitis.

Nasopharyngitis (common cold) is a frequent cause of URIs, and most patients with this diagnosis with present with nasal congestion (80%). Nasopharyngitis rarely presents with a fever. Causes are predictably viral, and determining the exact viral pathogen is usually unnecessary. Treatment of the common cold is symptomatic, and hand washing is the best prevention.

Sinusitis is a common diagnosis seen in primary care. The diagnosis and differentiation between bacterial and viral sinusitis is made clinically, based on the history and examination. Augmentin is the IDSA-preferred antibiotic for empiric treatment of bacterial sinusitis. Nasal steroids are highly effective for both viral and bacterial acute sinusitis.

Identifying the cause of pharyngitis, especially GABHS, is important in helping prevent potential life-threatening complications. GAS pharyngitis accounts for 15% to 30% of infections in children and 5% to 15% in adults. The Centor criteria are useful prediction rules for the evaluation and management of possible GAS pharyngitis. Penicillins are the drugs class of choice for streptococcal pharyngitis.

LTB is an infectious-induced inflammatory condition affecting the larynx, trachea, and bronchi. It occurs most often in children ages 6 months to 6 years, the peak age being 2 years. Recommended imaging for suspected croup includes anteriorposterior views of the neck, which show edematous subglottic walls converging to create a characteristic "steeple sign." The cornerstone of LTB medical management is nebulized epinephrine and dexamethasone.

REFERENCES

1. White C, Kolble R, Carlson R, et al. The effect of hand hygiene on illness rate among students in university residence halls. Am J Infect Control 2003;31: 364–70.
2. Makris AT, Morgan L, Gaber DJ, et al. Effect of a comprehensive infection control program on the incidence of infections in long-term care facilities. Am J Infect Control 2000;28(1):3–7.
3. Rotter M. Hand washing and hand disinfection [Chapter 87]. In: Mayhall CG, editor. Hospital epidemiology and infection control. 2nd edition. Philadelphia: Lippincott Williams & Wilkins; 1999. p. 1339–55.
4. Boyce JM. Scientific basis for handwashing with alcohol and other waterless antiseptic agents. In: Rutala WA, editor. Disinfection, sterilization and antisepsis:

principles and practices in healthcare facilities. Washington, DC: Association for Professionals in Infection Control and Epidemiology, Inc; 2001. p. 140–51.

5. Simasek M, Blandino D. Treatment of the common cold. Am Fam Physician 2007; 75(4):515–20.

6. Treating the common cold; an expert panel consensus recommendations for primary care providers. Available at: http://www.iafp.com/pdfs/common%20cold%20guideline%20final.pdf. Accessed February 28, 2013.

7. The common cold in children. Available at: http://www.uptodate.com/contents/the-common-cold-in-children-beyond-the-basics. Accessed May 1, 2013.

8. Zoorob R, Sidani MA, Fremont RD, et al. Antibiotic use in acute upper respiratory tract infections. Am Fam Physician 2012;86(9):817–22.

9. Pleis JR, Lucas J, Ward B. Summary health statistics for U.S. adults: National Health Interview Survey, 2008. Vital Health Stat 10 2009. National Center for Health Statistics. Available at: www.cdc.gov/nchs/data/series/sr_10/sr10_242.pdf. Accessed July 10, 2012.

10. Aring AM, Chan MM. Acute rhinosinusitis in adults. Am Fam Physician 2011; 83(9):1057–63.

11. Mandel R, Patel N, Ferguson BJ. Role of antibiotics in sinusitis. Curr Opin Infect Dis 2012;25:183–92.

12. Chow AW, Benninger MS, Brook I, et al. IDSA clinical practice guideline for acute bacterial rhinosinusitis in children and adults. Clin Infect Dis 2012;54(8):e72–112.

13. Gonzalez R, Bartlett JG, Besser RE, et al, American Academy of Family Physicians, Infectious Disease Society of America, Centers for Disease Control, American College of Physicians – American Society of Internal Medicine. Principles of appropriate antibiotic use for treatment of nonspecific upper respiratory tract infections in adults: background. Ann Intern Med 2001;134(6):490–4.

14. Health care guideline: diagnosis and treatment of respiratory illness in children and adults. 3rd edition. ICSI; 2011. Available at: http://www.icsi.org/guidelines_and_more/gl_os_prot/respiratory_illness_in_children_and_adults_guideline_respiratory_illness_in_children_and_adults_guideline_13110.html. Accessed July 4, 2012.

15. Falagas ME, Karageorgopoulos DE, Grammatikos AP, et al. Effectiveness and safety of short vs. long duration of antibiotic therapy for acute bacterial sinusitis: a meta-analysis of randomized trials. Br J Clin Pharmacol 2009;67(2):161–71.

16. Meltzer EO, Teper A, Danzig M. Intranasal corticosteroids in the treatment of acute rhinosinusitis. Curr Allergy Asthma Rep 2008;8(2):133–8.

17. Small CB, Bachert C, Lund VJ, et al. Judicious antibiotic use and intranasal corticosteroids in acute rhinosinusitis. Am J Med 2007;120(4):289–94.

18. Vincent MT, Celestin N, Hussain AN. Pharyngitis. Am Fam Physician 2004;69(6): 1465–70.

19. Bisno AL, Gerber MA, Gwaltney JM Jr, et al, Infectious Diseases Society of America. Practice guidelines for the diagnosis and management of group A streptococcal pharyngitis. Infectious Diseases Society of America. Clin Infect Dis 2002;35(2):113–25.

20. Hayes CS, Williamson H Jr. Management of Group A beta-hemolytic streptococcal pharyngitis. Am Fam Physician 2001;63(8):1557–64.

21. Baquero F, García-Rodríguez JA, de Lomas JG, et al. Antimicrobial resistance of 914 beta-hemolytic streptococci isolated from pharyngeal swabs in Spain: results of a 1-year (1996-1997) multicenter surveillance study. The Spanish Surveillance Group for Respiratory Pathogens. Antimicrob Agents Chemother 1999;43(1): 178–80.

22. Available at: http://internalmedicinejournal.blogspot.com/2008/08/acute-laryngo tracheobronchitis-croup.html. Accessed February 28, 2013.
23. Bickley LS, Szilagyi PG. Bates' guide to physical examination and history taking. 8th edition. Philadelphia: Lippincott, Williams & Wilkins; 2003. p. 687.
24. Domino FJ. The 5-minute clinical consult. 20th edition. Philadelphia: Lippincott, Williams & Wilkins; 2012. p. 320–1.
25. Everard ML. Acute bronchiolitis and croup. Pediatr Clin North Am 2009;56: 119–33, x–xi.
26. King L. Emergent management of croup. Available at: http://emedicine. medscape.com/article/800866-overview. Accessed February 28, 2013.
27. Cetinkaya F, Tufekci BS, Kutluk G. A comparison of nebulized budesonide and intramuscular and oral dexamethasone for treatment of croup. Int J Pediatr Oto-rhinolaryngol 2004;68:453–6.
28. Zoorob R, Sidani M, Murray J. Croup: an overview. Am Fam Physician 2011;83(9): 1067–73.

Index

Note: Page numbers of article titles are in **boldface** type.

A

Abacavir, for HIV infections, 604–608, 614
Abscess(es), MRSA, 645–646
Acetic acid, for otitis externa, 674–675
Acute gastroenteritis. *See* Gastroenteritis, acute.
Acute-phase reactants, in pneumonia, 659
Acyclovir, for herpes simplex virus infections, 570, 574, 714
Adenovirus infections, gastrointestinal, 728-729
Affirm test, for trichomoniasis, 564
Agammaglobulinemia, aseptic meningitis in, 711
AIDS. *See* Human immunodeficiency virus infections.
Aluminum acetate, for otitis externa, 674
Amikacin, for tuberculosis, 752
Amoxicillin
    for otitis media, 680
    for pneumonia, 663–664
    for tick-borne infections, 624, 626, 630
    for upper respiratory infections, 765
Amoxicillin-clavulanate
    for otitis media, 679–680
    for upper respiratory infections, 762
    for UTIs, 699
Ampicillin
    for bacterial meningitis, 722
    for pneumonia, 664–665
Analgesics
    for otitis externa, 674
    for otitis media, 679
    for upper respiratory infections, 763
Anaplasmosis, 621–625, 628–629
Antibiotic-associated diarrhea, *Clostridium difficile*, 731, 735–738
Anticholinergics, for common cold, 759
Antihistamines, for common cold, 760
Antimicrobial susceptibility testing
    for MRSA infections, 640
    for tuberculosis, 751
Antiretroviral agents, for HIV infections, 600–608
Antiretroviral Therapy Cohort Collaboration, 602
APTIMA test, for trichomoniasis, 564
Arthritis
    reactive, 578
    septic, MRSA, 648–649

http://dx.doi.org/10.1016/S0095-4543(13)00078-X
0095-4543/13/$ – see front matter © 2013 Elsevier Inc. All rights reserved. **primarycare.theclinics.com**

Printed and bound by CPI Group (UK) Ltd, Croydon, CR0 4YY

03/10/2024

01040390-0004